Surgical Techniques for Anterior Shoulder Instability

Ladislav Kovačič
Frank Martetschläger
Geoffroy Nourissat • Nuno Gomes
Editors

Surgical Techniques for Anterior Shoulder Instability

A Case and Video Based Guide

Springer

European Society of Sports Traumatology, Knee Surgery & Arthroscopy
ESSKA

Editors
Ladislav Kovačič
Arbormea - Artro Center
Ljubljana, Slovenia

Geoffroy Nourissat
Clinique Maussins Nollet
Clinique de l'épaule
Paris, France

Frank Martetschläger
German Center of Shoulder Surgery
Atos Clinic Munich
Munich, Bayern, Germany

Nuno Gomes
Orthopaedics Department
Hospital das Forças Armadas and
Hospital da Luz
Porto, Portugal

ISBN 978-3-662-73063-8 ISBN 978-3-662-73064-5 (eBook)
https://doi.org/10.1007/978-3-662-73064-5

This Springer imprint is published by the registered company Springer-Verlag GmbH, DE, part of Springer Nature.
The registered company address is: Heidelberger Platz 3, 14197 Berlin, Germany

To all who make my life beautiful and meaningful. To my family. Thank you.

Ladislav Kovačič

To my wife Andrea, to Aaron and Raphael. Thank you!

Frank Martetschläger

To my Family.

Nuno Gomes

Foreword

This book is intended to serve as a user-friendly and clinically relevant resource, providing up-to-date information on common aspects of anterior shoulder instability—an area that has undergone significant innovation in recent years.

Each chapter has been authored by a European expert with a specific interest in the topic addressed. The 32 chapters, organized into four sections, present key concepts essential for a comprehensive understanding of this condition. The contributing authors deserve recognition for sharing their experience and insights, which will enable readers to advance their clinical and surgical proficiency.

Ladislav Kovačič, Frank Martetschläger, Geoffroy Nourissat, and Nuno Gomes performed an outstanding job in organizing this volume under the auspices of the European Society of Sports Traumatology, Knee Surgery and Arthroscopy (ESSKA).

The information presented is cutting-edge, and the references are both relevant and valuable. This book offers an excellent resource for all those seeking to deepen their understanding of anterior shoulder instability, presented in a format that is both efficient and enjoyable.

Chief, Shoulder and Elbow Service, IOT-HSVP-UFFS Osvandré Lech
Passo Fundo, Brazil

5th Chair, International Board of Shoulder
and Elbow Surgery (IBSES)
Washington, DC, USA

Preface

The topic of anterior shoulder instability has been full of controversies for many years, even decades. It is well known that the optimal management of these patients remains a subject of extensive debate. Despite the growing body of scientific evidence, many questions regarding treatment decision-making are still unanswered.

For this reason, ESSKA-ESA Shoulder Section has devoted the last few years to this important field of shoulder pathology. One of the immense projects focusing on anterior shoulder instability was the ESSKA-ESA formal consensus on the specific management of these injuries in the focus of patient's age and time from injury. During discussions addressing highly relevant questions related to diagnosis, decision-making, and treatment of the patients with anterior shoulder instability, it became clear—not for the first time—that different surgical solutions can be applied to the same problem with comparable outcomes.

In light of this, a strong need for a specific and a dedicated educational resource was identified. We felt that a comprehensive overview and a practical guide for practitioners in their daily clinical practice was missing and would therefore be very welcome. We hope that the present ESSKA book fills this gap in the existing literature. Namely, the core of the book consists of detailed descriptions of surgical techniques, accompanied by video presentations. Additionally, solutions to specific clinical problems illustrated through clinical cases are proposed. Among them, complex and revision cases are presented by renowned experts, offering readers the opportunity to understand expert strategies and best practices.

We believe that this book represents a valuable educational resource for residents, fellows, and young surgeons in training. Furthermore, it provides advanced insights for experienced surgeons.

We are grateful to all the authors for sharing their experience and knowledge, as well as for their patience throughout the process. We also thank the ESSKA Board and ESSKA Office for their support of the project, and Springer for their professional assistance.

Ljubljana, Slovenia — Ladislav Kovačič
Munich, Germany — Frank Martetschläger
Paris France — Geoffroy Nourissat
Porto, Portugal — Nuno Gomes

Contents

List of Videos

Part I

Updates in Anterior Shoulder Instability

1 Physical Assessment in the Emergency Room, Safe Reduction, and Proper Examination in Outpatient Clinic

Marcello Motta, MacDonald Tedah Djemetio, Claudio Bertoli, and Maristella F. Saccomanno

Key Points

- Clinical examination in the E.R. mainly consists of neurovascular assessment pre- and post-reduction.
- X-rays pre and postop reduction are mandatory to rule out fractures.
- A CT scan can be performed immediately if an articular fracture is suspected.
- History and patient characteristics should be carefully investigated in the outpatient clinic.
- Clinical examination is important to confirm instability symptoms, but it must also include assessment of shoulder and generalized joint laxity.

1.1 Introduction

- The glenohumeral (GH) joint is one of the most common traumatically dislocated joints in the body [45].
- The natural history, treatment, and prognosis differ according to the diagnosis.
- Anterior GH dislocation accounts for 95% to 97% of all shoulder dislocations [32].
- The highest incidence of anterior GH dislocation is seen between the ages of 15 and 30, with a male-to-female ratio of 2.64 [16].
- In patients older than 40 years old, dislocations are often associated with rotator cuff tears [47].
- Etiology could be traumatic or atraumatic. A fall onto an outstretched arm or with the arm overreached in the elevated and externally rotated position is the most common mechanism [20].
- Closed reduction of acute dislocations should be performed in a timely manner. Further diagnostic workup and long-term management are guided by patient age, patient activity level, and mechanism of injury.

M. Motta · M. T. Djemetio · C. Bertoli
Department of Medical and Surgical Specialties, Radiological Sciences, and Public Health, University of Brescia, Brescia, Italy

M. F. Saccomanno (✉)
Department of Bone and Joint Surgery, Spedali Civili, Brescia, Italy

Department of Orthopedics, Fondazione Policlinico Univarsitario A Gemelli IRCSS, Rome, Italy

L. Kovačič et al. (eds.), *Surgical Techniques for Anterior Shoulder Instability*,
https://doi.org/10.1007/978-3-662-73064-5_1

1.2 Scientific Update

- Two main topics of debate are still ongoing: immobilization position after closed reduction; conservative or surgical management after first-time dislocation.
- Conservative management after first-time dislocation has been the mainstay of treatment for decades. It mainly consists of immobilization in a sling for at least three weeks, followed by rehabilitation. Immobilization in external rotation after closed reduction was proposed by Itoi et al. [18] in 2007 to reduce the risk of redislocation. Recent systematic reviews and meta-analyses confirmed this finding [17, 35, 46].
- Recent advances in imaging modalities and knowledge of natural history claimed a new role for surgical treatment after first-time dislocation [31].
  - A recent systematic review stated that operative management significantly reduces recurrence rates among the young and active population [23].
  - A Delphi consensus concluded that over 90% of shoulder instability experts recommend surgery after a first-time anterior GH dislocation for contact athletes aged >14 years at the end of the season with both apprehension and meaningful bone loss [38].

1.3 Assessment and Planning

1.3.1 Emergency Room Assessment

- *History:* Trauma with the arm in abduction and external rotation is most commonly encountered.
- *Clinical examination:*
  - Neurologic and vascular injuries should be first ruled out.
  - Anesthesia in the deltoid region should always be explored as a sign of axillary nerve injury.
  - In case of acute unreduced dislocation, the shoulder is squared-off, losing its rounded contour. The acromion becomes prominent.
- *Imaging:*
  - Plain radiographs are fundamental before reduction maneuvers to ascertain the presence and the direction of the dislocation as well as to rule out concomitant fractures.
  - Another X-ray must be executed after reduction to confirm the success of the operation and to rule out iatrogenic fractures.
  - In the emergency room, CT scan could be useful after reduction to exclude a bony Bankart lesion or any other articular fracture.

1.3.2 Outpatient Clinic

- *History:*
  - Patients usually report one or more dislocations and/or subluxations in a precise time period.
  - Onset, mechanism of injury, volition, number of dislocations and reduction maneuvers are mandatory questions to understand soft tissue and bone lesions.
  - Patient characteristics must be carefully investigated at this time in order to establish the decision-making algorithm:
    - Age
    - Functional request
    - Sport and work activities
    - Level of sport activities
- *Clinical examination* [43]:
  - Bilateral range of motion
  - Specific instability tests
    - Anterior (provocative): apprehension, relocation

    - Inferior: sulcus sign
    - Posterior: Kim's test
  - Specific tests for shoulder laxity [5]
    - Anterior: adduction/external rotation >85°
    - Inferior: Gagey's test
  - Specific tests for generalized joint hyperlaxity
    - Beighton score [3]
  - Specific test to rule out rotator cuff tears are not part of the usual workup, unless patient is older than 40 years old.
- *Imaging:*
  - CT scan: bi- and three-dimensional (3D) evaluation. Bipolar bone loss could be assessed as follows:
    - On-track/off-track method [11]. An off-track lesion is today a major indication for a bony procedure.
    - Hill-Sachs interval to glenoid width (H/G) ratio [44]. A ratio > 0.7, which defines a peripheral-track lesion, has been related to less satisfactory functional results after an arthroscopic Bankart repair [42].
  - MRI: indicated when a concomitant rotator cuff tears is suspected.

1.4 Treatment Option and Indication

1.4.1 Acute Management in Emergency Room: Closed Reduction

- Early reduction leads to lower risk of muscle spasm and damaging manipulation of neurovascular structures within the shoulder [16].
- Closed reduction is contraindicated in case of humeral head, neck, or shaft fracture to avoid fracture displacement.
- How to perform a safe closed reduction:
  - Sedation, as a combination of narcotics and benzodiazepines with or without the addition of propofol, is sometimes required for muscle relaxation.
  - Reduction maneuvers basically consist of traction, leverage, manipulation, or a combination of these. More than 20 methods on how to perform the reduction have been proposed [1] (Table 1.1).
- After reduction, the neurological status of the upper arm must be reassessed.
- If closed reduction is not possible even after sedation, open reduction should be considered.

Table 1.1 Reduction maneuvers divided by main mode of action

Reduction method	Mode of action	Description
Milch maneuver [29]	Leverage	The patient lies in a supine vertical position, with his shoulders slightly higher than his pelvic position. The doctor holds the patient's arm at the wrist, abducting it to an overhead position and externally rotating it to 90°. Subsequently, the doctor pushes the humeral head into a superior and lateral direction
Janecki's forward elevation technique [19]	Leverage	The patient lies in a supine position while the doctor holds his wrist and slowly and gradually lifts it to an overhead position with the arm externally rotated. The arm of the patient is then abducted while traction is applied, initiating reduction
Hanging arm technique [25]	Leverage	The patient lies in a prone position with a pillow beneath his head and chest with his affected arm hanging freely over the side of the examining table. The doctor holds the epicondyle with one hand and the medial part of the upper arm in the other hand. The patient's arm, slightly flexed, rests on the forearm of the doctor. Meanwhile, the doctor applies steady traction with abduction of the affected arm, forward flexion and internal rotation, initiating the reduction

(continued)

Table 1.1 (continued)

Reduction method	Mode of action	Description
Eskimo technique [33]	Leverage	The patient lies on the side of the unaffected shoulder. Two doctors lift the patient by the dislocated arm while the arm is abducted. By doing this, they elevate the patient slightly above the ground for a short time, initiating the reduction. If no reduction occurs, the doctor can place his hand in the axilla and apply pressure on the humeral head to reposition it in the glenoid rim
Bhan's reduction maneuver [4]	Traction–countertraction	The patient lies on the unaffected side, having the affected shoulder facing upward. The doctor then holds the humerus with both hands and applies upward traction perpendicular to the long axis of the humerus. A posterior traction is performed alongside the upward traction
Eachempati method (external rotation maneuver) [10]	Leverage	The patient lies in a supine position with his arm adducted to the thorax, the elbow flexed at 90°, and the shoulder flexed at 20°. The doctor, holding the hand of the patient in one arm and the elbow in the other arm, slowly externally rotates the arm of the patient till it is parallel to the body of the patient without providing traction, which will initiate the reduction
Kocher maneuver [21]	Leverage	The patient lies in supine position with his arm adducted to the thorax and his elbow flexed in 90°. The doctor then provides external rotation in the shoulder until resistance is felt. Then, the arm is flexed (lifted), retaining the external rotation in the shoulder, and adducted. The arm is then internally rotated, initiating the reduction
Hippocratic method [39]	Traction–countertraction	The patient lies in a supine position, while the doctor holds the affected limb by the forearm and hand. The doctor then places his heel in the axilla of the affected shoulder, acting as a fulcrum while the arm is adducted, initiating reduction
Spaso technique [30]	Traction–countertraction	The patient lies in a supine position with his shoulder flexed at 90° and the elbow in an extended position. The doctor should first initiate longitudinal traction until the patient is comfortable enough to tolerate the scapula touching the examination table. Then, the doctor should provide external rotation to the shoulder to facilitate reduction
Sitting method [28]	Scapular manipulation	The patient is seated while facing the doctor. The doctor then holds the forearm of the affected limb and flexes the shoulder to 90° while having the elbow of the patient slightly flexed. The patient should be fully relaxed during this maneuver. Then, the doctor places his other arm on the anterior chest wall at the side of the affected limb to control the glenoid tilt by manipulating a part of the scapula, such as the acromion or coracoid process. Finally, the doctor applies longitudinal traction to initiate the reduction
Stimson's maneuver [36]	Traction–countertraction	The patient lies in a prone position with his arm hanging beside the examining table. A downward traction to the arm is applied for 10–20 min by the doctor or by attaching weights to the wrist of the patient. Then, the weights are released, allowing the humerus to fall back into its position, thus reducing the glenohumeral joint
Chair method [41]	Traction–countertraction	The patient sits sideways on a chair, having the backrest of the chair in his axilla. A small bed sheet or a stiff pillow can be rested on the backrest of the chair to avoid complications. The doctor holds the hand of the patient in one hand and the elbow of the patient in the other while he ensures that the elbow of the patient is gently flexed. After calming the patient, downward traction is applied by the doctor or by an attached sling with weights, facilitating reduction
Aufmesser's method [13]	Traction–countertraction	The patient lies in a supine position. The doctor holds the hand of the patient in one hand and fixates the acromion of the patient with the other hand. The doctor performs axial traction of the affected arm while considering the muscular tension of the patient. Additionally, the doctor can use his body as a fulcrum to add more leverage

(continued)

Table 1.1 (continued)

Reduction method	Mode of action	Description
Surfer's method [37]	Traction–countertraction	The patient lies in a supine position with his affected arm adducted to his body. The doctor holds the wrist of the patient and leans back and away to provide axial traction and adduction of the arm. A clicking sound can be heard if the arm is reduced
Matsen's traction-countertraction maneuver [9]	Traction–countertraction	The patient lies in a supine position with a sheet around his thorax and also around the waist of the assistant standing at the contralateral side of the affected shoulder. Another sheet is wrapped around the waist and forearm of the doctor standing on the side of the dislocated shoulder near the waist of the patient while holding the elbow of the patient in 90° flexion and the shoulder in 90° abduction. The doctor applies traction to the affected arm by leaning back while the assistant provides countertraction
Bokor-Billmann's shoulder reduction technique [6]	Leverage	The patient sits upright with his back against a firm surface to minimize movements of the upper body. The doctor holds the wrist of the patient in one hand and the elbow in the other, maintaining 90° flexion of the elbow and 90° flexion of the shoulder. The arm is then adducted until it reaches the midline of the thorax. Maintaining the arm in the midline position the shoulder is internally rotated (Fig. 1.3). The doctor should maintain constant pressure to overcome this resistance, inducing reduction
Cunningham technique [8]	Traction–countertraction	The patient sits in a chair with his back straight and his arm adducted to the body with his arm in neutral position and his elbow in 90° flexion. The doctor kneels on the side of the affected arm facing the opposite direction. The doctor then slides his hand between the patients forearm and body having the hand of the patient resting on the upper arm of the doctor. The doctor applies gentle downward traction (if this initiates spasms or pain the doctor stops and starts over). The doctor should massage the trapezius, deltoid and biceps muscle sequentially with his other hand initiating the reduction
Scapular manipulation technique [22]	Scapular manipulation	The patient lies in a prone position with his shoulder flexed to 90° and his arm hanging in externally rotated position from an examining table. A downward traction is applied by hanging weights on the wrist of the patient or by having an assistant apply traction. Thereafter, the doctor pushes the tip of the inferolateral scapular edge medially, rotating upward, initiating the reduction
FAst, REliable, and Safe (FARES) method [34]	Traction–countertraction	The patient lies in a supine position with the doctor standing at the side of the dislocated shoulder. The doctor holds the wrist of the patient with both arms, keeping the elbow of the patient extended and the forearm in a neutral position. Then, the arm is slowly abducted in an oscillating movement (approximately 5 cm up- and downward movement) while constant longitudinal traction is applied. The arm is externally rotated when abducted beyond 90°
Legg maneuver [14]	Leverage	The patient is seated in a straight-backed chair to minimize movement while the assistant stabilizes the unaffected shoulder by applying downward pressure. The patient actively abducts his affected arm to 90°, with the help of the doctor as needed. Subsequently, the arm is externally rotated until the palm faces forward. The doctor then flexes the elbow to 90° and stabilizes the affected arm behind the patient's head. Then, the arm is adducted to the patient's side while fully flexing the elbow. The patient is then asked to internally rotate his arm across the chest
Manes' method [27]	Traction–countertraction	The patient is seated in a chair while the doctor stands behind him and places his flexed forearm in the axilla of the affected shoulder of the patient. He then presses the forearm in the axilla in a superolateral direction while applying gentle traction on the flexed forearm of the affected arm of the patient with his other hand

(continued)

Table 1.1 (continued)

Reduction method	Mode of action	Description
Walz method [40]	Traction–countertraction	The patient sits straight-backed on a chair while the doctor stands behind him. The doctor then places one hand in the axilla making a fist and having his thumb facing upward, making contact with the humeral head. With the other hand, the doctor holds the forearm of the patient and applies downward traction, usually initiating the reduction. If no reduction occurs, the doctor can rotate his hand externally in the axilla, pushing the humeral head laterally in the glenoid fossa
Boss-Holzach-Matter method [7]	Traction–countertraction	The patient sits on the examination table with his leg straight while his wrists are protected by cotton wool and bound together. The knee on the same side of the dislocated arm is then flexed to 90°, and the patient places his forearms around this knee. The head of the examination table is then lowered slowly, and the patient is asked to lean back, hyperextending his neck, providing anterior axial traction to the dislocated shoulder, and pushing the shoulders anteriorly, thus creating a rotational movement of the scapula in the vertical axis
Slump method [24]	Traction–countertraction	The patient sits in a chair leaning forward in a slumped position (leaning forward from the waist), letting the assistant support all of the body weight, which allows the assistant to assess the muscle tonus of the patient. When the patient is fully relaxed, the assistant gives a sign to the doctor to initiate the reduction maneuver. The doctor then holds the elbow of the affected arm and applies longitudinal traction together with external rotation if necessary. Additionally, the inferior tip of the scapula can be pushed medially by the forearm of the assistant

1.5 Decision-Making Algorithm

1.5.1 Emergency Room

- Neurovascular examination
- X-rays
- Reduction maneuver
- Neurovascular re-check and X-rays after reduction
- If there is any suspicion of an articular fracture, a CT scan should be performed
  - If a bony Bankart lesion is present, a surgical repair should be scheduled.
- Immobilization in a sling. At the moment, there is no clear evidence on the best type of immobilization among external rotation, neutral position, or internal rotation. Most of the time, the only immobilization available in the emergency department is a standard brace in internal rotation.

1.5.2 Outpatient Clinic

- Clinical examination.
- Imaging: CT scan is mandatory to assess bipolar lesions.
- Treatment options.
  - First-time dislocation: operative or conservative management should be carefully evaluated based on patient characteristics (age, functional request, etc.).
  - Recurrent dislocations: open or arthroscopic surgery should be evaluated based on the quantification of bipolar bone loss.

1.6 Clinical Case/Example

- A 16-year-old male presented to the emergency room. Parents described a left shoulder injury as the boy was playing soccer and fell with the arm abducted and externally rotated while he was trying to catch the ball. No previous episodes of glenohumeral dislocation were acknowledged.

- From a clinical standpoint, the boy presented with limited ROM associated with severe pain. No neurovascular injuries occurred.
- An X-ray was then undertaken and the suspicion of anterior glenohumeral dislocation was confirmed (Fig. 1.1).
- A Matsen's traction-countertraction maneuver was then attempted after sedation (Fig. 1.2). No neurological injuries were reported after reduction maneuver.
- X-rays confirmed the reduction, but also showed a double contour of the glenoid. A CT scan was therefore performed. 3D reconstructions showed a small Hill-Sachs lesion and a bony Bankart lesion (Fig. 1.3). Bipolar lesions were on-track with H/G ratio = 0.7.
- The arm was immobilized in a sling, and the patient was scheduled for an arthroscopic bony Bankart repair in a few days.
- Following surgery, the arm was immobilized in a sling with an abduction pillow for 4 weeks. After sling removal, an eight-week rehabilitation program was started. The patient was allowed to return to competitive sport activities six months after surgery.

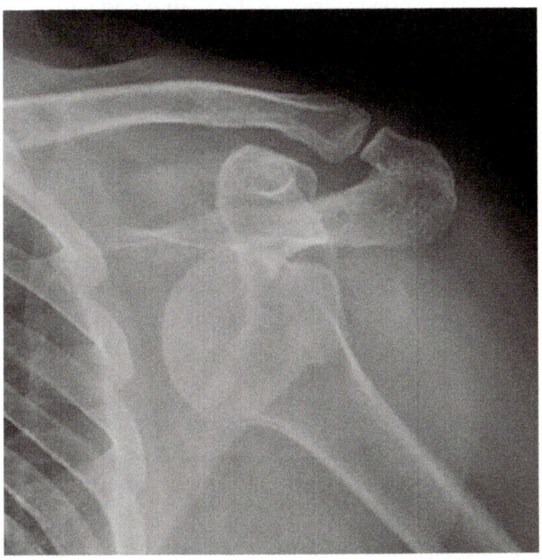

Fig. 1.1 Left shoulder. X-rays: anterior-inferior glenohumeral dislocation

Pearls and Pitfalls

- Timing and relaxation are key factors for successful reduction.
- Pre- and post-reduction checks of neurovascular integrity are mandatory.
- Pre- and post-reduction X-rays are fundamental to rule out concomitant fractures.
- Watch out for rotator cuff tears or rotator cuff tear arthropathy in older patients.

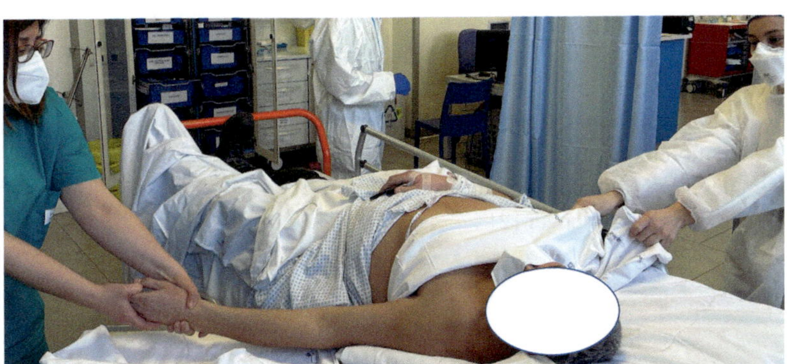

Fig. 1.2 Reduction maneuver: The patient lies in a supine position with a sheet around the thorax. The doctor, standing on the side of the dislocated shoulder, applies traction to the affected arm by leaning back, while the assistant provides countertraction

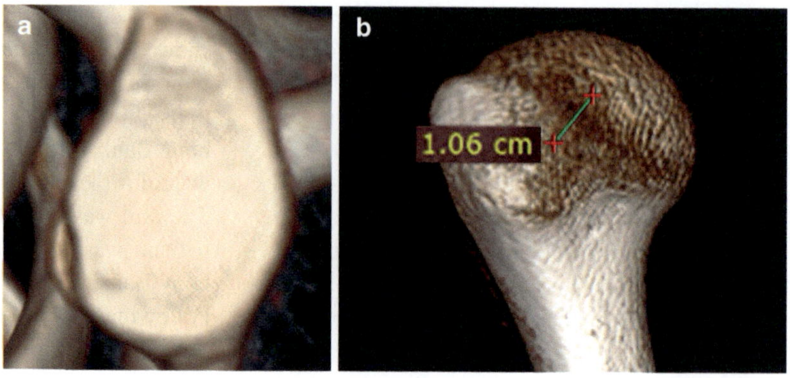

Fig. 1.3 3D-CT scan of the left shoulder showing a bony Bankart lesion (**a**) associated with a Hill-Sachs lesion (**b**)

1.7 Outcomes

- Approximately 75% of acute primary dislocations are sustained during sports and wilderness activities. Most are treated in the emergency department.
- No clear evidence exists regarding the superiority of one reduction technique over another [1, 12, 15]. Dong et al. [12] reported that traction–countertraction methods are less painful but slower than leverage methods, with no difference in complication rates.
- Recurrence after first-time dislocation treated conservatively ranges between 26% and 92% [26, 32].
- Kraeutler et al. [23] stated that operative management significantly reduces recurrence rates among the young and active population.

1.8 Potential Complication/Difficulties

- Axillary nerve injury is identified in about 42% of acute anterior shoulder dislocations. Nerve transection is rare, and traction injuries are more common [32].
- Glenoid or humeral fracture can occur during a reduction maneuver [2].

Take-Home Message

- Acute anterior shoulder dislocations are common injuries in the young and active population.
- A safe and early reduction in the emergency room is paramount to avoid neurological injuries due to prolonged traction.
- Patient characteristics and a careful clinical and imaging evaluation are fundamental in the outpatient clinic in order to establish a correct decision-making algorithm.

References

1. Alkaduhimi H, van der Linde JA, Flipsen M, van Deurzen DFP, van den Bekerom MPJ. A systematic and technical guide on how to reduce a shoulder dislocation. Turk J Emerg Med. 2016;16:155–68.
2. Beattie TF, Steedman DJ, McGowan A, Robertson CE. A comparison of the Milch and Kocher techniques for acute anterior dislocation of the shoulder. Injury. 1986;17:349–52.
3. Beighton P, Horan F. Orthopaedic aspects of the Ehlers-Danlos syndrome. J Bone Joint Surg Br. 1969;51:444–53.
4. Bhan S, Mehara AK. A simple and universal method for reduction of dislocation of the shoulder. Int Orthop. 1994;18:14.

5. Boileau P, Villalba M, Héry J-Y, Balg F, Ahrens P, Neyton L. Risk factors for recurrence of shoulder instability after arthroscopic Bankart repair. J Bone Joint Surg Am. 2006;88:1755–63.
6. Bokor-Billmann T, Lapshyn H, Kiffner E, Goos MF, Hopt UT, Billmann FG. Reduction of acute shoulder dislocations in a remote environment: a prospective multicenter observational study. Wilderness Environ Med. 2015;26:395–400.
7. Boss A, Holzach P, Matter P. A new self-repositioning technique for fresh, anterior-lower shoulder dislocation. Helv Chir Acta. 1993;60:263–5.
8. Cunningham N. A new drug free technique for reducing anterior shoulder dislocations. Emerg Med Australas. 2003;15:521–4.
9. Cunningham NJ. Techniques for reduction of anteroinferior shoulder dislocation. Emerg Med Australas. 2005;17:463–71.
10. Danzl DF, Vicario SJ, Gleis GL, Yates JR, Parks DL. Closed reduction of anterior subcoracoid shoulder dislocation. Evaluation of an external rotation method. Orthop Rev. 1986;15:311–5.
11. Di Giacomo G, Itoi E, Burkhart SS. Evolving concept of bipolar bone loss and the Hill-Sachs lesion: from "engaging/non-engaging" lesion to "on-track/off-track" lesion. J Arthrosc. 2014;30:90–8.
12. Dong H, Jenner EA, Theivendran K. Closed reduction techniques for acute anterior shoulder dislocation: a systematic review and meta-analysis. Eur J Trauma Emerg Surg. 2021;47:407–21.
13. Dreu M, Aufmesser W, Aufmesser H, Dolcet C, Feigl G, Sadoghi P. A simple and gentle technique for reduction after anterior shoulder dislocation. Arch Orthop Trauma Surg. 2015;135:1379–84.
14. Dyck DD, Porter NW, Dunbar BD. Legg reduction maneuver for patients with anterior shoulder dislocation. J Am Osteopath Assoc. 2008;108:571–3.
15. Fennelly JT, Gourbault L, Neal-Smith G, Pradhan A, Gade V, Baxter JA. A systematic review of prehospital shoulder reduction techniques for anterior shoulder dislocation and the effect on patient return to function. Chin J Traumatol Zhonghua Chuang Shang Za Zhi. 2020;23:295–301.
16. Hasebroock AW, Brinkman J, Foster L, Bowens JP. Management of primary anterior shoulder dislocations: a narrative review. Sports Med. 2019;5:31.
17. Hurley ET, Fried JW, Alaia MJ, Strauss EJ, Jazrawi LM, Matache BA. Immobilisation in external rotation after first-time traumatic anterior shoulder instability reduces recurrent instability: a meta-analysis. J ISAKOS Jt Disord Orthop Sports Med. 2021;6:22–7.
18. Itoi E, Hatakeyama Y, Sato T, Kido T, Minagawa H, Yamamoto N, Wakabayashi I, Nozaka K. Immobilization in external rotation after shoulder dislocation reduces the risk of recurrence. A randomized controlled trial. J Bone Joint Surg Am. 2007;89:2124–31.
19. Janecki CJ, Shahcheragh GH. The forward elevation maneuver for reduction of anterior dislocations of the shoulder. Clin Orthop. 1982:177–80.
20. Khiami F, Gérometta A, Loriaut P. Management of recent first-time anterior shoulder dislocations. Orthop Traumatol Surg Res. 2015;101:S51–7.
21. Kocher T. Eine neue Reductions methode fur Srchulter verrenkung. Berl Kiln Wchnschr. 1870;7:101–5.
22. Kothari RU, Dronen SC. Prospective evaluation of the scapular manipulation technique in reducing anterior shoulder dislocations. Ann Emerg Med. 1992;21:1349–52.
23. Kraeutler MJ, Belk JW, Carver TJ, McCarty EC, Khodaee M. Traumatic primary anterior Glenohumeral joint dislocation in sports: a systematic review of operative versus nonoperative management. Curr Sports Med Rep. 2020;19:468–78.
24. Kuah DEK. An alternative slump reduction technique of anterior shoulder dislocations: a 3-year prospective study. Clin J Sport Med. 2000;10:158–61.
25. Lacey T, Crawford HB. Reduction of anterior dislocations of the shoulder by means of the Milch abduction technique. J Bone Joint Surg Am. 1952;34-A:108–9.
26. Longo UG, Papalia R, Ciapini G, De Salvatore S, Casciaro C, Ferrari E, Cosseddu F, Novi M, Piergentili I, Parchi P, Scaglione M, Denaro V. Instability severity index score does not predict the risk of shoulder dislocation after a first episode treated conservatively. Int J Environ Res Public Health. 2021;18:12026.
27. Manes HR. A new method of shoulder reduction in the elderly. Clin Orthop. 1980:200–2.
28. Matsumoto K, Itoh Y, Fukuta M, Itokazu M, Shimizu K. Anterior dislocation of the shoulder: a simple and sitting method for reduction. Curr Orthop Pract. 2009;20:281–4.
29. Milch H. The treatment of recent dislocations and fracture-dislocations of the shoulder. J Bone Joint Surg Am. 1949;31A:173–80.
30. Miljesic S, Kelly A-M. Reduction of anterior dislocation of the shoulder: the Spaso technique. Emerg Med. 2009;10:173–5.
31. Novakofski KD, Melugin HP, Leland DP, Bernard CD, Krych AJ, Camp CL (2021) Nonoperative management of anterior shoulder instability can result in high rates of recurrent instability and pain at long-term follow-up. J Shoulder Elbow Surg S1058-2746(21):00632–7.
32. Pak T, Kim AM. Anterior Glenohumeral joint dislocation. In: StatPearls. Treasure Island: StatPearls Publishing; 2021.
33. Poulsen SR. Reduction of acute shoulder dislocations using the Eskimo technique: a study of 23 consecutive cases. J Trauma Inj Infect Crit Care. 1988;28:1382–3.
34. Sayegh FE, Kenanidis EI, Papavasiliou KA, Potoupnis ME, Kirkos JM, Kapetanos GA. Reduction of acute anterior dislocations: a prospective ran-

domized study comparing a new technique with the Hippocratic and Kocher methods. J Bone Jt Surg-Am Vol. 2009;91:2775–82.
35. Shinagawa K, Sugawara Y, Hatta T, Yamamoto N, Tsuji I, Itoi E. Immobilization in external rotation reduces the risk of recurrence after primary anterior shoulder dislocation: a meta-analysis. Orthop J Sports Med. 2020;8:2325967120925694.
36. Stimson LA. An easy method of reducing dislocations of the shoulder and hip. Med Rec. 1900;57:356.
37. Summers A. Shoulder dislocation: reduction without sedation in the emergency department. Emerg Nurse. 2007;15:24–8.
38. Tokish JM, Kuhn JE, Ayers GD, Arciero RA, Burks RT, Dines DM, Duralde XA, ElAttrache NS, Millett PJ, St Pierre P, Provencher MT, Tibone JE, Ticker JB, Cordasco FA. Decision making in treatment after a first-time anterior glenohumeral dislocation: a Delphi approach by the Neer Circle of the American Shoulder and Elbow Surgeons. J Shoulder Elb Surg. 2020;29:2429–45.
39. Ufberg JW, Vilke GM, Chan TC, Harrigan RA. Anterior shoulder dislocations: beyond traction-countertraction. J Emerg Med. 2004;27:301–6.
40. Walz M, Kolbow B, Auerbach F. A painless technique for reposition of anterior shoulder dislocation. Unfallchirurg. 2006;109:551–5.
41. Westin CD, Gill EA, Noyes ME, Hubbard M. Anterior shoulder dislocation: a simple and rapid method for reduction. Am J Sports Med. 1995;23:369–71.
42. Yamamoto N, Shinagawa K, Hatta T, Itoi E. Peripheral-track and central-Track Hill-Sachs lesions: a new concept of assessing an on-track lesion. Am J Sports Med. 2020;48:33–8.
43. Yang S, Kim TU, Kim DH, Chang MC. Understanding the physical examination of the shoulder: a narrative review. Ann Palliat Med. 2021;10:2293–303.
44. Yang T-C, Chen K-H, Chiang E-R, Chang M-C, Ma H-L. Using the "Hill-Sachs interval to glenoid track width ratio" for prediction of recurrent instability after arthroscopic Bankart repair. Orthop Traumatol Surg Res OTSR. 2018;104:797–801.
45. Zacchilli MA, Owens BD. Epidemiology of shoulder dislocations presenting to emergency departments in the United States. J Bone Joint Surg Am. 2010;92:542–9.
46. Zhang B, Sun Y, Liang L, Yu X, Zhu L, Chen S, Wei Y, Wen G. Immobilization in external rotation versus internal rotation after shoulder dislocation: a meta-analysis of randomized controlled trials. Orthop Traumatol Surg Res OTSR. 2020;106:671–80.
47. Zhou R, Prasad G, Robinson S, Shahane S, Sinha A. The significance of urgent ultrasound scan for shoulder dislocation in patients above the age of 40: a prospective British Elbow and Shoulder Society pathway implementation study. Shoulder Elb. 2021;13:303–10.

2 Bony Defects: From Imaging Workup to Intraoperative Assessment

Dominik Szymski, Stefan Greiner, and Andreas Voss

Key Points to Assess Bony Defects

- When using CT for preoperative assessment, having contralateral shoulder images available is useful for accurate comparison.
- Ensure parasagittal images (CT or MRI) of the glenoid are parallel to its surface to avoid false calculations of defect size.
- In acute cases, intraarticular liquid (e.g., blood) aids in generating high contrast for MRI assessments. Arthro-MRI may be necessary in chronic cases.
- Always consider patient expectations, age, and activity level.
- Do not rely solely on radiological information to decide on therapy.

2.1 Introduction

- Instability of the shoulder joint is a commonly diagnosed condition with frequent indication for operative treatment [20, 26].
- Both acute and chronic instability of the glenohumeral joint are associated with glenoid bone loss. In patients with persistent shoulder instability, bone loss of the glenoid has been reported in up to 90% of the cases [10, 12, 17], while after primary dislocations it is found in up to 41% of the cases [5, 17].
- The "normal" glenoid articulating pear-shaped surface can lose articulating surface on the anterior part of the glenoid, reducing its function as a static restraint for the shoulder [25]. Subsequent off-axis forces and a reduction of shear-force resistance lead to persistent instability and accelerated degeneration [17]. In abduction and external rotation, a significant increase in instability with increasing bone loss was found [15].
- Preoperative evaluation of bone loss size is relevant for the further therapeutic procedure. Bone loss of more than 20% of the glenoid surface is associated with a high rate of failure using a soft-tissue reconstruction only, and even with a 13.5% bony defect zone, a significantly worse outcome was found [24, 28]. For this reason, patients with glenohumeral insta-

D. Szymski · S. Greiner · A. Voss (✉)
Sporthopaedicum Regensburg, Regensburg, Germany

Department of Trauma Surgery, University Medical Center Regensburg, Regensburg, Germany
e-mail: Dominik.Szymski@sporthopaedicum.de; greiner@sporthopaedicum.de; voss@sporthopaedicum.de

L. Kovačič et al. (eds.), *Surgical Techniques for Anterior Shoulder Instability*,
https://doi.org/10.1007/978-3-662-73064-5_2

bility require detailed diagnostics and precise preoperative planning to prevent possible treatment failure.

2.2 Scientific Update

- The evaluation of critical size of bone loss and indications for bone grafting procedures is highly discussed in the literature. While 20% bone loss has often been described as the critical bone loss [17, 24], recent publications have shown that even a 13.5% defect size may lead to a significant decrease in outcomes after an isolated soft-tissue procedure [28]. Shin et al. defined 17.3% of bone loss as the critical size for recurrent instability and the need for revision surgery [29].
- Stillwater et al. compared the bone defect size in 3D-MRI and 3D-CT scans in patients with glenohumeral instability and found no significant difference in bone loss size between the two methods [30], while using 2D imaging showed significant variations [7].
- The growing availability of 3D-MRI allows comprehensive examination of both bone defects and soft-tissue pathologies with reduced radiation.
- Superior results for 3D CT scans compared to 2D CT have been published, but a definitive validation of the commonly used "best-fit circle" measuring method is still lacking [17]. 3D CT, however, provides accurate and reliable images for the quantification of bone loss [27].
- Arthroscopic evaluation, on the other hand, is not sufficient and can show an overestimaten bone loss by up to 55% compared with 3D CT imaging [2].
- Moroder et al., with their investigation of the biomechanical effects of bony lesions, have challenged the current bone loss measurement methods. In their study, smaller glenoid defects might have a higher biomechanical effect than larger osseous defects [21].
- Still, all current treatment concepts are based on the classification of the bony lesion size and, therefore, this must be properly evaluated.

2.3 Assessment and Planning

- An accurate history and clinical examination are essential for the assessment of bone loss in patients with shoulder instability.
- Acute bone loss often results from axial high-energy impact on the glenoid surface [6]. During shoulder examination, attention should be given to the function of the axillary nerve and distal arm paresthesia, as well as apprehension tests in all directions [3, 26].
- Patients with bone loss describe instability with increasing frequency, and, particularly, early abduction and external rotation worsen the symptoms [3, 18, 26].
- Balg and Boileau published the *Instability Severity Index Score (ISIS),* a simple tool for evaluation of contraindications for an arthroscopic Bankart repair in patients with shoulder instability, considering several risk factors such as age, activity level, hyperlaxity, and bony lesions on X-rays [3, 19].
- Giacomo et al. went further by using 3D CT imaging—the gold standard for the evaluation and sizing of glenoid bone loss [7, 16]—instead of conventional X-ray, classifying the Hill-Sachs lesion as an "on-track" or "off-track" injury of the glenoid track (*Glenoid Track Instability Management Score—GTIMS*) [9].
- In daily routine, one of the most commonly used methods for measurement is the ratio method or "best fit circle," described by Sugaya et al. [17, 31]. Thereby a circle was created following the orientation of the posteroinferior glenoid contour, and the maximum diameter was measured (=A). Subsequently, the distance between the anterior rim and the anterior part of the circle was measured (=B) (see Fig. 2.1). The defect size is calculated as follows [17, 31]:

$$\text{Bone defect size}(\%) = \text{B} / \text{A} \times 100$$

- If available, images of the healthy shoulder can be used for comparison and measurement of the diameter.

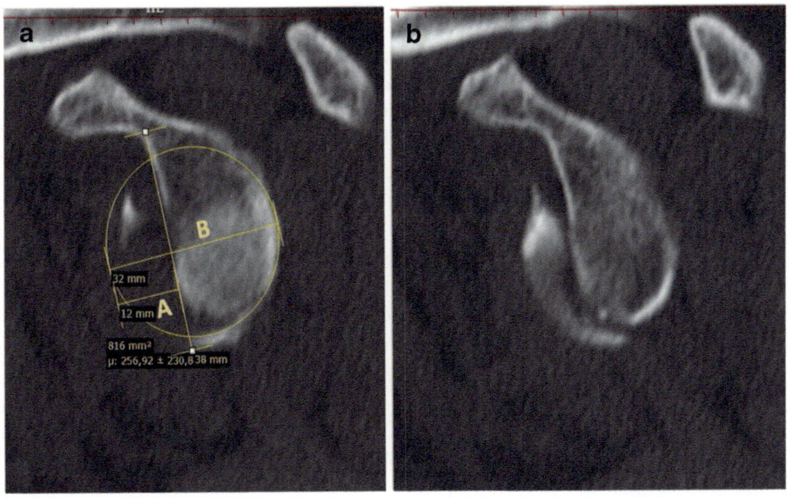

Fig. 2.1 (**a**) Assessment of glenoid bone loss after traumatic primary shoulder dislocation in an 2D-CT with approximately 37% of bone loss, (**b**) Medialized bony Bankart fragment

- Simultaneously, along with the evaluation of osseous defects, also soft-tissue pathologies must also be assessed. MRI imaging is here the gold standard and provides, in acute situations with blood in the joint or in chronic cases with contrast arthrography, the possibility for a more detailed assessment of soft tissues [26].

2.4 Treatment Options and Indications

- After detailed measurement and localization of the bony fragment, different treatment options are available [14].
- Conservative treatment is not recommended for younger and active patients due to progression of cartilage and osseous damage. Only for older patients with lower demands and only minor glenoidal bone loss does conservative treatment with physiotherapy offer an option [26].
- Minor bone loss in younger and active patients is an indication for arthroscopic or open Bankert repair, with or without remplissage [26].
- In patients with anterior shoulder instability, the usage of a soft-tissue stabilization procedure was less effective with great bone loss [23]. Dependent on activity level, already a bone loss of 13.5% seems to be critical for the outcome of only soft-tissue Bankert repair [28], while a defect size of more than 20% was a predictor for persistent instability after isolated soft-tissue Bankert repair [24].
- For patients with extensive bone loss, different autologous bone grafting techniques are available. The aim of these techniques is always to restore the bony defect and rebuild the glenoidal surface.
- On the one hand, coracoid transfer procedures use the proc. coracoideus with the attached tendons to stabilize the shoulder using the combination of sling effect and bone graft. In the Latarjet procedure, a common coracoid transfer procedure, the coracoid is moved to the anterior bone defect zone of the glenoid through a persistent horizontal split of the subscapularis [11, 23, 33].
- On the other hand, free bone grafting procedures, e.g., the iliac crest bone graft transfer or the Eden-Hybinette procedure, use an autologous iliac bone graft to reconstruct the glenoid concavity. The graft is here transferred through a temporary split of the subscapularis to the anterior rim of the glenoid [1, 22, 23].
- Stabilization of the shoulder is thereby generated by the restoration of glenoidal bone structure [23, 32]. In a prospective randomized study, both procedures were compared in regard to clinical and radiologic outcomes up to 2 years after surgery and showed no significant differences except for sensory disorders in the iliac crest group and poorer internal rotation in the Latarjet group [23].
- Defects of more than 40% of the glenoid surface could also lead to an endoprosthetic treatment [4].

2.5 Decision-Making Algorithm

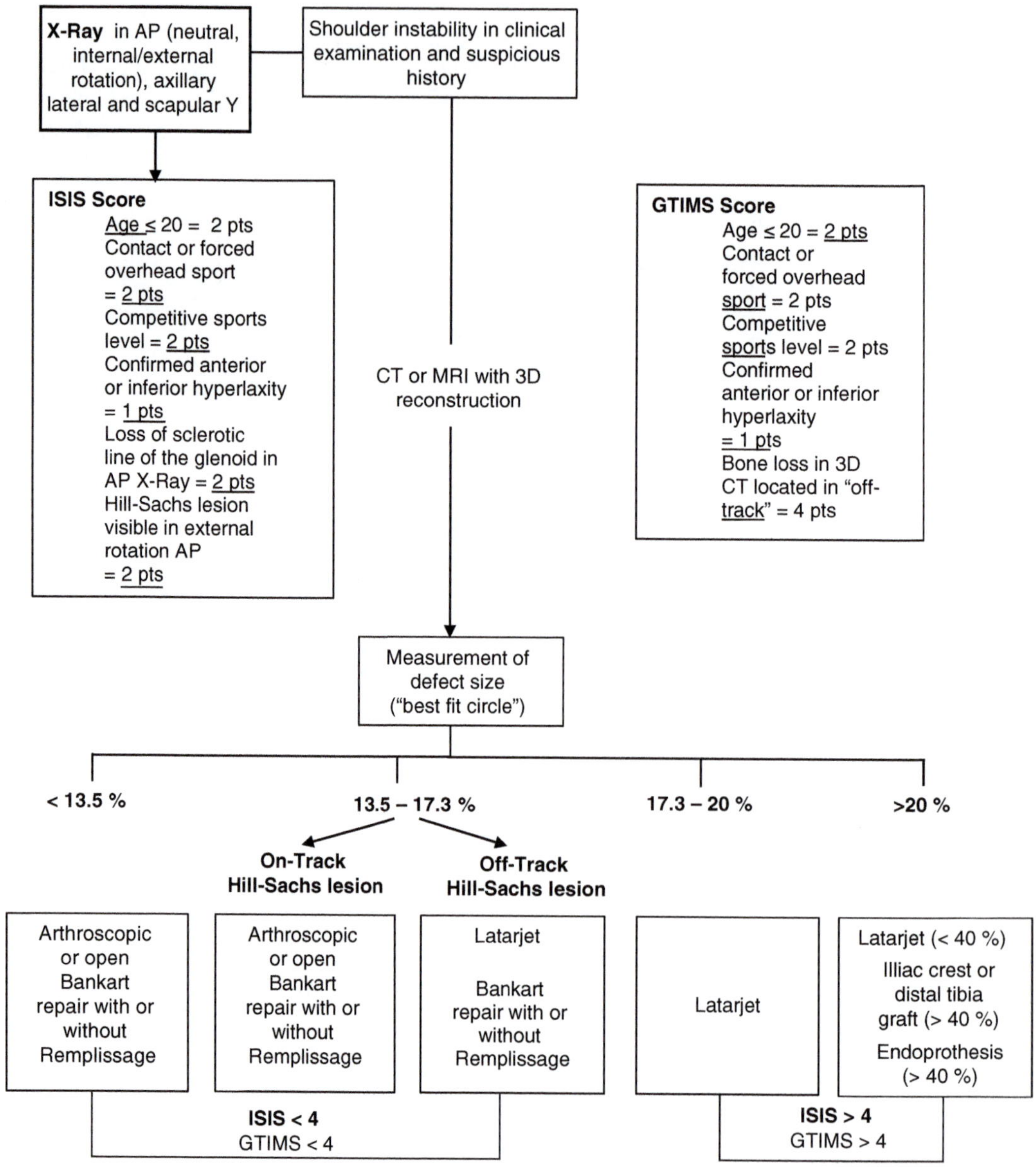

Adapted from Rabinowitz et al. 2017; Balg and Boileau 2007; Di Giacomo et al. 2020 [3, 9, 26]

Pearls and Pitfalls

- Usage of 2D-CT imaging could lead to under- or overestimation of lesion size.
- Arthroscopic measurement is not sufficient due to a high rate of overestimation of bone loss.
- Activity level, age and the patient's expectation must be part of the therapeutic decision-making—Only bone loss size is not a sufficient marker.

2.6 Outcomes

- For the treatment of glenoidal bone loss, different operative techniques are available depending on bone loss sizes and patient activity level.
- Especially decisions exclusively based on lesion size have to been questioned critically due to latest research revealing that lesion size does not correlate with biomechanical impact [21].
- For small bone loss defects arthroscopic Bankart repair and open Bankart repairs show equal results, with faster recovery in arthroscopically treated patients [6].
- Bigger lesions are an indication for bone grafting procedures as the Latarjet or iliac bone graft transplantation surgery. Between both procedures clinical and radiologic no significant differences were registered in 2 year follow-up examinations [23].
- The commonly used Latarjet procedure does also improve glenohumeral stability with a sling effect of the conjoint coracoidal tendon loading [11].
- Temporary oversizing of glenoidal depth and concavity after bone transplantation procedures could appear with these surgical techniques, but in the course of time a normalization will adjust due to remodeling processes [22].

2.7 Potential Complications/ Difficulties

- Although the "best fit circle" method is commonly used in clinical practice and in scientific literature, validation is still lacking [8, 17]. Yet the 3D CT is a reliable method for the quantification of glenoid bone lesions [27].
- The size of bone loss in radiographic examination should not be used as the only predictor of a treatment, but patient-specific aspects such as age, activity level and demand on the joint need to be included in decision-making.
- Another potential source of error is the orientation of the radiographic reconstructions. In 3D-MRI or 3D-CT reconstructions, the images have to be adjusted parallel to the glenoid surface to minimize the risk of undersizing or oversizing [13].
- Usage of 2D imaging leads to significant differences and leads in up to one-third of the cases to an incorrect treatment for the actual size of the lesion [7].
- As well, arthroscopic measurement of glenoidal bone defect shows significant overestimation and is not suitable for the indication of therapy [2].

2.8 Expert Recommendation

- The title "Bony Defects—from Imaging Workup to Intraoperative Assessment" suggests an intraoperative evaluation of the glenoid bone loss. Since the intraoperative assessment of glenoid bone loss is not as accurate and reliable as the preoperative assessment using CT or MRI data, the authors cannot recommend using this technique [2].
- The most important thing before surgery is to know what kind of surgical procedure to perform (open vs. arthroscopic or soft tissue vs. bony augmentation procedure) and should be clear and not be related to the intraoperative finding alone.

- However, the intraoperative findings can add additional information regarding tissue quality.

2.9 Remaining Questions

- The size for critical bone loss was reduced in recent years from over 20% to 17.3%.
- Between 13.5% and 17.3% of subcritical bone loss with no clear determination of optimal treatment is found [24, 28]. Here a patient-specific consideration of soft-tissue repair only or the usage of a bone transfer procedure must be carried out.
- The basic relevance of bone loss size has been discussed recently, because measurements of the size are unable to provide information on biomechanical effects. The relation between the biomechanical effect and osseous defect size is non-linear and challenges the classification of treatment indication by bone loss size [21]. Detailed considerations of treatment have to be obtained, and a new classification has to be discussed based on this work.
- In recent years the availability of Cone-beam CT (CBCT) has been rising continuously and offers a method with significant reduction of radiation compared to a conventional CT.
- So far, no comparison between conventional CT, MRI and CBCT is made, but it could be a possible aspect in future diagnosis.

Take Home Message

- 3D-CT for patients with shoulder instability is the best way for assessment of bone loss injuries.
- Always consider the patient's activity level for decision-making of operative technique.
- Bone loss size does not always correlate with biomechanical impact and is not sufficient as an exclusive parameter for decision-making.

References

1. Auffarth A, Schauer J, Matis N, et al. The J-bone graft for anatomical glenoid reconstruction in recurrent posttraumatic anterior shoulder dislocation. Am J Sports Med. 2008;36:638–47. https://doi.org/10.1177/0363546507309672.
2. Bakshi NK, Patel I, Jacobson JA, et al. Comparison of 3-dimensional computed tomography-based measurement of glenoid bone loss with arthroscopic defect size estimation in patients with anterior shoulder instability. Arthroscopy. 2015;31:1880–5. https://doi.org/10.1016/j.arthro.2015.03.024.
3. Balg F, Boileau P. The instability severity index score. A simple pre-operative score to select patients for arthroscopic or open shoulder stabilisation. J Bone Joint Surg Br. 2007;89:1470–7. https://doi.org/10.1302/0301-620X.89B11.18962.
4. Baudi P, Campochiaro G, Rebuzzi M, et al. Assessment of bone defects in anterior shoulder instability. Joints. 2013;1:40–8.
5. Bois AJ, Fening SD, Polster J, et al. Quantifying glenoid bone loss in anterior shoulder instability: reliability and accuracy of 2-dimensional and 3-dimensional computed tomography measurement techniques. Am J Sports Med. 2012;40:2569–77. https://doi.org/10.1177/0363546512458247.
6. Burkhart SS, De Beer JF. Traumatic glenohumeral bone defects and their relationship to failure of arthroscopic Bankart repairs: significance of the inverted-pear glenoid and the humeral engaging Hill-Sachs lesion. Arthroscopy: The Journal of Arthroscopic & Related Surgery. 2000;16:677–94. https://doi.org/10.1053/jars.2000.17715.
7. Chalmers PN, Christensen G, O'Neill D, Tashjian RZ. Does bone loss imaging modality, measurement methodology, and Interobserver reliability Alter treatment in glenohumeral instability? Arthroscopy. 2020;36:12–9. https://doi.org/10.1016/j.arthro.2019.06.025.
8. De Filippo M, Saba L, Negrini G, et al. Inter-observer agreement of CT measurement of the glenoid bone surface by the CT Pico method: comparison with laser in a cadaveric model. Skeletal Radiol. 2015;44:1491–7. https://doi.org/10.1007/s00256-015-2199-0.
9. Di Giacomo G, Peebles LA, Pugliese M, et al. Glenoid track instability management score: radiographic modification of the instability severity index score. Arthroscopy. 2020;36:56–67. https://doi.org/10.1016/j.arthro.2019.07.020.
10. Edwards TB, Boulahia A, Walch G. Radiographic analysis of bone defects in chronic anterior shoulder instability. Arthroscopy. 2003;19:732–9. https://doi.org/10.1016/s0749-8063(03)00684-4.
11. Giles JW, Boons HW, Elkinson I, et al. Does the dynamic sling effect of the Latarjet procedure improve shoulder stability? A biomechanical evalua-

tion. J Shoulder Elb Surg. 2013;22:821–7. https://doi.org/10.1016/j.jse.2012.08.002.
12. Griffith JF, Antonio GE, Yung PSH, et al. Prevalence, pattern, and spectrum of glenoid bone loss in anterior shoulder dislocation: CT analysis of 218 patients. AJR Am J Roentgenol. 2008;190:1247–54. https://doi.org/10.2214/AJR.07.3009.
13. Gross DJ, Golijanin P, Dumont GD, et al. The effect of sagittal rotation of the glenoid on axial glenoid width and glenoid version in computed tomography scan imaging. J Shoulder Elb Surg. 2016;25:61–8. https://doi.org/10.1016/j.jse.2015.06.017.
14. Heitmann DM, Frosch DK-H, Wittner DB Posttraumatische Schulterinstabilität. AWMF online:32.
15. Itoi E, Lee SB, Berglund LJ, et al. The effect of a glenoid defect on anteroinferior stability of the shoulder after Bankart repair: a cadaveric study. J Bone Joint Surg Am. 2000;82:35–46. https://doi.org/10.2106/00004623-200001000-00005.
16. Kwon YW, Powell KA, Yum JK, et al. Use of three-dimensional computed tomography for the analysis of the glenoid anatomy. J Shoulder Elbow Surg. 2005;14:85–90. https://doi.org/10.1016/j.jse.2004.04.011.
17. Lacheta L, Herbst E, Voss A, et al. Insufficient consensus regarding circle size and bone loss width using the ratio—"best fit circle"—method even with three-dimensional computed tomography. Knee Surg Sports Traumatol Arthrosc. 2019;27:3222–9. https://doi.org/10.1007/s00167-019-05391-9.
18. Lazarus MD, Sidles JA, Harryman DT, Matsen FA. Effect of a chondral-labral defect on glenoid concavity and glenohumeral stability. A cadaveric model. J Bone Joint Surg Am. 1996;78:94–102. https://doi.org/10.2106/00004623-199601000-00013.
19. Loppini M, Delle Rose G, Borroni M, et al. Is the instability severity index score a valid tool for predicting failure after primary arthroscopic stabilization for anterior glenohumeral instability? Arthroscopy. 2019;35:361–6. https://doi.org/10.1016/j.arthro.2018.09.027.
20. Lynch JR, Clinton JM, Dewing CB, et al. Treatment of osseous defects associated with anterior shoulder instability. J Shoulder Elbow Surg. 2009;18:317–28. https://doi.org/10.1016/j.jse.2008.10.013.
21. Moroder P, Damm P, Wierer G, et al. Challenging the current concept of critical glenoid bone loss in shoulder instability: does the size measurement really tell it all? Am J Sports Med. 2019;47:688–94. https://doi.org/10.1177/0363546518819102.
22. Moroder P, Hitzl W, Tauber M, et al. Effect of anatomic bone grafting in post-traumatic recurrent anterior shoulder instability on glenoid morphology. J Shoulder Elb Surg. 2013;22:1522–9. https://doi.org/10.1016/j.jse.2013.03.006.
23. Moroder P, Schulz E, Wierer G, et al. Neer Award 2019: Latarjet procedure vs. iliac crest bone graft transfer for treatment of anterior shoulder instability with glenoid bone loss: a prospective randomized trial. J Shoulder Elb Surg. 2019;28:1298–307. https://doi.org/10.1016/j.jse.2019.03.035.
24. Nacca C, Gil JA, Badida R, et al. Critical glenoid bone loss in posterior shoulder instability. Am J Sports Med. 2018;46:1058–63. https://doi.org/10.1177/0363546518758015.
25. Piasecki DP, Verma NN, Romeo AA, et al. Glenoid bone deficiency in recurrent anterior shoulder instability: diagnosis and management. J Am Acad Orthop Surg. 2009;17:482–93. https://doi.org/10.5435/00124635-200908000-00002.
26. Rabinowitz J, Friedman R, Eichinger JK. Management of glenoid bone loss with anterior shoulder instability: indications and outcomes. Curr Rev Musculoskelet Med. 2017;10:452–62. https://doi.org/10.1007/s12178-017-9439-y.
27. Saliken DJ, Bornes TD, Bouliane MJ, et al. Imaging methods for quantifying glenoid and Hill-Sachs bone loss in traumatic instability of the shoulder: a scoping review. BMC Musculoskelet Disord. 2015;16:164. https://doi.org/10.1186/s12891-015-0607-1.
28. Shaha JS, Cook JB, Song DJ, et al. Redefining "critical" bone loss in shoulder instability: functional outcomes worsen with "subcritical" bone loss. Am J Sports Med. 2015;43:1719–25. https://doi.org/10.1177/0363546515578250.
29. Shin S-J, Kim RG, Jeon YS, Kwon TH. Critical value of anterior glenoid bone loss that leads to recurrent glenohumeral instability after arthroscopic Bankart repair. Am J Sports Med. 2017;45:1975–81. https://doi.org/10.1177/0363546517697963.
30. Stillwater L, Koenig J, Maycher B, Davidson M. 3D-MR vs. 3D-CT of the shoulder in patients with glenohumeral instability. Skeletal Radiol. 2017;46:325–31. https://doi.org/10.1007/s00256-016-2559-4.
31. Sugaya H, Moriishi J, Dohi M, et al. Glenoid rim morphology in recurrent anterior glenohumeral instability. J Bone Joint Surg Am. 2003;85:878–84. https://doi.org/10.2106/00004623-200305000-00016.
32. Yamamoto N, Muraki T, Sperling JW, et al. Stabilizing mechanism in bone-grafting of a large glenoid defect. J Bone Joint Surg Am. 2010;92:2059–66. https://doi.org/10.2106/JBJS.I.00261.
33. Young AA, Maia R, Berhouet J, Walch G. Open Latarjet procedure for management of bone loss in anterior instability of the glenohumeral joint. J Shoulder Elb Surg. 2011;20:S61–9. https://doi.org/10.1016/j.jse.2010.07.022.

3 Decision-Making According to Age

Adrian Błasiak, Mikołaj Podsiadło, and Roman Brzóska

Abbreviations

3D CT	Three-dimensional computed tomography
AP	Anteroposterior
APP	Apprehension
IGHL	Inferior gleno-humeral ligament
MRI	Magnetic resonance imaging
ROM	Range of motion

Key Points

- Age is a relevant factor in decision-making regarding treatment of patients with shoulder instability.
- Two age groups are specific: patients younger than 18 years old, mainly because of high redislocation rate, and patients older than 40 years old, mainly because of concomitant injuries, predominantly rotator cuff tears.
- Operative treatment of patients younger than 18 years old should be taken into consideration if predictors of recurrent instability are present, such as: male sex, age 14 years and over, contact or collision sport athlete, closed humeral physis, injured shoulder dominance, significant Hill-Sachs lesion.
- Patients aged 40 years and more who sustained anterior shoulder dislocation should be assessed for concomitant injuries. The practitioner should exclude rotator cuff tear, nerve palsy, and/or fracture.

3.1 Introduction / Background

- Eight to twenty-six per 100 k persons per year suffer primary shoulder dislocation.
- Eleven to fifty-six per 100 k persons per year suffer shoulder dislocation episodes.
- When compared to a younger population (below 20 years of age), the recurrence rate of shoulder dislocation is much lower between the ages of 23 and 29 and even lower in patients over 30 years of age (27–30%) [1].
- Through aging and morphologic changes encompassing static and dynamic shoulder stabilizers, an ongoing stiffening takes place due to collagen structure changes in the capsular complex. In addition, changes in daily life routine and sport activities also affect

A. Błasiak (✉) · M. Podsiadło · R. Brzóska
St. Luke's Hospital Bielsko-Biała,
Bielsko-Biała, Poland

L. Kovačič et al. (eds.), *Surgical Techniques for Anterior Shoulder Instability*,
https://doi.org/10.1007/978-3-662-73064-5_3

the decreasing recurrence rate according to age [2, 3].

- In the age group above 40, first-time dislocators may suffer additional injuries such as rotator cuff tear (63–90%), a neurologic deficiency (including brachial plexus or isolated axillary nerve) in up to 65%, or fractures in up to 74% of the cases [4–7].

3.2 Scientific Updates

- Among 14- to 16-year-old patients, the rate of recurrent shoulder dislocation reflects that of high-risk adults aged 17–20 and equals up to 95% (Fig. 3.1) [1, 8–14].
- Among patients aged 12 years or less, primary dislocations are rare (Fig. 3.2) [2, 8].

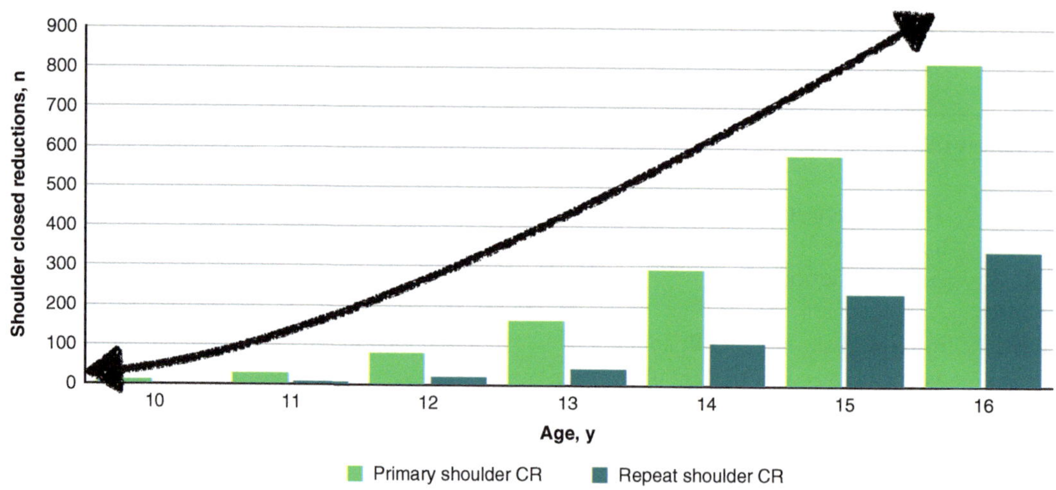

Fig. 3.1 Primary and secondary shoulder dislocations in adolescents. Age-specific distribution of primary and repeat shoulder closed reduction (CR) procedures. The rate of repeat shoulder CR was defined as the proportion of patients who underwent repeat shoulder CR compared with the number who underwent primary shoulder CR. (Adapted from Leroux et al. [8])

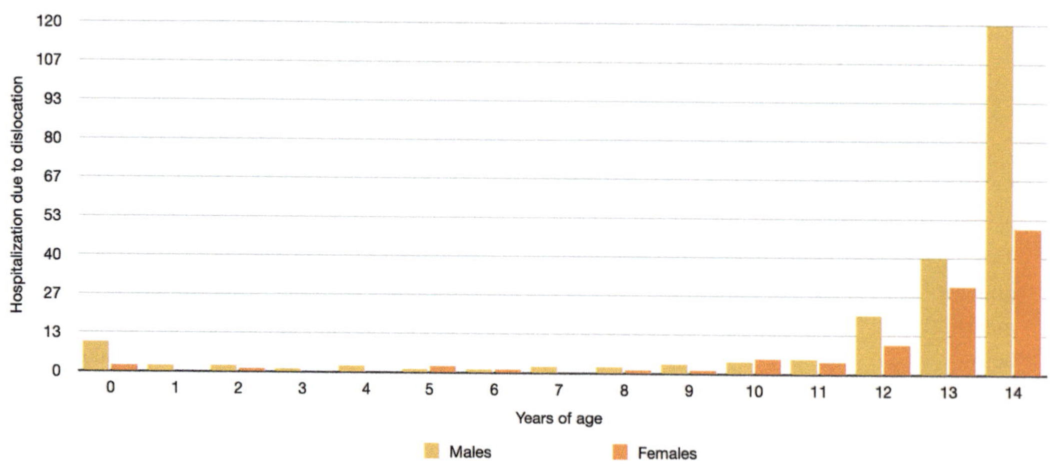

Fig. 3.2 Epidemiology of primary shoulder dislocation in children and adolescents. Hospitalizations in the 2001–2014 timespan, stratified by patient age when hospitalization due to shoulder dislocation was performed. (Adapted from Longo et al. [1]. Reproduced under the terms and conditions of the Creative Commons Attribution (CC BY) license (http://creativecommons.org/licenses/by/4.0/)

- When considering conservative treatment, there is no significant difference in terms of recurrent dislocation based on the position (internal or external rotation) or its duration when applying immobilization after the first dislocation [15].

3.3 Assessment and Planning

- The pathoanatomic explanation for a lower primary dislocation rate in children is that the insertion of the capsule on the glenoid is more lateral in the skeletally immature patient and, therefore, with a smaller anterior-inferior recess [16].
- Ligaments in the skeletally immature patient are up to seven times stronger than bone, resulting in fractures being more common than ligamentous ruptures in children.
- Typically, the inciting incident comprises a translational event without true subluxation, a subluxation with spontaneous reduction (transient subluxation), or a complete dislocation that requires manual closed reduction.
- Careful examination with range of motion, general laxity, and apprehension assessment is mandatory after either a first-time dislocation or a redislocation.
- After a shoulder dislocation episode, an X-ray with AP and Y views is mandatory.
- In the age group with higher risk of redislocation (14–25 years), an MRI is highly recommended, because it allows assessment of concomitant lesions, such as HAGL, ALPSA, and Bankart lesions, which make the patients more vulnerable to recurrent anterior dislocation.
- Three-dimensional CT is the best option for bony defect assessment, because it allows measurement of the bony glenoid loss and helps decide whether to stabilize the joint using a soft tissue or bony procedure.
- Careful history taking, including patients' demands, expectations, sport activity level, and number of redislocations, is of high importance in deciding the best treatment option.

3.4 Treatment Options and Indications

- Operative treatment should be taken into consideration in the group of young active patients with concomitant positive predictors of recurrent instability such as: male sex, age 14 years and over, contact or collision sport athlete, closed humeral physis, injured shoulder dominance, and a significant Hill-Sachs lesion [13, 17, 18].
- Conservative treatment (immobilization in a sling or brace) and a consecutive rehabilitation protocol with anterior shoulder stabilizer strengthening should be indicated in patients after a first time dislocation with no additional redislocation risk predictors or in the age group >25 years [19].

3.5 Decision-Making Algorithm

- Patients aged 13 years and less are typically treated conservatively after the first dislocation; after the second dislocation, operative treatment is considered depending on the risk factors [1, 20].
- Patients aged 14–40 years without risk factors are treated conservatively after the first dislocation; after the second dislocation, operative treatment is considered depending on the risk factors (operative treatment is recommended because of high redislocation rate) [13, 15, 20, 21].
- In patients aged over 40 years, after the first dislocation one must exclude nerve palsy, fracture, and/or cuff tear. If no concomitant injury is present, patients are treated conservatively. If fracture or cuff tear is present, operative treatment is considered. In patients after the second dislocation, operative treatment is considered depending on risk factors [3, 5–7, 22, 23].
- After third dislocation—point of no return—operative treatment is recommended because of anterior labrum lesion and/or bony Bankart and anterior capsule laxity, which make physi-

cal therapy ineffective in terms of stabilizing the joint, giving over 90% risk of redislocation.

Pearls and Pitfalls

- In skeletally immature patients, there is typically no capsulolabral disruption on MRI [16].
- In skeletally immature patients, the anatomy of the physis might be mistaken for a Hill-Sachs lesion.
- In patients over 40, start rehabilitation within 1–2 weeks after dislocation [24].
- In patients over 40, rule out fracture, nerve palsy, or cuff tear if recovery is too slow [24].
- A third dislocation is considered to be a point of no return in terms of shoulder dislocation recurrence.

3.6 Outcomes

- A high redislocation rate is expected after conservative treatment, regardless of applying immobilization, in adolescents between 14 and 18 years of age [20].
- Relatively high redislocation rates (23%) have been reported after surgical stabilization for adolescents (89% treated with closed or open Bankart repair) [15, 20].
- Patients below 18 years old undergoing an open Latarjet procedure had a significantly lower positive apprehension test (25% vs 60%; $p = 0.01$), lower radiologically proven dislocation postoperatively (7% vs 56%; $p < 0.05$), and a higher return to pre-injury level of sport (75% vs 36%) versus non-operative treatment [19].

3.7 Potential Complications/Difficulties

- The instability recurrence results in progressive labro-ligamentous injury and degeneration of anterior passive stabilizers, anterior hinge loss with labrum and IGHL tear, irreversible ligament, and capsule elongation with plastic deformation [17].

3.8 Expert Recommendation

When to consider operative treatment:

- Individual indications for each patient.
- Recurrent shoulder instability in the age group of 14–25 years.
- Anterior glenoid or Hill-Sachs fracture.
- Professional athletes.
- Active patients (contact sports).
- Patients with hyperlaxity but not MDI.

3.9 Remaining Questions

- Length of the rehabilitation protocol after first-time dislocation in the population of young athletes older than 14 years old.
- Indication for operative treatment in patients above 14 years old with higher risk of redislocation even after first-time dislocation.

Take Home Message

- Primary dislocations among patients aged 12 years old or less are rare [1].
- Consider treating immature patients aged 14–18 years similarly to the group of patients aged 18–25, taking into consideration risk factors and imaging stud-

(continued)

ies, because of the similar redislocation rate in these groups [1].

- A third dislocation is considered to be a point of no return in terms of shoulder dislocation recurrence because of redislocation rate exceeding 90% and coexistence of lesions that preclude shoulder joint stability [7].
- In recurrent shoulder dislocation, an operative treatment is the method of choice because of inability to stabilize the joint by means of conservative treatment.

References

1. Longo UG, Salvatore G, Locher J, Ruzzini L, Candela V, Berton A, Stelitano G, Schena E, Denaro V. Epidemiology of paediatric shoulder dislocation: a nationwide study in Italy from 2001 to 2014. Int J Environ Res Public Health. 2020;17(8):2834.
2. Franklin CC, Weiss JM. The natural history of pediatric and adolescent shoulder dislocation. J Pediatr Orthop. 2019;39(6, Suppl 1):S50–2.
3. Hovelius L, Olofsson A, Sandström B, Augustini BG, Krantz L, Fredin H, Tillander B, Skoglund U, Salomonsson B, Nowak J, Sennerby U. Nonoperative treatment of primary anterior shoulder dislocation in patients forty years of age and younger. A prospective twenty-five-year follow-up. J Bone Joint Surg Am. 2008;90(5):945–52.
4. Avis D, Power D. Axillary nerve injury associated with glenohumeral dislocation: a review and algorithm for management. EFORT Open Rev. 2018;3(3):70–7.
5. de Beer J, Bhatia DN. Shoulder instability in the middle-aged and elderly patients: pathology and surgical implications. Int J Shoulder Surg. 2010;4(4):87.
6. Gutkowska O, Martynkiewicz J, Urban M, Gosk J. Brachial plexus injury after shoulder dislocation: a literature review. Neurosurg Rev. 2020;43(2):407–23.
7. Kao JT, Chang CL, Su WR, Chang WL, Tai TW. Incidence of recurrence after shoulder dislocation: a nationwide database study. J Shoulder Elb Surg. 2018;27(8):1519–25. https://doi.org/10.1016/j.jse.2018.02.047. Epub 2018 Apr 25. PMID: 29705013.
8. Leroux T, Ogilvie-Harris D, Veillette C, Chahal J, Dwyer T, Khoshbin A, Henry P, Mahomed N, Wasserstein D. The epidemiology of primary anterior shoulder dislocations in patients aged 10 to 16 years. Am J Sports Med. 2015;43(9):2111–7.
9. Robinson CM, Howes J, Murdoch H, Will E, Graham C. Functional outcome and risk of recurrent instability after primary traumatic anterior shoulder dislocation in young patients. J Bone Joint Surg Am. 2006;88(11):2326–36.
10. Chalidis B, Sachinis N, Dimitriou C, Papadopoulos P, Samoladas E, Pournaras J. Has the management of shoulder dislocation changed over time? Int Orthop. 2007;31(3):385–9.
11. Zacchilli MA, Owens BD. Epidemiology of shoulder dislocations presenting to emergency departments in the United States. J Bone Joint Surg Am. 2010;92(3):542–9.
12. Liavaag S, Svenningsen S, Reikerås O, Enger M, Fjalestad T, Pripp AH, Brox JI. The epidemiology of shoulder dislocations in Oslo. Scand J Med Sci Sports. 2011;21(6):e334–40.
13. Olds M, Donaldson K, Ellis R, Kersten P. In children 18 years and under, what promotes recurrent shoulder instability after traumatic anterior shoulder dislocation? A systematic review and meta-analysis of risk factors. Br J Sports Med. 2016;50(18):1135–41.
14. Postacchini F, Gumina S, Cinotti G. Anterior shoulder dislocation in adolescents. J Shoulder Elbow Surg. 2000;9(6):470–4.
15. Gigis I, Heikenfeld R, Kapinas A, Listringhaus R, Godolias G. Arthroscopic versus conservative treatment of first anterior dislocation of the shoulder in adolescents. J Pediatr Orthop. 2014;34(4):421–5.
16. Li X, Ma R, Nielsen NM, Gulotta LV, Dines JS, Owens BD. Management of shoulder instability in the skeletally immature patient. J Am Acad Orthop Surg. 2013;21(9):529–37.
17. Carpinteiro EP, Barros AA. Natural history of anterior shoulder instability. Open Orthop J. 2017;11:909–18.
18. Deitch J, Mehlman CT, Foad SL, Obbehat A, Mallory M. Traumatic anterior shoulder dislocation in adolescents. Am J Sports Med. 2003;31(5):758–63.
19. Khan A, Samba A, Pereira B, Canavese F. Anterior dislocation of the shoulder in skeletally immature patients: comparison between non-operative treatment versus open Latarjet's procedure. Bone Joint J. 2014;96-B(3):354–9.
20. Leland DP, Bernard CD, Keyt LK, Krych AJ, Dahm DL, Sanchez-Sotelo J, Camp CL. An age-based approach to anterior shoulder instability in patients under 40 years old: analysis of a US population. Am J Sports Med. 2020;48(1):56–62.
21. Milewski MD, Nissen CW. Pediatric and adolescent shoulder instability. Clin Sports Med. 2013;32(4):761–79.
22. Paxton ES, Dodson CC, Lazarus MD. Shoulder instability in older patients. Orthop Clin North Am. 2014;45(3):377–85.
23. Robinson CM, Shur N, Sharpe T, Ray A, Murray IR. Injuries associated with traumatic anterior glenohumeral dislocations. J Bone Joint Surg Am. 2012;94(1):18–26.
24. Alentron-Geli E, Kovacic L et al. Age and time specific management of traumatic anterior shoulder instability the ESSKA-ESA formal consensus. ESSKA Academy.

507461_1_En

Soft Tissue or Bony Reconstruction: Is There a Gold Standard Today?

4

Bartlomiej Kordasiewicz, Michal Janyst, and Andrzej Boszczyk

Key Points

- Decision between soft tissue reconstruction or a bony procedure in the treatment of anterior shoulder instability remains one of the most difficult and debatable questions.
- In the step-by-step decision-making process, evaluation of bone loss of the anterior glenoid rim and the humeral head is the first and crucial step.
- Proper patient assessment is necessary to evaluate patient "at risk."
- Adequate shoulder stabilization procedure is on an "à la carte" basis.
- None of the procedures are 100% safe and reliable, therefore patients must be informed about the potential risk of complications and recurrence.

Supplementary Information The online version contains supplementary material available at https://doi.org/10.1007/978-3-662-73064-5_4.

B. Kordasiewicz (✉) · A. Boszczyk
Idea Ortopedia, Warsaw, Poland

M. Janyst
Trauma and Orthopedics Department, SPSK im. A. Grucy, Otwock, Poland

4.1 Introduction

- Soft tissue reconstruction or bony procedure—this is probably one of the most crucial questions in the surgery of anterior shoulder instability.
- Unfortunately, the answer remains not clear, and the updated literature does not bring a simple solution.
- There are some guidelines, but it is hard to announce it a gold standard.

4.2 Scientific Update

- Glenohumeral joint anatomy is responsible for the largest range of motion in the human body, but it is related to the highest risk of instability. Only 25% of the humeral head is covered by the socket. This poor ratio makes any additional bone deficiencies hard to compensate [1].
- Bone deficits represented by the glenoid anterior rim and the humeral head side—Hill-Sachs lesion (HSL)—are believed to be crucial in the evaluation of a shoulder instability [2].
- Burkhart et al. revealed that glenoid bone loss above 25% required bone grafting [2, 3].
- Itoi et al. proved that glenoid defect of 21% of superior-inferior glenoid length would

L. Kovačič et al. (eds.), *Surgical Techniques for Anterior Shoulder Instability*, https://doi.org/10.1007/978-3-662-73064-5_4

increase the failure rate of Bankart procedure [4]. Sang-Jin Shin et al., in their anatomical study, expanded bone block indications to 15% of the glenoid bone loss [5]. Boileau and Balg recommend using bone block stabilization in glenoid defect ≥10% [6].

- Burkhart et al. first introduced the term "engaging Hill-Sachs," which means that its size and position create engagement with the anterior glenoid rim in the position of abduction and external rotation [7].
- Kurokawa et al. presented "true engaging HSL"—it occurs during arthroscopic examination even after Bankart repair or when it extends over the glenoid track. Width and depth of engaging lesions were larger and more horizontal than non-engaging ones. The authors proposed two types of engaging HSL: type wide and large and type, and narrow but medially located [8].
- Hardy et al. reported the importance of measuring of HSL parameters, particularly the depth of the lesion. The authors analyzed the ratio of the depth of the lesion to the humeral head radius and showed that patients with a ratio > 15% had significantly more recurrence after arthroscopic Bankart repair [9].
- Four out of five patients with recurrent anterior instability present bipolar lesion, so the dynamic interplay between the Hill-Sachs lesion (HSL) and the anterior glenoid rim bone loss seems to be the crucial factor for instability.
- Yamamoto et al. presented the concept of the glenoid track, which is a contact zone between the glenoid and the humeral head. The authors introduced the term on-track, when the HSL stays on the glenoid track without engagement, and therefore without dislocation, and the term off-track, when the HSL engages with the glenoid rim, causing dislocation [10].
- Omori et al. calculated this zone as 83% of the glenoid width [11]. Yamamoto et al. also showed that patients after Bankart repair with on-track lesions but with ≥75% of Hill-Sachs occupancy had a significantly worse Western Ontario Shoulder Instability Index score [12].
- The remaining problem is the exact evaluation of the on-track/off-track concept. Schneider et al. reported a poor level of interobserver reliability of this classification (72%) and a poor level of agreement between observers (65%) regarding treatment classification [13].
- Additionally, Moroder et al. studied the critical bone loss of the glenoid on the printed models of patients with glenoid bone loss—the authors also evaluated the glenoid concavity shape. The authors concluded that current glenoid bone loss methods were unable to provide the biomechanical effect of a glenoid defect, because this relationship is nonlinear and because patients with shoulder instability had smaller glenoid concavity compared to healthy individuals. It was also noticed that the same glenoid bone loss resulted in a higher loss of stability ratio in patients with more concave glenoids [14].
- Other risk factors are related to patients' age, constitution (laxity), and activity.
- Balg and Boileau introduced the Instability Severity Index Score (ISIS), which helps to put these factors together and to identify the patients at risk of recurrence before the surgery. The authors reported that a score > 6 was associated with a 70% risk of recurrence after arthroscopic Bankart repair [15]. Phadnis et al. confirmed that this score was a valid preoperative tool but reported a 70% recurrence of instability after arthroscopic Bankart repair in patients scoring ≥4 [16]. Thomazeau et al., in 2010, also suggested that an ISIS ≤4 was more suitable for arthroscopic Bankart repair [17].
- In 2019, Thomazeau et al. again investigated the Instability Severity Index Score in patients treated with isolated Bankart repair, without bony lesions. The overall recurrence rate at 9-year follow-up was 23% and 42% in patients <20 years old at the time of surgery. The authors reported that patients with preoperative ISIS ≤2 had a recurrence rate of 10% versus 35.6% in patients with ISIS 3 or 4 [18].
- Lopini et al. interviewed by telephone 670 patients after Bankart repair and divided patients into 3 groups depending on ISIS score

regarding the success rate: group A (≤ 3 points)—93.7%, group B (≤ 6 points)—85.7% and group C (> 6 points)—54.6%. The authors found that the most important risk factors for predicting recurrence after a soft tissue procedure were glenoid bone loss and contact or forced overhead sports [19].

- In an editorial commentary, Boileau and Lemmex stated that an important risk of recurrence after Bankart repair exists if the score is >3 [20].
- Balg and Boileau reported that radiographic evaluation of the bone defects remains difficult on plain radiographs [15]. Many authors suggested using 3D CT as the most useful tool for evaluation of bone loss [21, 22].
- In 2020, Di Giacomo et al. modified the ISIS into GTIMS (Glenoid Track Instability Management Score), introducing the glenoid track concept (Table 4.1) [23]. 3D CT evaluation of glenoid bone loss and HSL was used instead of plain radiographs. When an off-track lesion was confirmed, 4 points were added to the score. The indication for Latarjet stabilization was ≥4 points. In this study, the authors concluded that exact bone loss evaluation permits lowering the number of Latarjet stabilizations: 14.3% of patients underwent Latarjet stabilization in the GTIMS group versus 69.4%. The results seemed to be relatively comparable; however, the average follow-up was 33 months, so further conclusions should be drawn very carefully [23].
- In 2021, Dekker et al. stated that the ISIS score had no correlation with the outcomes after arthroscopic Bankart repair [24]. In another editorial commentary, Boileau and Balg discussed this study, recommending using their score with 3D CT diagnostics [6].
- To conclude, using this guideline, not including the bony status of the joint, the term "patient at risk" could be introduced—it concerns patient with age under 20, laxity, and involved in professional or contact or high risk of injury sports.

Table 4.1 Glenoid track instability management score (GTIMS)—modification of ISIS

GTIMS Prognostic Factors	Score
Age at surgery	
< 20	2
> 20	0
Type of sport	
Contact or forced overhead	1
Other	0
Level of competition in sport	
Competitive	2
Recreational or none	0
Shoulder hyperlaxity	
Confirmed anterior or inferior hyperlaxity	1
Normal laxity	0
Evaluation of bone loss on 3D CT	
On-track	0
Off-track	4
Total GTIMS	10

4.3 Treatment Options and Indications

- Surgical techniques of stabilization are numerous, and a detailed discussion concerning their advantages and modifications largely exceeds this chapter. Nevertheless, it is important to put these techniques in some order and to use them "à la carte" if necessary.
- To date, there is no consensus in the literature concerning clear guidelines on which techniques should be used in a particular case. Reconstructive procedures can be divided into 2 groups:
  1. Concerning anterior compartment (anterior glenohumeral wall: anterior glenoid rim, labrum, and capsule), including anterior bony procedures and anterior soft tissue procedures,
  2. Concerning humeral head lesion (fulfilling the HSL: remplissage technique or osteochondral grafts).
- All these techniques could be also divided into bony and soft tissue procedures listed below with a short comment.

4.3.1 Soft Tissue Procedures

- Anterior wall reconstruction—arthroscopic Bankart repair, a classic reconstruction of the labrum with capsular shift [25].
- Anterior wall reinforcement
  - BLS technique, using medial glenohumeral ligament augmentation or one of the subscapularis cords [26].
  - Augmentation technique using the long head of the biceps tendon (LHB) as a sling (dynamic anterior stabilization—DAS) [27].
  - Glenohumeral Inferior ligament reconstruction using the palmaris longus tendon [28].
  - Bankart-Plus technique—a Bankart procedure is associated with small bone graft reconstruction [29].
  - Hill-Sachs procedure—remplissage [30].

4.3.2 Bone Block Procedures

- Anterior glenoid ream reconstruction
  - Latarjet stabilization—open or arthroscopic; it is important to remember that the Latarjet procedure is not only a bone block procedure, but also the dynamic sling effect plays an important role in a shoulder stabilization [31–33].
  - Iliac crest graft procedures: Eden-Hybinette, J-graft, distal tibia allograft [34–36].
- Hill-Sachs procedure—osteochondral graft [37–39].

4.4 Assessment and Planning

- Patient evaluation is based on clinical information (age, laxity, level of apprehension, number of instability episodes, and sport).
- Computed tomography (CT) evaluation is focused on glenoid and humeral head lesions, as bony lesions are principal risk factors for instability. 3D reconstruction CT allows precise evaluation of bony lesions and calculation of HSL engagement is possible.
- In older group of patients, or if clinical examination suggests, MRI could be useful to evaluate rotator cuff injuries.
- Surgery is planned concerning the type of bony lesions and the presence of all data reported as "patient at risk."
- The surgery should be focused on the type of anterior compartment problem as well as the type of humeral head lesion.
- In our institution, surgical planning starts from with evaluation of glenoid bone loss. The bone loss can be divided into small, medium, and minimal. We believe that only minimal glenoid defect ($\leq 10\%$) could be an indication for an anterior soft tissue procedure. If the glenoid bone loss is >10%, a bone block procedure should be considered, especially if other risk factors are present.
- According to the presence of Hill-Sachs lesion and qualification as "patient at risk," the proper procedure is chosen "à la carte." The diagnostic algorithm is proposed in Table 4.2.

A Clinical Case is presented in Fig. 4.1.

Table 4.2 Algorithm in shoulder instability. Patient at risk—patient with laxity, age < 20 and professional or high-risk sport activity

Instability → Glenoid bone loss

	No or minimal (<10%)	Medium 10-20%	Large (>20%)
No HSL or on-track	Bankart repair + anterior reinforcement (LHB) if patient at risk[a]	Bankart repair or bone block if patient at risk	Bone block
Off-track HSL	Bankart repair + HS procedure	Bankart repair + HS procedure or Bone block if patient at risk	Bone block +/- HS procedure if patient at risk[a]

[a]Authors preferred method, not proven scientifically

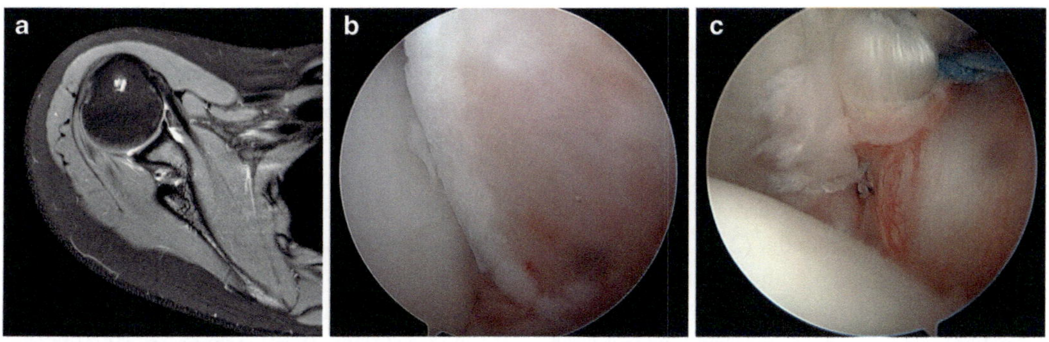

Fig. 4.1 Case report. 20-year-old woman, R-handed, physiotherapist, volleyball player—very active. 5 years earlier, at the age of 15—fall whilst volleyball, possible subluxation. 2 years ago—dislocation during serve in volleyball, since that moment—painful shoulder. Clinical examination: good ROM, apprehension test positive at 120° abduction, relocation+, Gagey—apprehension from 110°, laxity +. (**a**) MRI—no anterior glenoid bone loss (in such a case—if no doubts about the quality of anterior glenoid rim—no complementary CT is performed), small HSL—10% of humeral head diameter. (**b**) Non-engaging HSL, camera in posterior portal, beach chair position. (**c**) Anterior soft tissue—Bankart reconstruction with LHB augmentation was chosen—Milenin's technique [27]. No indication for bony procedure, remplissage was abandoned due to risk of external rotation loss

Pearls and Pitfalls

Proposed guidelines for workup and treatment:

1. Glenoid bone loss evaluation is preferably done with a 3D CT scan.
2. Thorough history and clinical examination are important to identify "patient at risk."
3. In the case of minimal glenoid bone loss (≤ 10%), soft tissue stabilization could be augmented by HSL—remplissage or LHB (DAS) in patients at risk.
4. In the case of medium glenoid bone loss (10–20%), bone block stabilization could be performed in patients at risk. In low-risk patients, Bankart alone or Bankart and remplissage could be performed.
5. In the case of glenoid bone loss (> 20%), a bone block procedure could be augmented by remplissage (or osteochondral graft) in massive HSL in patients at risk.

4.5 Outcomes

- Arthroscopic Bankart repair is the most popular stabilization procedure. Nevertheless, the recurrence rate reaches up to 29% or even 42%, with an average ratio of 8.9% [40–42].
- In 2014, Wolf and Arinjam reported only a 4.4% (2 patients) of recurrence rate at a mean follow-up of 58 months (2 to 10 years) in a group of 45 patients after Bankart and remplissage stabilization. Except for these 2 patients, no complications and no revisions were reported [43].
- Cavalier et al. evaluated 133 patients with a mean follow-up of 4 years after arthroscopic Bankart repair and the remplissage technique. The recurrence rate was 7.5%, but was significantly higher in the group of patients with subcritical glenoid bone loss of 10% to 20%. Another risk factor for recurrence was age < 23 years. Seventy-eight percent of patients could return to sport, but only 65% returned to practicing high-risk sports [44].
- Only a few studies report the outcomes after Bankart repair combined with the reinforcement techniques. Brzoska et al. presented a 14% of recurrence rate in their group with an average follow-up of 83 months [26]. Garcia et al. evaluated 20 patients after a minimum of 24 months following the DAS procedure using LHB reinforcement. The authors reported excellent results with no recurrence and no complications [45]. Azavedo and Angelo reported one redislocation (6.7%) out of 15 patients followed-up for a minimum of 1 year after DAS stabilization [46].
- Latarjet stabilization remains one of the most effective procedures in anterior shoulder instability. Bhatia et al. reported a recurrence rate between 0 and 8% [47].
- Arthroscopic and open techniques seem to be comparable; however, precise graft position, arthrolysis of the superior part of the graft, and loss of external rotation with the arm at the side remained problems to be solved in the future in arthroscopic stabilization [48–50].
- In 2015, Cho et al. reported the results comparing arthroscopic Bankart repair with associated remplissage and Latarjet stabilization. The authors concluded that the results in both groups were similar, but the number of complications was significantly higher in the Latarjet group (14.3% versus 0%) [51]. Yang et al. also compared the results of Latarjet stabilization in 91 patients versus arthroscopic Bankart repair and remplissage in 98 cases, after a mean follow-up of 3.2 years. The authors reported no difference between the 2 groups in revision rate neither in recurrence, but higher pain scores and more limited internal rotation in abduction in the remplissage group, and higher complication rates in the Latarjet group. However, in revision cases, in patients with glenoid bone loss >10%, and in collision and contact athletes, patients in the Latarjet group had better results; therefore, in these

cases, the authors recommended a Latarjet stabilization instead [52].

- Boehm et al. presented the results of arthroscopic iliac crest bone grafting in 17 patients evaluated after a minimum 5-years follow-up. The authors reported an apprehension sign in 2 patients (14%)—1 had traumatic dislocation (7%), and 1 was revised with arthroscopic capsular plication due to a feeling of instability [53]. However, in another study, Boehm et al. concluded that this procedure did not accomplish an anatomic reconstruction of the glenoid concavity due to excessive graft resorption [54].
- Some studies present the results of grafting the Hill-Sachs lesion using allografts or autografts, but most of them showed relatively short-term follow-up results or described a surgical technique [37–39, 55]. Zhuo et al. published the results of 19 patients with osteochondral allograft transplantation for large Hill-Sachs lesion s(> 30% of the articular surface) at a mean follow-up of 28 months. None of these patients had recurrence, the overall satisfaction rate was 95%, but the rate of graft resorption was 43% [56].
- Very promising results were reported after stabilization using fresh-frozen distal tibial allograft, also in cases of revision after failed Latarjet procedure, but the use of these grafts in Europe remains more complex [36, 57, 58].

4.6 Potential Complications/Difficulties

4.6.1 Bankart Repair

- The most probable problem after arthroscopic Bankart repair remains recurrence of instability.
- Yian et al. reported that 30% of patients following primary arthroscopic Bankart repair, with an average follow-up of 6.2 years developed symptomatic recurrent instability. Some predictive factors following surgical treatment were found: age under 21, "off-track" lesions, intact anterior articular arc <150°, and glenoid bone loss of at least 10%. Glenoid bone loss of 10% and greater was the most predictive variable for recurrence [59].
- Also, Zimmerman et al. reported that 41.7% of patients after Bankart repair, at an average 10-year follow-up, presented some recurrence, defined as any type of subjective instability: apprehension, subluxation, or dislocation. Interestingly, 20% of the first recurrences occurred no earlier than 91 months postoperatively [42].
- Flinkkila et al. presented results of 186 shoulders with arthroscopic Bankart repair after minimum 10-year follow-up. Thirty percent of patients had recurrence with 18% of revision surgery. The authors reported a 54% failure rate in patients younger than 20 years old [60].
- Ernstbrunner et al. compared the results of the arthroscopic Bankart repair at a mean follow-up of 13.2 years and open Latarjet stabilization at a mean follow-up of 11 years in patients older than 40 years. The authors reported significantly higher rates of redislocation and subluxation compared with the open Latarjet procedure and significantly lower simple shoulder value in the Bankart group. The authors reported no significant differences in the final arthropathy and revision rate between both groups [61].

4.6.2 Remplissage

- Reported outcomes seem to be satisfactory, as it has already been mentioned. However, Merola et al. reported significant limitation of external rotation compared to the healthy shoulder [62]. Gouveia et al. compared patients treated with arthroscopic Bankart repair with remplissage and bone block augmentation. The authors stated that patients with glenoid bone loss >10% who underwent arthroscopic Bankart repair with remplissage may have a higher risk of failure than patients treated with bone block augmentation. However, the number of complications in bone block procedures was reported to be up to 66.7%, compared to 2.3% in arthroscopic Bankart repair and remplissage [63].

4.6.3 DAS (Dynamic Anterior Stabilization with LHB Tendon)

- This relatively new technique seems to be very effective, as it is based on a sling effect without complications related to the bone block fixation. There are many technical options for LHB tendon preparation and fixation; however, very few studies report the outcomes [27, 64, 65]. It seems to be less technically demanding than an arthroscopic bone block procedure; however, the thorough knowledge of "pericoracoid arthroscopic anatomy" is necessary. This procedure could fulfill the gap between the bony procedures and simple Bankart repair, but more studies reporting the results are necessary to prove its efficacy.

4.6.4 Latarjet

- In a systematic review concerning complications, Williams et al. showed that arthroscopic bone block procedures had the highest rate of complications (13.6%) [66]. Arthroscopic soft tissue repair had a complication rate of 1.6% and open bone block stabilization 7.2%. Nevertheless, the group of patients treated with an arthroscopic soft tissue procedure had the highest recurrence rate (16.4%) [66]. Ernstbrunner et al. studied 39 patients (40 shoulders) older than 40 years old after Latarjet stabilization at a mean follow-up of 11 years. The authors reported no dislocation, subluxation in 8% and persistent apprehension in 13% of patients. Eighteen percent of patients had reoperation, mainly due to persistent pain. The authors also showed that lateral positioning of the graft (> +1 mm) was correlated with the development of dislocation arthropathy, whereas medial positioning of the graft (> 4 mm) was correlated with apprehension and subluxation. The risk of dislocation arthropathy also increased with higher age and existing joint degeneration at the time of stabilization surgery. Other authors also confirmed that complications related to bone block procedures concern mainly hardware and graft problems [67, 68].

4.7 Expert Recommendation

- The problem of performing soft tissue reconstruction or a bone block procedure remains the most important question when anterior shoulder stabilization is planned.
- The bony status of the patient's glenohumeral joint should be carefully analyzed, preferably, on 3D CT, as it seems to be a crucial risk factor.
- Anterior soft tissue procedures, based on Bankart stabilization alone, should be proposed if the glenoid bone loss is minimal (≤ 10%).
- In larger glenoid defects, also analyzing other patient-related risk factors, all other procedures should be considered, including also bony procedures.
- If the glenoid deficit is >20%, bone block stabilization should be strongly recommended. Latarjet stabilization is recommended in this condition, as this is not only a bony procedure but also a dynamic one due to its "sling effect." If Latarjet stabilization is done arthroscopically (as in our institution), a final decision could be made after initial arthroscopic inspection in "border line" cases—it allows to evaluate soft tissue quality and "live" interplay between HSL and the anterior glenoid rim to confirm or exclude an off-track lesion.

Take Home Message

The important steps before the decision on the type of stabilization in anterior shoulder instability should be the following:

1. Bone deficiency evaluation, using preferentially 3D CT.
2. Patient evaluation—be aware of "patient at risk."
3. In case of glenoid bone loss > 10%, consider a bone block procedure if the patient is at risk.
4. Use all procedures "à la carte" depending on the combination of all risk factors.
5. Tell the patients about the risk of failure.

References

1. Turkel SJ, Panio MW, Marshall JL, Girgis FG. Stabilizing mechanisms preventing anterior dislocation of the glenohumeral joint. J Bone Joint Surg Am. 1981;63:1208–17.
2. Burkhart SS, Debeer JF, Tehrany AM, Parten PM. Quantifying glenoid bone loss arthroscopically in shoulder instability. Arthroscopy. 2002;18:488–91.
3. Ochoa E, Burkhart SS. Bone defects in anterior instability of the shoulder: diagnosis and management. Oper Tech Orthop. 2008;18:68–78.
4. Itoi E, Lee SB, Berglund LJ, Berge LL, An KN. The effect of a glenoid defect on anteroinferior stability of the shoulder after Bankart repair: a cadaveric study. J Bone Joint Surg Am. 2000;82:35–46.
5. Shin S-J, Koh YW, Bui C, Jeong WK, Akeda M, Cho NS, McGarry MH, Lee TQ. What is the critical value of glenoid bone loss at which soft tissue Bankart repair does not restore glenohumeral translation, restricts range of motion, and leads to abnormal humeral head position? Am J Sports Med. 2016;44:2784–91.
6. Boileau P, Balg F. Editorial Commentary: Should We Condemn the Shoulder Instability Severity Index Scoring System? Not at All!... Can We Improve Its Radiographic Component? Yes, We Can! Arthroscopy: The Journal of Arthroscopic & Related Surgery. 2021;37:1392–6.
7. Burkhart SS, De Beer JF. Traumatic glenohumeral bone defects and their relationship to failure of arthroscopic Bankart repairs: significance of the inverted-pear glenoid and the humeral engaging Hill-Sachs lesion. Arthroscopy. 2000;16:677–94.
8. Kurokawa D, Yamamoto N, Nagamoto H, Omori Y, Tanaka M, Sano H, Itoi E. The prevalence of a large hill-Sachs lesion that needs to be treated. J Shoulder Elb Surg. 2013;22:1285–9.
9. Hardy P, Lopes R, Bauer T, Conso C, Gaudin P, Sanghavi S. New quantitative measurement of the Hill–Sachs lesion: a prognostic factor for clinical results of arthroscopic glenohumeral stabilization. Eur J Orthop Surg Traumatol. 2012;22:541–7.
10. Yamamoto N, Itoi E, Abe H, Minagawa H, Seki N, Shimada Y, Okada K. Contact between the glenoid and the humeral head in abduction, external rotation, and horizontal extension: a new concept of glenoid track. J Shoulder Elb Surg. 2007;16:649–56.
11. Omori Y, Yamamoto N, Koishi H, Futai K, Goto A, Sugamoto K, Itoi E. Measurement of the glenoid track in vivo as investigated by 3-dimensional motion analysis using open MRI. Am J Sports Med. 2014;42:1290–5.
12. Yamamoto N, Shinagawa K, Hatta T, Itoi E. Peripheral-track and central-track Hill-Sachs lesions: a new concept of assessing an on-track lesion. Am J Sports Med. 2020;48:33–8.
13. Schneider AK, Hoy GA, Ek ET, Rotstein AH, Tate J, Taylor DM, Evans MC. Interobserver and intraobserver variability of glenoid track measurements. J Shoulder Elb Surg. 2017;26:573–9.
14. Moroder P, Damm P, Wierer G, Böhm E, Minkus M, Plachel F, Märdian S, Scheibel M, Khatamirad M. Challenging the current concept of critical glenoid bone loss in shoulder instability: does the size measurement really tell it all? Am J Sports Med. 2019;47:688–94.
15. Balg F, Boileau P. The instability severity index score. A simple pre-operative score to select patients for arthroscopic or open shoulder stabilisation. J Bone Joint Surg Br. 2007;89:1470–7.
16. Phadnis J, Arnold C, Elmorsy A, Flannery M. Utility of the instability severity index score in predicting failure after arthroscopic anterior stabilization of the shoulder. Am J Sports Med. 2015;43:1983–8.
17. Thomazeau H, Courage O, Barth J, et al. Can we improve the indication for Bankart arthroscopic repair? A preliminary clinical study using the ISIS score. Orthop Traumatol Surg Res. 2010;96:S77–83.
18. Thomazeau H, Langlais T, Hardy A, Curado J, Herisson O, Mouton J, Charousset C, Courage O, Nourissat G. Long-term, prospective, multicenter study of isolated Bankart repair for a patient selection method based on the instability severity index score. Am J Sports Med. 2019;47:1057–61.
19. Loppini M, Delle Rose G, Borroni M, Morenghi E, Pitino D, Domínguez Zamora C, Castagna A. Is the instability severity index score a valid tool for predicting failure after primary arthroscopic stabilization for anterior glenohumeral instability? Arthroscopy. 2019;35:361–6.
20. Boileau P, Lemmex DB. Editorial commentary: which patients are likely to undergo Redislocation after an arthroscopic Bankart repair? Preoperative instability

severity index scoring over 3 points-the game is over! Arthroscopy. 2019;35:367–71.

21. Kubicka AM, Stefaniak J, Lubiatowski P, Długosz J, Dzianach M, Redman M, Piontek J, Romanowski L. Reliability of measurements performed on two dimensional and three dimensional computed tomography in glenoid assessment for instability. Int Orthop. 2016;40:2581–8.
22. Stefaniak J, Kubicka AM, Wawrzyniak A, Romanowski L, Lubiatowski P. Reliability of humeral head measurements performed using two- and three-dimensional computed tomography in patients with shoulder instability. Int Orthop. 2020;44:2049–56.
23. Di Giacomo G, Peebles LA, Pugliese M, Dekker TJ, Golijanin P, Sanchez A, Provencher MT. Glenoid track instability management score: radiographic modification of the instability severity index score. Arthroscopy: The Journal of Arthroscopic & Related Surgery. 2020;36:56–67.
24. Dekker TJ, Peebles LA, Bernhardson AS, Golijanin P, Di Giacomo G, Hackett TR, Provencher MT. Limited predictive value of the instability severity index score: evaluation of 217 consecutive cases of recurrent anterior shoulder instability. Arthroscopy. 2021;37:1381–91.
25. Lubiatowski P, Długosz J, Ślęzak M, Ogrodowicz P, Stefaniak J, Walecka J, Romanowski L. Effect of arthroscopic techniques on joint volume in shoulder instability: Bankart repair versus capsular shift. Int Orthop. 2017;41:149–55.
26. Brzóska R, Laprus H, Michniowski P, Solecki W, Klon W, Błasiak A. Novel and effective arthroscopic extra-capsular stabilization technique for anterior shoulder instability-BLS. Knee Surg Sports Traumatol Arthrosc. 2019;27:3897–904.
27. Milenin O, Toussaint B. Labral repair augmentation by labroplasty and simultaneous trans-subscapular transposition of the long head of the biceps. Arthrosc Tech. 2019;8:e507–12.
28. Arenas-Miquelez A, Karargyris O, Zumstein M. All-arthroscopic, 270° reconstruction of the inferior glenohumeral ligament with palmaris longus autograft. Arthrosc Tech. 2019;8:e1145–51.
29. Moroder P, Böhm E, Scheibel M. The arthroscopic Bankart-plus procedure for treatment of anterior shoulder instability with small to intermediate glenoid defects. Arthrosc Tech. 2018;7:e379–84.
30. Purchase RJ, Wolf EM, Hobgood ER, Pollock ME, Smalley CC. Hill-sachs "remplissage": an arthroscopic solution for the engaging hill-sachs lesion. Arthroscopyy. 2008;24:723–6.
31. Latarjet M. Treatment of recurrent dislocation of the shoulder. Lyon Chir. 1954;49:994–7.
32. Lafosse L, Lejeune E, Bouchard A, Kakuda C, Gobezie R, Kochhar T, Sc M, Tr FRCS. The arthroscopic Latarjet procedure for the tratment of anterior shoulder instability. Arthroscopy. 2007;23:1242e1–5.
33. Lafosse L, Boyle S. Arthroscopic Latarjet procedure. J Shoulder Elb Surg. 2010;19:2–12.
34. Moroder P, Blocher M, Auffarth A, Hoffelner T, Hitzl W, Tauber M, Resch H. Clinical and computed tomography-radiologic outcome after bony glenoid augmentation in recurrent anterior shoulder instability without significant glenoid bone loss. J Shoulder Elb Surg. 2014;23:420–6.
35. Anderl W, Kriegleder B, Heuberer PR. All-arthroscopic implant-free iliac crest bone grafting: new technique and case report. Arthroscopy: The Journal of Arthroscopic & Related Surgery. 2012;28:131–7.
36. Provencher MT, Frank RM, Golijanin P, Gross D, Cole BJ, Verma NN, Romeo AA. Distal tibia allograft glenoid reconstruction in recurrent anterior shoulder instability: clinical and radiographic outcomes. Arthroscopy: The Journal of Arthroscopic & Related Surgery. 2017;33:891–7.
37. Yagishita K, Thomas BJ. Use of allograft for large Hill-Sachs lesion associated with anterior glenohumeral dislocation. A case report. Injury. 2002;33:791–4.
38. Saltzman BM, Riboh JC, Cole BJ, Yanke AB. Humeral head reconstruction with osteochondral allograft transplantation. Arthroscopy. 2015;31:1827–34.
39. Snir N, Wolfson TS, Hamula MJ, Gyftopoulos S, Meislin RJ. Arthroscopic anatomic humeral head reconstruction with osteochondral allograft transplantation for large hill-sachs lesions. Arthrosc Tech. 2013;2:e289–93.
40. Hobby J, Griffin D, Dunbar M, Boileau P. Is arthroscopic surgery for stabilisation of chronic shoulder instability as effective as open surgery? A systematic review and meta-analysis of 62 studies including 3044 arthroscopic operations. J Bone Joint Surg Br. 2007;89:1188–96.
41. van der Linde JA, van Kampen DA, Terwee CB, Dijksman LM, Kleinjan G, Willems WJ. Long-term results after arthroscopic shoulder stabilization using suture anchors: an 8- to 10-year follow-up. Am J Sports Med. 2011;39:2396–403.
42. Zimmermann SM, Scheyerer MJ, Farshad M, Catanzaro S, Rahm S, Gerber C. Long-term restoration of anterior shoulder stability: a retrospective analysis of arthroscopic Bankart repair versus open Latarjet procedure. J Bone Joint Surg Am. 2016;98:1954–61.
43. Wolf EM, Arianjam A. Hill-Sachs remplissage, an arthroscopic solution for the engaging Hill-Sachs lesion: 2- to 10-year follow-up and incidence of recurrence. J Shoulder Elb Surg. 2014;23:814–20.
44. Cavalier M, Johnston TR, Tran L, Gauci M-O, Boileau P. Glenoid erosion is a risk factor for recurrent instability after Hill-Sachs remplissage. Bone Joint J. 2021;103-B:718–24.
45. Garcia JJC, Yukie Nakano Schincariol C, Mendes RB, Muzy PC. Dynamic anterior stabilization of the shoulder using buttons. JSES Int. 2024;8:1169–74.
46. de Campos AC, Ângelo AC. Onlay dynamic anterior stabilization with biceps transfer for the treatment of anterior glenohumeral instability produces good clinical outcomes and successful healing at a minimum

1 year of follow-up. Arthrosc Sport Med Rehabil. 2023;5:e445–57.
47. Bhatia S, Frank RM, Ghodara NS, Hsu AR, Romeo AA, Bach BR Jr, Boileau P, Provencher MT. The outcomes and surgical techniques of the Latarjet procedure. Arthroscopy. 2014;30:227–35.
48. Nourissat G, Neyton L, Metais P, Clavert P, Villain B, Haeni D, Walch G, Lafosse L. Functional outcomes after open versus arthroscopic Latarjet procedure: a prospective comparative study. Orthop Traumatol Surg Res. 2016;102:S277–9.
49. Kordasiewicz B, Malachowski K, Kicinski M, Chaberek S, Pomianowski S. Comparative study of open and arthroscopic coracoid transfer for shoulder anterior instability (Latarjet)-clinical results at short term follow-up. Int Orthop. 2017;41:1023–33.
50. Kordasiewicz B, Kicinski M, Malachowski K, Wieczorek J, Chaberek S, Pomianowski S. Comparative study of open and arthroscopic coracoid transfer for shoulder anterior instability (Latarjet)-computed tomography evaluation at a short term follow-up. Part II. Int Orthop. 2018;42:1119–28.
51. Cho NS, Yoo JH, Rhee YG. Management of an engaging Hill-Sachs lesion: arthroscopic remplissage with Bankart repair versus Latarjet procedure. Knee Surg Sports Traumatol Arthrosc. 2016;24:3793–800.
52. Yang JS, Mehran N, Mazzocca AD, Pearl ML, Chen VW, Arciero RA. Remplissage versus modified Latarjet for off-track Hill-Sachs lesions with subcritical glenoid bone loss. Am J Sports Med. 2018;46:1885–91.
53. Boehm E, Minkus M, Moroder P, Scheibel M. Arthroscopic iliac crest bone grafting in recurrent anterior shoulder instability: minimum 5-year clinical and radiologic follow-up. Knee Surg Sports Traumatol Arthrosc. 2021;29:266–74.
54. Boehm E, Minkus M, Moroder P, Scheibel M. Massive graft resorption after iliac crest allograft reconstruction for glenoid bone loss in recurrent anterior shoulder instability. Arch Orthop Trauma Surg. 2020;140:895–903.
55. Capito NM, Owens BD, Sherman SL, Smith MJ. Osteochondral allografts in shoulder surgical procedures. JBJS Rev. 2016; https://doi.org/10.2106/JBJS.RVW.16.00001.
56. Zhuo H, Xu Y, Zhu F, Pan L, Li J. Osteochondral allograft transplantation for large Hill-Sachs lesions: a retrospective case series with a minimum 2-year follow-up. J Orthop Surg Res. 2019;14:344.
57. Frank RM, Romeo AA, Richardson C, Sumner S, Verma NN, Cole BJ, Nicholson GP, Provencher MT. Outcomes of Latarjet versus distal tibia allograft for anterior shoulder instability repair: a matched cohort analysis. Am J Sports Med. 2018;46:1030–8.
58. Provencher MT, Peebles LA, Aman ZS, Bernhardson AS, Murphy CP, Sanchez A, Dekker TJ, LaPrade RF, Di Giacomo G. Management of the failed Latarjet procedure: outcomes of revision surgery with fresh distal Tibial allograft. Am J Sports Med. 2019;47:2795–802.
59. Yian EH, Weathers M, Knott JR, Sodl JF, Spencer HT. Predicting failure after primary arthroscopic Bankart repair: analysis of a statistical model using anatomic risk factors. Arthroscopy. 2020;36:964–70.
60. Flinkkilä T, Knape R, Sirniö K, Ohtonen P, Leppilahti J. Long-term results of arthroscopic Bankart repair: minimum 10 years of follow-up. Knee Surg Sports Traumatol Arthrosc. 2018;26:94–9.
61. Ernstbrunner L, De Nard B, Olthof M, Beeler S, Bouaicha S, Gerber C, Wieser K. Long-term results of the arthroscopic Bankart repair for recurrent anterior shoulder instability in patients older than 40 years: a comparison with the open Latarjet procedure. Am J Sports Med. 2020;48:2090–6.
62. Merolla G, Paladini P, Di Napoli G, Campi F, Porcellini G. Outcomes of arthroscopic Hill-Sachs remplissage and anterior Bankart repair: a retrospective controlled study including ultrasound evaluation of posterior capsulotenodesis and infraspinatus strength assessment. Am J Sports Med. 2015;43:407–14.
63. Gouveia K, Abidi SK, Shamshoon S, Gohal C, Madden K, Degen RM, Leroux T, Alolabi B, Khan M. Arthroscopic Bankart repair with remplissage in comparison to bone block augmentation for anterior shoulder instability with bipolar bone loss: a systematic review. Arthroscopy. 2021;37:706–17.
64. Collin P, Lädermann A. Dynamic anterior stabilization using the long head of the biceps for anteroinferior glenohumeral instability. Arthrosc Tech. 2018;7:e39–44.
65. Tang J, Zhao J. Arthroscopic transfer of the long head of the biceps brachii for anterior shoulder instability. Arthrosc Tech. 2017;6:e1911–7.
66. Williams HLM, Evans JP, Furness ND, Smith CD. It's not all about redislocation: a systematic review of complications after anterior shoulder stabilization surgery. Am J Sports Med. 2019;47:3277–83.
67. Shah AA, Butler RB, Romanowski J, Goel D, Karadagli D, Warner JJP. Short-term complications of the Latarjet procedure. J Bone Joint Surg Am. 2012;94:495–501.
68. Kordasiewicz B, Malachowski K, Kicinski M, Chaberek S, Boszczyk A, Marczak D, Pomianowski S. Intraoperative graft-related complications are a risk factor for recurrence in arthroscopic Latarjet stabilisation. Knee Surg Sports Traumatol Arthrosc. 2019;27:3230–9.

The Latarjet Procedure: Open or Arthroscopic?

5

Berte Bøe, Kaare S. Midtgaard, and Gilbert Moatshe

Key Points

- The instability diagnosis should be based on the history and the clinical exam.
- Imaging is beneficial to support the diagnosis.
- Both glenoid and humeral bone loss are recognized as important contributors to recurrent instability.
- Age < 25, competitive athletes, and bone loss are the most important risk factors for recurrent instability.
- Open and arthroscopic techniques have proven similar clinical outcomes and complication rates.

5.1 Introduction/Background

- The significance of glenoid bone loss (GBL) cannot be overstated in regard to recurrence of anterior shoulder instability.
- Historically, restoration of GBL has been reserved in patients with 20–25% of GBL [1]. The concept of the glenoid track has also emphasized the significance of the Hill-Sachs lesion (HSL) when assessing the clinical implication of GBL. Thus, clinicians must not only consider the size of the GBL but also the size, depth, and location of the HSL.
- Recent publications have demonstrated that inferior clinical outcomes can be expected with GBL > 13.5%, and the critical amount of GBL that can be accepted seems to be diminishing, especially in young, active high-demand individuals [2].
- There are several graft options available to restore GBL. Recent publications reporting on

Supplementary Information The online version contains supplementary material available at https://doi.org/10.1007/978-3-662-73064-5_5.

B. Bøe (✉)
Oslo University Hospital, Division of Orthopaedic Surgery, Oslo, Norway

K. S. Midtgaard
Oslo University Hospital, Division of Orthopaedic Surgery, Oslo, Norway

Norwegian Armed Forces Joint Medical Services, Oslo, Norway

G. Moatshe
Oslo University Hospital, Division of Orthopaedic Surgery, Oslo, Norway

Oslo Sports Trauma Research Center, Norwegian School of Sports Sciences, Oslo, Norway

L. Kovačič et al. (eds.), *Surgical Techniques for Anterior Shoulder Instability*, https://doi.org/10.1007/978-3-662-73064-5_5

the use of iliac crest autografts (Eden-Hybinette, J-graft) have demonstrated good results, although donor site morbidity can be expected in up to 26% [3]. Distal clavicle autograft is not widely used; however, it is a viable option that offers the advantage of a cartilage covered bone restoration [4]. Fresh frozen distal tibia allograft offers restoration of the native glenoid with a cartilage-covered surface but is expensive and reserved for severe GBL or salvage procedures [5].

- Today, the most widely used technique for restoration of GBL is coracoid autograft transfer. Different variations of coracoid autografts have been described in the literature, but the procedure is associated with the French surgeon Michel Latarjet, who described the technique in 1958 [6]. It has been hypothesized that the Latarjet procedure improves anterior shoulder stability by three mechanisms: (1) the bone block restores the attritional glenoid surface, (2) repair of the anterior capsule to the stump of the coracoacromial ligament creates a bumper, and (3) the new position of the conjoined tendon acts as a sling preventing anteroinferior translation of the humeral head [1].
- Since the introduction of the Latarjet procedure, the technique has undergone numerous advancements, and the procedure can now be performed arthroscopically. In this chapter, we present our considerations and experience from converting from open to arthroscopic procedure.

5.2 Scientific Update

- Although the Latarjet procedure is considered the initial surgical option in the treatment of anterior shoulder instability in certain patient populations, the majority reserve this procedure for revision of failed Bankart procedures or in patients with moderate to severe GBL (20–25%). However, recent publications have demonstrated that a lower threshold for bone augmentation should be considered [2, 7].
- Shin et al. performed a study of 169 patients with anterior glenoid erosion and reported that the critical amount of GBL that led to recurrence following arthroscopic Bankart repair was 17.3%. In a high-demand population, it has been demonstrated that GBL > 13.5% resulted in a clinically significant decrease in patient-reported outcomes [2, 7, 8].
- In the last decade, focus has been on defining the critical amount of GBL. Although the amount of GBL leading to higher risk of recurrence and inferior clinical results seems to be lower than 20–25%, surgeons must be cognizant that the concave glenoid has a complex three-dimensional architecture and there are individual differences [9]. Furthermore, it is increasingly becoming apparent that the amount and location of bone loss on the humeral head influences the glenoid track and overall glenohumeral joint stability. Thus, when evaluating glenohumeral joint instability and bone loss, both the glenoid and the humerus should be evaluated together.
- With the focus on restoring GBL and several reports demonstrating excellent outcomes following the Latarjet procedure, there is some concern regarding the complications associated with the Latarjet procedure. The most frequently reported complications are non-union, infection, hardware-related problems, and nerve damage [10–13]. Some authors have advocated for arthroscopically performed Latarjet procedure, and that this would yield less stiffness and wound complications and potentially quicker recovery. However, the Latarjet procedure is considered a technically challenging procedure when performed as open surgery, and it is likely that the complexity increases when performed arthroscopically [14, 15]. In a systematic review, Hurley et al. compared outcomes following open and arthroscopic Latarjet procedure and found similar recurrence (2.0% vs 2.4%, $P = 0.75$), revision (2.4% vs. 5.4%, $P = 0.06$), and complication rates (13.8% vs. 11.9%, $P = 0.50$), respectively [13]. Of note, the authors recommended that arthroscopic Latarjet procedures

should be reserved for high-volume centers given the learning curve with arthroscopic procedure.

5.3 Assessment and Planning

- For most orthopedic surgeons, the Latarjet is a revision procedure or a procedure for cases with severe GBL. In these cases, there should always be a preoperative evaluation of the amount of bone loss. We prefer three-dimensional (3D) computed tomography (CT) scans to assess both GBL and the size of the HSL. Best-fit circle is an easy and reproducible method to measure the percentage of bone defect on the anterior glenoid (Fig. 5.1). On-track/Off-track is another well-known method of measurement described by DiGiacomo in 2014 [16]. This method also brings the humeral bone defect into consideration. In a systematic review by Longo et al. in 2013 evaluating 1801 patients with traumatic anterior shoulder dislocations, the authors found a bony glenoid defect in 18% of the patients, 30% had defects in the humeral head, and 22% had a combination of both [17]. They concluded that even though the principle of recognizing and treating glenoid and humeral bone defects in patients with traumatic anterior glenohumeral instability is widely accepted, few studies are available to accurately describe which bone defects should be treated with bony procedures. Later, a study by Nakamura et al. reported nearly 60% of bipolar defects in 153 shoulders [18].
- When the indication of Latarjet is made, the operating team should work together to optimize the success of the procedure and minimize the risk of complications. When the team is prepared, everybody in the room understands the challenge and tries to contribute in their way. Especially in an arthroscopic procedure, the surgeon is dependent on low bleeding and benefits from cooperation with the anaesthesiologist. Muscular relaxation, tranexamic acid, and low systolic blood pressure might be key points to succeed. For the beach-chair position, the use of monitors for cerebral blood flow can contribute to safe and stable low-pressure anaesthesia. When the beach-chair position is used, the operating table can be flattened when the arthroscope is moved from the posterior to an anterior portal.

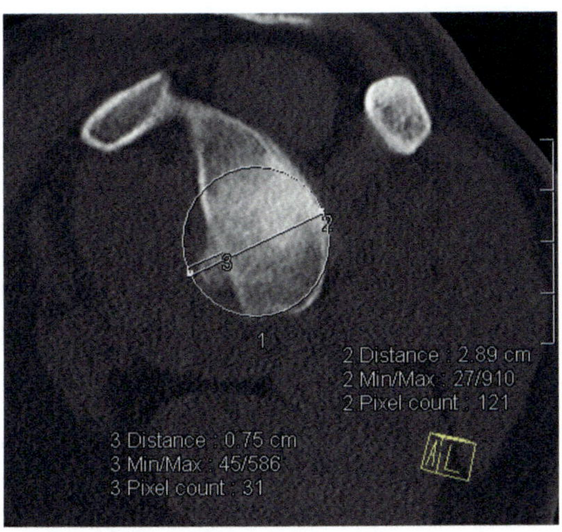

Fig. 5.1 Measuring glenoid bone loss using a best-fit circle method on a sagittal plane view of a CT. On sagittal view, the image best showing the glenoid is found, and a circle that best fits on the glenoid is drawn (1). The diameter of the circle is measured (2). The distance from the edge of the circle to the glenoid where there is bone loss (3) is measured, and this represents the amount of glenoid bone loss. This is presented as a ratio (percentage): distance 3/distance 2

5.4 Treatment Options and Indications

- Large HSLs will increase the possibility for engaging or off-track situations. Some orthopedic surgeons have argued that Latarjet represents an unanatomical procedure and favor Bankart with different possibilities of reinforcement such as Remplissage or different subscapularis procedures. With Remplissage, the intra-articular bone defect is “filled” with the infraspinatus tendon and converted to an extra-articular defect. The fixation of the tendon is done with suture anchors medially in the defect of the humeral head. The consequences of this nonanatomic repair are reported to be loss of external rotation [19]. For overhead athletes, a restriction in range of motion can be crucial when it comes to return to play. Other authors have reported excellent results and no loss in range of motion, especially no loss of external rotation, after the same procedure [20].

- Subscapularis augmentation is another supplementary possibility. Maiotti et al. have published a technique where the upper third of the subscapularis is fixed to the anterior glenoid in a tenodesis in combination with Bankart repair in patients with GBL. The results were reported to be promising according to recurrence rates after 3 years, but this is short follow-up for instability surgery, and the external rotation was reduced by 8 degrees [21]. Another novel technique taking advantage of the upper subscapularis is the sling operation described by Vagstad et al. [22] In this biomechanical study, the shoulders were stabilized by making a sling around the subscapularis tendon with a semitendinosus autograft, and the anterior rim of the glenoid was enhanced with the same tendon. The same group has also published on the sling technique utilizing quadriceps tendon-bone graft [23].
- Injuries often seen in combination with instability include superior or posterior labral injuries. Concomitant injuries are easily repaired in an arthroscopic procedure. If Latarjet is performed openly, inspection of the posterior part of the joint is difficult.

5.5 Decision-Making Algorithm

Flow chart

Pearls and Pitfalls

Drilling a guide pin in the glenoid before the graft is fixed to the guide.	Excessive use of a shaver increases the risk of bleeding and reduced visualization.
Positioning of the arm makes the dissection easier; flexion releases tension on the anterior structures. External rotation moves the axillary nerve medially.	Wide portals increase leaking and decrease visualization.
Elastic band and muscle relaxation can be used to lift the superior part of the subscapularis muscle when placing the graft.	Fracture of the graft.
Chiseling from inferior before osteotomy of the coracoid to avoid spike formation.	Lateral placement of the graft.

5.6 Outcomes

- Both the open and the arthroscopic Latarjet result in significant improvements when it comes to patient outcome scores and rates of recurrent instability. The open procedure has been the gold standard, and the development of the novel arthroscopic technique is under continuous evaluation with the aim of keeping safety for the patients and limiting the expenses. Orthopaedic surgeons with long arthroscopic experience have recognized the arthroscopic Latarjet procedure to be a technically demanding and time-consuming procedure. Some authors have published on their learning curve where they have meticulously evaluated the safety and possible benefits of this novel technique [24, 25].

- In a paper from Nourissat et al. and the French Arthroscopy Society, the authors prospectively compared the results from open and arthroscopic procedures 12 months after surgery [26]. They found that the patients operated on with the arthroscopic procedure had less pain in the first week after the operation compared to patients operated on with the open procedure. They found no other early differences between the arthroscopic and open groups. Regarding recurrence of instability, 12 months is short observational time.
- In a systematic review from Hurley et al., the open and arthroscopic procedures resulted in comparable rates of total recurrent instability, revision procedures, and total complications [13]. Outcomes evaluated were also the Rowe score and external rotation, with no significant difference. The only parameter that was different between the techniques was persistent apprehension. Following open surgery, 10% had persistent apprehension compared to 35% in the arthroscopic surgery group.
- The patients operated on with the Latarjet procedure, either open or arthroscopic, are patients with a high risk of recurrence because of bone loss, age, hyperlaxity, and/or activity level. Despite of this, the overall recurrence rate is low after the Latarjet procedure.

5.7 Potential Complications/Difficulties

- *Bleeding and reduced visualization.*
  When performing a technically demanding arthroscopic procedure, excellent visualization is crucial. The anaesthesiologist needs to be a part of the pre-operative planning to make sure the blood pressure is kept low and stable during the entire procedure. Cerebral oximetry and tranexamic acid might be additional tools to maintain visualization and avoid bleeding.
- *Injury to the nerves*
  Nerve injuries are the feared and critical complications in a Latarjet procedure. Nerves are at risk in both techniques, and the safest approach is to seek them out to know exactly where they are. The musculocutaneous and axillary nerves are most at risk in the Latarjet procedure. These nerves are also at risk in the glenohumeral dislocation.
- *Placement of the graft.*
  Lateral placement will most probably lead to early osteoarthritis, which will be a disaster for a young patient. Medial placement is more forgiving but can result in recurrent instability and/or apprehension for the patient. Too high opens the possibility for dislocations under the graft. Too low makes it possible to dislocate superiorly to the graft, and the fixation might be inadequate to the glenoid. The position of the graft relative to the glenoid is an issue some authors have argued is easier arthroscopically, and others argue it is easier and more reliable with open surgery. In the arthroscopic procedure, the technical trick is to use a switching stick from the posterior portal and position it to be parallel to the joint surface. If you move the stick superiorly and inferiorly, it will touch the bone graft if the graft is positioned too laterally. The arthroscopic procedure has been shown to result in a higher rate of persistent apprehension compared to the open procedure [13].

  For both arthroscopic and open Latarjet procedures, the authors recommend performing a post-operative CT scan. With this routine, the surgeon has the possibility to reoperate on patients with unacceptable placement of the graft before it is too late.
- *Fracture of the graft.*
  In the arthroscopic procedure, there might be difficulties in dealing with a fracture of the graft. There are one or two holes burred in the coracoid for placement of screws or but-

tons. This is a weakness of the graft when you later perform the osteotomy. Two holes and chiseling probably have a higher risk than one hole and sawing of the osteotomy. When chiseling in hard bone, it might strike cracks that go into the holes. The coracoid can also break during fixation. If you still have one hole intact, you could in most cases accept fixation in only one hole, but if the cracks affect both holes, it will be difficult to go through with a solid fixation arthroscopically. Fixation with suture anchors and sutures through the proximal part of the conjoined tendon can be achieved, but experienced surgeons have recognized that this event requires open surgery.

- *Removal of screws*
  Screw fixation of the coracoid graft appears solid. Graft resorption post-operatively might lead to prominence of the screw head and pain because of irritation of subscapularis. Reoperations will always represent a new risk for complications, including nerve injuries.
- *Osteoarthritis*
  Regardless of surgical procedure, nearly half of patients having surgery for anterior shoulder instability will develop radiographic glenohumeral arthritis [27].

5.8 Expert Recommendation

- Planning is essential.
  Latarjet procedure is technically demanding, and attention to details is crucial. Previously, arthroscopic Latarjet was considered experimental surgery; however, more centers are reporting on outcomes when performing this procedure. Current data has not shown any significant difference between open and arthroscopic Latarjet in terms of outcomes, recurrence, and complications. However, arthroscopic Latarjet has been demonstrated to have a longer learning curve, longer surgery time, and requires expensive instruments. Arthroscopic Latarjet provides an opportunity to evaluate the glenohumeral joint and address concomitant injuries.

5.9 Remaining Questions

- Is it beneficial for patients to be operated arthroscopically?
  Surgeons should be cautious when adopting new techniques, especially those with potentially high risk of complications such as the arthroscopic Latarjet. Such procedures should ideally be performed in a systematic way with patient follow-up and documentation of outcomes and complications. Several studies have demonstrated that arthroscopic Latarjet is technically challenging, has a long learning curve, and is time-consuming. Therefore, it is reasonable to reserve arthroscopic Latarjet to high-volume centers and surgeons capable of performing open Latarjet procedures in case converting to open surgery is needed. It should also be noted that there was skepticism when arthroscopic Bankart procedures and arthroscopic rotator cuff repairs were introduced, and they are now standard approaches. The need to adopt new techniques, advance the field of surgery, and improve outcomes should be balanced with the costs and complications associated with the procedures. Arthroscopic Latarjet is not inferior to open Latarjet and has been demonstrated to be a safe procedure. Arthroscopic Latarjet procedure is a good technique and a good option for both patients and surgeons; however, it is not for all patients and not for all surgeons.

Take Home Message

- Prepare thoroughly before you start doing the Latarjet procedure arthroscopically
- Optimize visualization (low BP, Tranexamic acid)
- Experienced assistant is beneficial
- Dissect the nerves (axillary and musculocutaneous) to make sure you avoid injuries
- CT scan post-operatively to avoid lateral placement of graft

References

1. Provencher MT, Midtgaard KS, Owens BD, Tokish JM. Diagnosis and management of traumatic anterior shoulder instability. J Am Acad Orthop Surg. 2021;29(2):e51–61.
2. Shaha JS, Cook JB, Song DJ, Rowles DJ, Bottoni CR, Shaha SH, et al. Redefining "critical" bone loss in shoulder instability: functional outcomes worsen with "subcritical" bone loss. Am J Sports Med. 2015;43(7):1719–25.
3. Silber JS, Anderson DG, Daffner SD, Brislin BT, Leland JM, Hilibrand AS, et al. Donor site morbidity after anterior iliac crest bone harvest for single-level anterior cervical discectomy and fusion. Spine. 2003;28(2):134–9.
4. Kwapisz A, Fitzpatrick K, Cook JB, Athwal GS, Tokish JM. Distal clavicular osteochondral autograft augmentation for glenoid bone loss: a comparison of radius of restoration versus Latarjet graft. Am J Sports Med. 2018;46(5):1046–52.
5. Provencher MT, Peebles LA, Aman ZS, Bernhardson AS, Murphy CP, Sanchez A, et al. Management of the failed Latarjet procedure: outcomes of revision surgery with fresh distal tibial allograft. Am J Sports Med. 2019;47(12):2795–802.
6. van der Linde JA, van Wijngaarden R, Somford MP, van Deurzen DF, van den Bekerom MP. The Bristow-Latarjet procedure, a historical note on a technique in comeback. Knee Surg Sports Traumatol Arthrosc. 2016;24(2):470–8.
7. Shin SJ, Kim RG, Jeon YS, Kwon TH. Critical value of anterior glenoid bone loss that leads to recurrent Glenohumeral instability after arthroscopic Bankart repair. Am J Sports Med. 2017;45(9):1975–81.
8. Dickens JF, Owens BD, Cameron KL, DeBerardino TM, Masini BD, Peck KY, et al. The effect of subcritical bone loss and exposure on recurrent instability after arthroscopic Bankart repair in intercollegiate American football. Am J Sports Med. 2017;45(8):1769–75.
9. Moroder P, Damm P, Wierer G, Bohm E, Minkus M, Plachel F, et al. Challenging the current concept of critical glenoid bone loss in shoulder instability: does the size measurement really tell it all? Am J Sports Med. 2019;47(3):688–94.
10. Hardy A, Sabatier V, Laboudie P, Schoch B, Nourissat G, Valenti P, et al. Outcomes after Latarjet procedure: patients with first-time versus recurrent dislocations. Am J Sports Med. 2020;48(1):21–6.
11. Frank RM, Gregory B, O'Brien M, Bernardoni E, Verma NN, Cole BJ, et al. Ninety-day complications following the Latarjet procedure. J Shoulder Elb Surg. 2019;28(1):88–94.
12. Moroder P, Schulz E, Wierer G, Auffarth A, Habermeyer P, Resch H, et al. Neer Award 2019: Latarjet procedure vs. iliac crest bone graft transfer for treatment of anterior shoulder instability with glenoid bone loss: a prospective randomized trial. J Shoulder Elb Surg. 2019;28(7):1298–307.
13. Hurley ET, Lim Fat D, Farrington SK, Mullett H. Open versus arthroscopic Latarjet procedure for anterior shoulder instability: a systematic review and meta-analysis. Am J Sports Med. 2019;47(5):1248–53.
14. Leuzinger J, Brzoska R, Metais P, Clavert P, Nourissat G, Walch G, et al. Learning curves in the arthroscopic Latarjet procedure: a multicenter analysis of the first 25 cases of 5 international surgeons. Arthroscopy. 2019;35(8):2304–11.
15. Bonnevialle N, Thelu CE, Bouju Y, Vogels J, Agout C, Duriez P, et al. Arthroscopic Latarjet procedure with double-button fixation: short-term complications and learning curve analysis. J Shoulder Elbow Surg. 2018;27(6):e189–e95.
16. Di Giacomo G, Itoi E, Burkhart SS. Evolving concept of bipolar bone loss and the Hill-Sachs lesion: from "engaging/non-engaging" lesion to "on-track/off-track" lesion. Arthroscopy. 2014;30(1):90–8.
17. Longo UG, Loppini M, Rizzello G, Romeo G, Huijsmans PE, Denaro V. Glenoid and humeral head bone loss in traumatic anterior glenohumeral instability: a systematic review. Knee Surg Sports Traumatol Arthrosc. 2014;22(2):392–414.
18. Nakagawa S, Ozaki R, Take Y, Iuchi R, Mae T. Relationship between glenoid defects and Hill-Sachs lesions in shoulders with traumatic anterior instability. Am J Sports Med. 2015;43(11):2763–73.
19. Garcia GH, Park MJ, Zhang C, Kelly JDt, Huffman GR. Large Hill-Sachs lesion: a comparative study of patients treated with arthroscopic Bankart repair with or without remplissage. HSS J. 2015;11(2):98–103.
20. Brilakis E, Avramidis G, Malahias MA, Stathellis A, Deligeorgis A, Chiotis I, et al. Long-term outcome of arthroscopic remplissage in addition to the classic Bankart repair for the management of recurrent anterior shoulder instability with engaging Hill-Sachs lesions. Knee Surg Sports Traumatol Arthrosc. 2019;27(1):305–13.
21. Maiotti M, Massoni C, Russo R, Schroter S, Zanini A, Bianchedi D. Arthroscopic subscapularis augmentation of Bankart repair in chronic anterior shoulder instability with bone loss less than 25% and capsular deficiency: clinical multicenter study. Arthroscopy. 2017;33(5):902–9.
22. Vagstad T, Klungsoyr PJ, Drogset JO, Nebel D, Ferle M, Hurschler C, et al. The novel arthroscopic subscapular sling procedure grants better stability than an arthroscopic Bankart repair in a cadaveric study. Knee Surg Sports Traumatol Arthrosc. 2020;28(7):2316–24.
23. Klungsoyr JA, Vagstad T, Ferle M, Drogset JO, Hoff SR, Dalen AF, et al. The novel arthroscopic subscapular quadriceps tendon-bone sling procedure provides increased stability in shoulder cadavers with severe glenoid bone loss. Knee Surg Sports Traumatol Arthrosc. 2021;29(1):170–80.

24. Valsamis EM, Kany J, Bonnevialle N, Castricini R, Ladermann A, Cunningham G, et al. The arthroscopic Latarjet: a multisurgeon learning curve analysis. J Shoulder Elb Surg. 2020;29(4):681–8.
25. Kordasiewicz B, Kicinski M, Malachowski K, Boszczyk A, Chaberek S, Pomianowski S. Arthroscopic Latarjet stabilization: analysis of the learning curve in the first 90 primary cases: early clinical results and computed tomography evaluation. Arthroscopy. 2019;35(12):3221–37.
26. Nourissat G, Neyton L, Metais P, Clavert P, Villain B, Haeni D, et al. Functional outcomes after open versus arthroscopic Latarjet procedure: a prospective comparative study. Orthopaed Traumatol Surg Res. 2016;102(8S):S277–S9.
27. Rollick NC, Ono Y, Kurji HM, Nelson AA, Boorman RS, Thornton GM, et al. Long-term outcomes of the Bankart and Latarjet repairs: a systematic review. Open Access J Sports Med. 2017;8:97–105.

The Role of 3D Planning and New Technologies

6

Philip Joseph Rosinsky, Ron Gilat,
Ira Bachar-Avnieli, Omri Lubovsky, and Ehud Atoun

Key Points

- 3D planning has become the standard of care for the preoperative assessment of anterior shoulder instability.
- Glenoid and humeral bone loss can be underestimated without appropriate 3D planning, which may result in failure of arthroscopic labral repair.
- New technologies are being introduced, which may deepen our understanding of anterior shoulder instability and optimize appropriate patient-specific treatment selection.

6.1 Introduction

- Treatment of anterior shoulder instability can be complex and challenging, particularly when associated with glenoid and humeral bone deficiency [1]. It has been reported that glenoid bone loss can be found in approximately 22% of primary shoulder dislocations and 90% of recurrent dislocations [2].
- Arthroscopic labral repair has been the typical primary procedure to address anterior shoulder instability. However, increased failure rates of arthroscopic labral repair have been reported in patients with glenoid bone loss as low as 13.5% and in patients with an Instability Severity Index Score (ISIS) ≥ 4 even without glenoid bone loss [3–6]. These findings highlight the need to critically assess bone deficiency and deformity prior to selecting the optimal primary or revision procedure to manage anterior shoulder instability.
- 3D reconstructions of computerized tomography (CT) or magnetic resonance imaging (MRI) have become the standard of care in selecting and planning the appropriate treatment modality.

6.2 Computerized Tomography (CT) 3D Reconstructions

- Three-dimensional CT scan using 3D volume-rendering reconstructions has become readily available for most surgeons for the assessment of bone deficiency prior to anterior shoulder stabilization surgery. Humeral subtraction is

P. J. Rosinsky · I. Bachar-Avnieli · O. Lubovsky
E. Atoun (✉)
Barzilai Medical Center, Ashkelon, Israel

Ben-Gurion University, Beer-Sheba, Israel

R. Gilat
Sourasky Medical Center, Tel Aviv, Israel

Sackler Faculty of Medicine, Tel Aviv University, Tel Aviv, Israel

L. Kovačič et al. (eds.), *Surgical Techniques for Anterior Shoulder Instability*,
https://doi.org/10.1007/978-3-662-73064-5_6

particularly valuable to quantify glenoid bone loss via an *en face* view of the glenoid [7–9].

- Kubicka et al. found 3D CT reconstructions to be more reliable in assessing glenoid bone loss when compared to 2D CT [10].
- Moroder et al. compared the value of 3D CT imaging versus 2D MRI for preoperative surgical planning in recurrent anterior shoulder instability in 48 patients. They found 3D CT provided better prediction of the necessity for open versus arthroscopic surgery and a significantly more accurate prediction of glenoid bone loss. They concluded that CT imaging proved to be more important for preoperative planning by prevailing in the detection of glenoid defects. They also recommended the replacement of MRI as preoperative imaging standard with CT imaging [11]. On the other hand, Markenstein et al. found sagittal MRA to be reliable and valid for measuring bony defects of the glenoid. Studying 35 patients, they found good to excellent intra- and moderate to good inter-observer correlations in quantifying glenoid bone loss using sagittal MRA when compared to 3D CT [12].
- Measurement of humeral bone loss (Hill-Sachs lesion) may be more difficult and more prone to inter-observer variability. Currently, there is no standard method available to make a precise evaluation of the Hill–Sachs lesion and/or predict engagement prior to stabilization surgery [13].
- Ho et al. used nine polyurethane humerus bone substitutes to create Hill-Sachs lesions of varying sizes, with a combination of varying lesion depth and width. They found 3D CT imaging to be effective and reproducible in determining lesion size. They also reported that Hill-Sachs interval width is also reliable when it is applied to the glenoid track concept. Importantly, they also concluded that measured values on 3D and 2-dimensional imaging using a conventional CT scanner may slightly underestimate true measurements [14].
- A more recent systematic review by Maio et al. found that while 3D CT is helpful for evaluation of bone loss, there were no significant differences between 3D CT and 3D MRI measurements of Hill-Sachs lesions [13].
- To summarize, true CT 3D reconstruction is the gold standard for identification and quantification of glenoid and humeral bone loss [7, 15]. It is also useful in the assessment of the on/off track relationship between a Hill–Sachs lesion and the anterior glenoid bone defect [15].
- Importantly, 3D CT may also aid in preoperative surgical planning and affect intraoperative decisions by predicting screw length and optimal location in a Latarjet or Eden-Hybinette procedure [16]. Other important considerations include glenoid version, prior hardware/anchor location, coracoid morphology and size, and many more.

6.3 Magnetic Resonance Imaging (MRI) 3D Reconstructions

- MRI and magnetic resonance arthrography (MRA) are commonly used to evaluate soft tissue injuries and concomitant pathologies prior to selecting an anterior shoulder stabilization procedure.
- Stillwater et al. compared 3D-MR osseous reformats of the shoulder with 3D CT osseous reformats in patients with glenohumeral instability [17]. They assessed 12 patients with glenohumeral instability who underwent CT and MRI and found 3D MR osseous models of the shoulder using a 3D isotropic volumetric interpolated breath-hold examination (VIBE) sequence to be equivalent to 3D CT, with no statistically significant differences between the two modalities [17].
- Gyftopoulos et al. aimed to assess the ability of 3D MR shoulder reconstructions to accurately quantify glenoid bony deficiency in the clinical setting using arthroscopy as the gold standard [18]. They retrospectively reviewed 15 patients and compared 3D MR to intraoperative glenoid bone loss measurements. They found that 3D MR reconstructions of the

shoulder can be used to accurately measure glenoid bone loss, with less than 2.21% true mean absolute error compared to intraoperative measurements [18].

- In regards to Hill-Sachs lesions, 3D MRI reconstructions have yielded similar results to 3D CT reconstructions as reported by Maio et al. in their systematic review [13]. They also concluded that the on/off track algorithm using MRI allows prediction of the engaging lesions with good accuracy [13].
- The use of 3D MRI/MRA in the evaluation of bone loss is developing increasingly and, in the future, may provide an equally accurate measurement tool for bone assessment while avoiding excessive radiation exposure for the patient [15].

6.4 The Role of New Technologies in Surgery for Shoulder Instability

- Besides the use of digital 3D models as described previously, physical reconstruction of these models using 3D printing has been utilized for preoperative and intraoperative planning. These models have the added benefit of not only visualizing and assessing the bony lesions but also evaluating the interaction between glenoid and humerus, including the exact anatomical position in which the lesions may interact [19]. Use of 3D printing to create a patient-specific titanium implant has been demonstrated in a cadaver model to restore glenohumeral morphology and stability. The 3D-printed anatomic implant and Latarjet procedure also achieved similar results with regard to the translational forces needed to dislocate the humerus 10 mm anteriorly on the glenoid [20].
- Some of the most exciting innovations in the realm of orthopedic surgery have come in the form of navigation- and robotic-assisted surgery. However, implementation of these in the shoulder, and specifically in shoulder arthroscopy, have been limited.
- Jung et al. presented a validity study for navigation-assistance in placement of anchors in shoulder arthroscopy [21]. The study simulated placement of anchors for rotator-cuff surgery in a phantom model as well as a cadaveric study. Although the authors simulated use for rotator cuff surgery, the implementation for placement of anchors for labral repair is plausible in the near future.
- A further innovation in arthroscopic surgery has been the expanding use of needle arthroscopy as a diagnostic tool and as a method for single-portal surgery. As a diagnostic tool for shoulder pathology, needle arthroscopy has shown comparable accuracy to MRI, with the advantage of hastening the diagnostic process as well as potentially reducing costs [22, 23]. Furthermore, needle arthroscopy has been shown to perform better at "ruling-in" pathology (high specificity and positive predictive value), rather than "ruling-out" pathologies (lower sensitivity and negative predictive value).
- However, the clinical use of needle arthroscopy still needs to be determined, especially in cases of labral tear, for which the accuracy is suboptimal [24].
- Recently, Lavender et al. demonstrated a labral repair using one working portal and a viewing portal with only the percutaneously inserted needle arthroscope (NanoScope, Arthrex) [25]. The authors propose that use of the needle arthroscopy for viewing provides several advantages, including faster recovery, less postoperative pain, less risk for surgical site infections, and less patient morbidity. Conversely, the authors acknowledge the limitations of this technique, including limited visibility and technical difficulties stemming from use of a 0-degree arthroscope to view the inferior glenoid.
- Lastly, as in the use of acellular dermal allografts for rotator cuff repair, these have been used for reconstruction of the anterior and posterior capsules in shoulder stability surgery [26, 27]. Use of acellular dermal allograft may be especially advantageous in

patients with multidirectional instability in the presence of connective tissue disorder. In these patients, the native capsule is patulous and redundant, and use of an autograft or capsular plication has a high likelihood of failure due to the innate properties of their connective tissue.

Pearls and Pitfalls

Pearls:

- Use 3D CT reconstruction with an *en face* view of the glenoid.
- Engagement of lesions is best assessed intraoperatively, so always be prepared for remplissage.
- 3D reconstructions can aid in planning screw size and location, assessment of prior hardware, coracoid morphology, glenoid version and bone stock, and more.

Pitfalls:

- Hill-Sachs measurements may have variable inter-observer reliability.
- MRI reconstruction may underappreciate bone deficiency.
- Needle arthroscopy has limited visualization capability when compared to traditional arthroscopy due to the angle of view.

Take Home Message

- Always use 3D CT reconstructions when glenoid or humeral bone loss is suspected or when a bony augmentation procedure is planned.
- 3D MRI reconstructions may be beneficial as well and as accurate as a 3D CT.
- Keep an eye out for new technologies in the field to optimize surgical procedure selection and planning.
- 3D printing can be used to enhance understanding of the existing bony lesions on the glenoid (Bankart) and humerus (Hill-Sachs), as well as the interaction between them.
- Minimally invasive shoulder stabilization surgery can take a further step by incorporation of needle arthroscopy.

References

1. Provencher MT, Ghodadra N, LeClere L, Solomon DJ, Romeo AA. Anatomic osteochondral glenoid reconstruction for recurrent glenohumeral instability with glenoid deficiency using a distal tibia allograft. Arthroscopy. 2009;25:446–52.
2. Sayegh ET, Mascarenhas R, Chalmers PN, Cole BJ, Verma NN, Romeo AA. Allograft reconstruction for glenoid bone loss in glenohumeral instability: a systematic review. Arthroscopy. 2014;30:1642–9.
3. Shaha JS, Cook JB, Song DJ, et al. Redefining "critical" bone loss in shoulder instability: functional outcomes worsen with "subcritical" bone loss. Am J Sports Med. 2015;43:1719–25.
4. Balg F, Boileau P. The instability severity index score: a simple pre-operative score to select patients for arthroscopic or open shoulder stabilisation. J Bone Joint Surg. 2007;89:1470–7.
5. Phadnis J, Arnold C, Elmorsy A, Flannery M. Utility of the instability severity index score in predicting failure after arthroscopic anterior stabilization of the shoulder. Am J Sports Med. 2015;43:1983–8.
6. Loppini M, Delle Rose G, Borroni M, et al. Is the Instability Severity Index Score a valid tool for predicting failure after primary arthroscopic stabilization for anterior glenohumeral instability? Arthroscopy. 2019;35:361–6.
7. Rerko MA, Pan X, Donaldson C, Jones GL, Bishop JY. Comparison of various imaging techniques to quantify glenoid bone loss in shoulder instability. J Shoulder Elb Surg. 2013;22:528–34.
8. Bishop JY, Jones GL, Rerko MA, Donaldson C, Group MS. 3-D CT is the most reliable imaging modality when quantifying glenoid bone loss. Clin Orthop Relat Res. 2013;471:1251–6.
9. Barchilon VS, Kotz E, Ben-Av MB, Glazer E, Nyska M. A simple method for quantitative evaluation of the missing area of the anterior glenoid in anterior instability of the glenohumeral joint. Skeletal Radiol. 2008;37:731–6.
10. Kubicka AM, Stefaniak J, Lubiatowski P, et al. Reliability of measurements performed on two dimensional and three dimensional computed tomography in glenoid assessment for instability. Int Orthop. 2016;40:2581–8.

11. Moroder P, Resch H, Schnaitmann S, Hoffelner T, Tauber M. The importance of CT for the pre-operative surgical planning in recurrent anterior shoulder instability. Arch Orthop Trauma Surg. 2013;133:219–26.
12. Markenstein JE, Jaspars KC, van der Hulst VP, Willems WJ. The quantification of glenoid bone loss in anterior shoulder instability; MR-arthro compared to 3D-CT. Skeletal Radiol. 2014;43:475–83.
13. Maio M, Sarmento M, Moura N, Cartucho A. How to measure a Hill–Sachs lesion: a systematic review. EFORT Open Rev. 2019;4:151–7.
14. Ho A, Kurdziel MD, Koueiter DM, Wiater JM. Three-dimensional computed tomography measurement accuracy of varying Hill-Sachs lesion size. J Shoulder Elb Surg. 2018;27:350–6.
15. Stefaniak J, Lubiatowski P, Kubicka AM, Wawrzyniak A, Wałecka J, Romanowski L. Clinical and radiological examination of bony-mediated shoulder instability. EFORT Open Rev. 2020;5:815–27.
16. Hardy A, Gerometta A, Granger B, et al. Preoperative CT planning of screw length in arthroscopic Latarjet. Knee Surg Sports Traumatol Arthrosc. 2018;26:24–30.
17. Stillwater L, Koenig J, Maycher B, Davidson M. 3D-MR vs. 3D-CT of the shoulder in patients with glenohumeral instability. Skeletal Radiol. 2017;46:325–31.
18. Gyftopoulos S, Beltran LS, Yemin A, et al. Use of 3D MR reconstructions in the evaluation of glenoid bone loss: a clinical study. Skeletal Radiol. 2014;43:213–8.
19. Sheth U, Theodoropoulos J, Abouali J. Use of 3-dimensional printing for preoperative planning in the treatment of recurrent anterior shoulder instability. Arthrosc Tech. 2015;4:e311–6.
20. Willemsen K, Berendes TD, Geurkink T, et al. A novel treatment for anterior shoulder instability: a biomechanical comparison between a patient-specific implant and the Latarjet procedure. J Bone Joint Surg Am. 2019;101:e68.
21. Jung K, Kim H, Kholinne E, et al. Navigation-assisted anchor insertion in shoulder arthroscopy: a validity study. BMC Musculoskelet Disord. 2020;21:1–9.
22. Voigt JD, Mosier M, Huber B. In-office diagnostic arthroscopy for knee and shoulder intra-articular injuries its potential impact on cost savings in the United States. BMC Health Serv Res. 2014;14:1–9.
23. McMillan S, Schwartz M, Jennings B, Faucett S, Owens T, Ford E. In-office diagnostic needle arthroscopy: understanding the potential value for the US healthcare system. Am J Orthop. 2017;46:252–6.
24. Wagner ER, Woodmass JM, Zimmer ZR, et al. Needle diagnostic arthroscopy and magnetic resonance imaging of the shoulder have comparable accuracy with surgical arthroscopy: a prospective clinical trial. Arthroscopy. 2021.
25. Lavender C, Lycans D, Kopiec A, Sayan A. Nanoscopic single-incision anterior labrum repair. Arthrosc Tech. 2020;9:e297–301.
26. Karpyshyn J, Gordey EE, Coady CM, Wong IH. Posterior glenohumeral capsular reconstruction using an acellular dermal allograft. Arthrosc Tech. 2018;7:e739–45.
27. Gallagher F, Wong IH-B. Anterior capsule augmentation and posterior glenohumeral capsular reconstruction with human dermal allograft for multidirectional shoulder instability. Arthrosc Tech. 2020;9:e657–62.

Part II

Surgical Techniques

Arthroscopic Capsulolabral Repair. Surgical Technique

7

Miguel A. Ruiz Ibán, Raquel Ruiz Díaz,
Ignacio de Rus Aznar, and Jorge Díaz Heredia

Key Point

- Arthroscopic Bankart repair is a successful and widely used surgical technique for the management of anterior shoulder instability.
- The best indication for this procedure is a young subject with low-demand activities that presents with recurrent anterior shoulder instability with a clear capsulolabral lesion and no significant bony defects in the glenoid. The role in subjects with glenoid bone defects is disputed.
- The procedure should start with identification of the labral injury and an extensive detachment of the capsulolabral tissue, so it can be mobilized as needed. This is usually attained with visualization from the anterosuperior portal.
- The objective of the repair is to bring the labrum and capsule to the glenoid edge. But the tissue does not only have to be displaced back to the glenoid in a mediolateral direction; a shift from inferior to superior, restoring the tension of the anteroinferior capsule, is necessary.
- At least three anchors placed in the glenoid rim are needed to obtain a secure fixation.
- The surgeon should consider possible extensions of the labral injury to the posterioinferior labrum and address those.
- If only milder injuries of the labrum are present, a HAGL tear should be suspected and ruled out.
- If there is a significant humeral defect, a remplissage procedure is a good addition to the Bankart repair.

Supplementary Information The online version contains supplementary material available at https://doi.org/10.1007/978-3-662-73064-5_7.

M. A. Ruiz Ibán (✉) · R. R. Díaz · I. de Rus Aznar
J. D. Heredia
Shoulder and Elbow Unit, Hospital Universitario
Ramon y Cajal, Madrid, Spain

L. Kovačič et al. (eds.), *Surgical Techniques for Anterior Shoulder Instability*,
https://doi.org/10.1007/978-3-662-73064-5_7

7.1 Introduction/Background

- In 1923 Arthur Bankart reported that the essential lesion in traumatic anterior shoulder instability was an injury to the anteroinferior capsulolabral complex [3]. An injury that is commonly referred to as the Bankart lesion.
- He also proposed a surgical procedure to manage it: a direct repair of the injury. The Bankart procedure evolved to a repair of the damaged labrum to the glenoid and became widely popular during the twentieth century, especially in the English-speaking world, where it was considered the gold standard for recurrent anterior instability management.
- There are different pathoanatomical variations of the labral lesion (Fig. 7.1): the typical Bankart lesion (the labrum is torn from the glenoid and the periosteum medially is also torn, leaving the labrum free from the glenoid), the Perthes lesion (the labrum is detached from the glenoid but there is periosteal continuity and the labrum is not completely detached from the anterior glenoid), the ALPSA lesion (Anterior Labral Periosteal Sleeve Avulsion, the labrum and periosteum are detached from the glenoid, become displaced medially and reattached in a medial position), or the GLAD lesion (glenolabral articular disruption, the labral tear includes part of the chondral surface of the glenoid).
- The introduction of advanced instrumentation and new anchor technology in the nineties allowed for the development of the arthroscop-

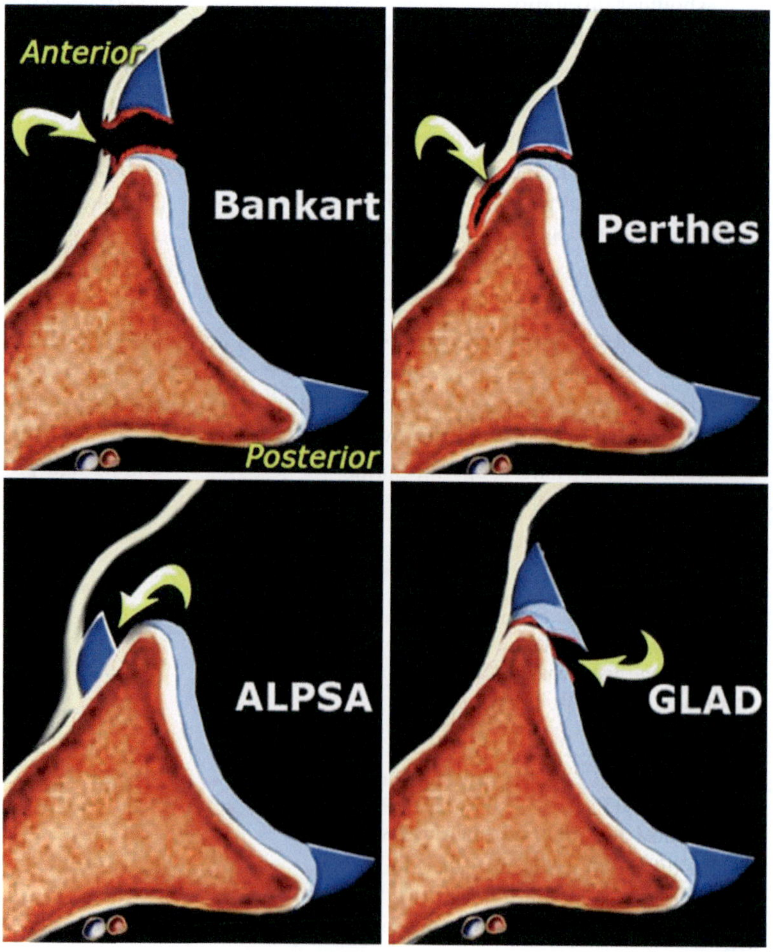

Fig. 7.1 The four most common labral injury types in anterior shoulder instability

ically assisted Bankart capsulolabral repair, a procedure that gradually replaced the open procedure [1].

- There is strong controversy on which patients will benefit most from an arthroscopic capsulolabral repair, as the recurrence rate, especially when assessed in the mid- or long-term, is relatively high [7].
- There is controversy on how other factors affect the chances of failure of an arthroscopic capsulolabral repair. Associated hyperlaxity, younger age and participation in contact sports are factors that increase the failure rate of a capsulolabral repair [2], but these factors will also negatively affect the outcome of any other procedure used.

7.2 Indications

- The perfect patient for an arthroscopic capsulolabral repair is a young subject with low-demand activities that presents with recurrent anterior shoulder instability with a clear capsulolabral lesion in the magnetic resonance study and no significant bony defects in the glenoid or humerus on a computed tomogram study.
- Subjects with glenoid defects larger than 20% or combined humeral and glenoid (bipolar) off-track lesions are considered poor candidates for this procedure due to high rates of recurrence [4].
- It is unclear which size of the glenoid defect precludes the use of this arthroscopic soft tissue procedure. Lesions larger than 20% constitute a clear formal contraindication, but smaller defects (larger than 8–13.5% of the surface of the glenoid, so-called subcritical defects) are considered by some authors to be relevant enough to preclude the use of this technique.
- With respect to humeral defects, it is widely accepted that associating a remplissage procedure can reduce the recurrence rate to acceptable levels in subjects with medium- or large-sized humeral Hill-Sachs lesions [5].
- The presence of a bony Bankart lesion is not a formal contraindication for a capsulolabral repair, as techniques to repair the bony fragment to the anterior labrum (as described by Sugaya and others) can restore the bone defect and allow for a low recurrence rate [9].
- The different pathoanatomical variations of the labral lesion can all be managed with an arthroscopic capsulolabral repair.

7.3 Clinical Evaluation

7.3.1 History

- In a subject with recurrent anterior shoulder instability, the surgeon should get precise data on the first dislocation episode. When did it happen, and whether it happened after a traumatic incident, during a forced movement or in a non-forced movement.
- The number of dislocations and the circumstances of the last episodes should also be taken into account.
- The dominance, the work and sport functional requirements of the subject, and the degree of current impairment should also be noted.

7.3.2 Physical Findings

- A thorough exam of the active and passive range of motion should be performed. Usually, no significant impairment is found, but occasionally some voluntary restriction of external rotation in abduction can be expected.
- The *apprehension test* should be performed in the supine position (Fig. 7.2a, b) with the shoulder in neutral rotation and the elbow flexed. The arm is brought to 90° of abduction, and progressive passive external rotation of the shoulder is done by the examiner. The patient should be warned that this maneuver will eventually cause either discomfort or apprehension (defined as the subjective perception of imminent risk of dislocation). In GLAD lesions, this maneuver might cause more discomfort than apprehension.

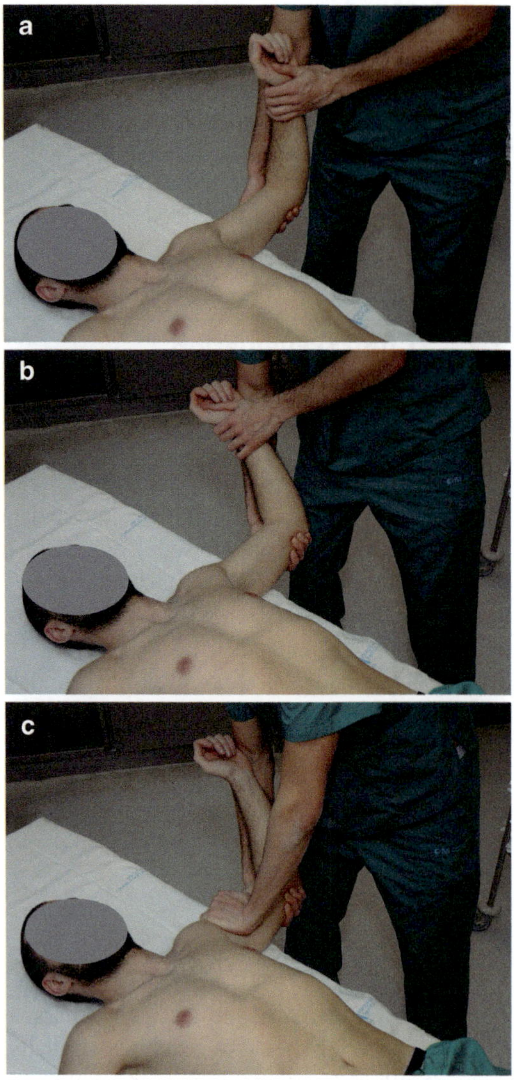

Fig. 7.2 The apprehension test (**a**, **b**) and the relocation test (**c**)

- If the apprehension test is positive, the *relocation test* (Fig. 7.2c) confirms the diagnosis: the examiner brings the rotated arm to a degree of external rotation in which mild apprehension or discomfort is perceived and, with the contralateral hand, applies a posterior force on the proximal third of the subject's arm, causing relief of symptoms.
- It is essential to assess for possible combined posterior instability using the *posterior apprehension test.*
- The *sulcus test* allows to defining the association with hyperlaxity, specifically when performed at 30° of external rotation. The test can be performed supine or sitting. With the arm in 0° of abduction and either 0° or 30° of external rotation, the examiner pulls the arm inferiorly. Displacement of the humeral head inferiorly with a noticeable dimple in the deltoid mass is considered a positive test. If the sulcus test elicits apprehension, a significant injury to the inferior glenohumeral ligament is present, and a HAGL (humeral avulsion of the glenohumeral ligaments) should be suspected (Fig. 7.3).
- The presence of local or generalized hyperlaxity should always assessed in subjects with instability. The Gagey hyperabduction test (isolated glenohumeral abduction greater than 95°) and the Beighton criteria are useful tools.

7.3.3 Imaging

- There is strong controversy over what is the best combination of imaging techniques for the assessment of shoulder instability: simple X-rays, CT scans, MRI, and arthrography are often used in combination.
- Simple X-rays provide confirmation of dislocation and reduction and can show gross bony defects. Specific projections for the assessment of bony injury are probably unnecessary, as CT scans have become more readily available.
- CT scans allow for precise assessment of bone defects both at the glenoid and the humerus. The most reproducible methods for assessing the magnitude of these defects and for addressing the importance of bipolar lesions use CT scans. If there is doubt about the real magnitude of a bony injury in a specific subject, a CT scan evaluation is compulsory.
- MRI identifies soft tissue injuries reliably, but its efficacy in assessing bony defects is limited. ArthroMRI will allow for better definition of labral injuries and other, more unusual injuries such as HAGL and GLAD lesions.

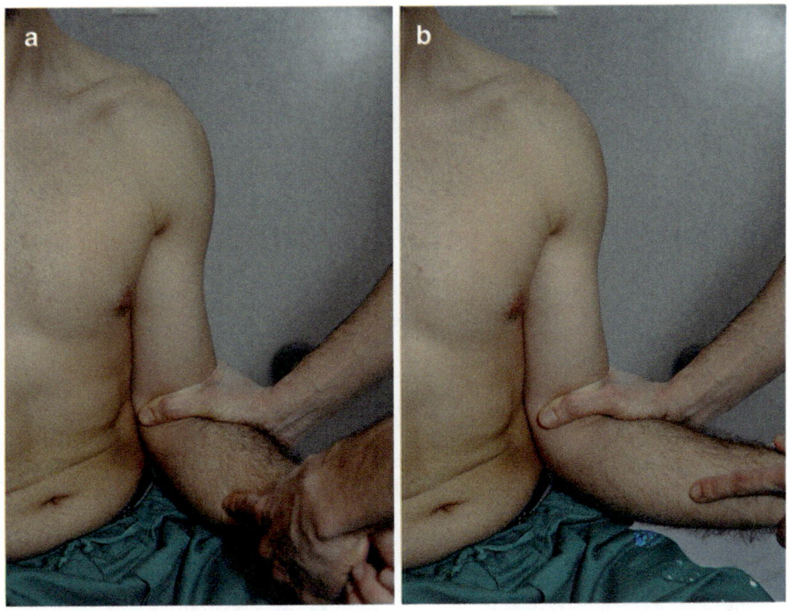

Fig. 7.3 The Sulcus test in 0° of external rotation (**a**) and 30° of external rotation (**b**)

7.4 Surgical Technique

7.4.1 Equipment

- A standard shoulder arthroscopy set with a 30° scope, motorized shaver, and radiofrequency device is needed.
- All-suture glenoid anchors and impacted non-metallic glenoid anchors can be used. The former are smaller and allow for less bone resection at the glenoid; the latter, especially those made with biocomposite materials, avoid cyst formation at the expense of larger bone resection and the risk of anchor protrusion.
- The use of curved anchor inserters makes things easier for the surgeon and improves anchor placement, allowing for more perpendicular insertion at the lower glenoid using the anterior portal.
- There are different devices available that allow suture passage through the antero-inferior capsule and glenoid. Single-use indirect suture-passing devices with pig-tail configurations of the tip allow for easier passage, as being single-use, they are always sharp. Furthermore, the curvature of the tip is higher than in direct suture-passing devices.
- The use of cannulas is disputed. Placing cannulas in the three portals used will give a soft-tissue seal that will prevent fluid from extravasating outside the glenohumeral joint, allowing for a more stable environment.

7.4.2 Positioning and portals

- Both lateral decubitus and beach chair positions are widely used. It is the preference of the authors to use the lateral decubitus position, with a traction device that allows for two-axis traction: in line with the arm and perpendicular to it, so as to allow for increased lateral distraction of the joint.
- In a typical case, three portals are used: the standard posterior portal; an anterior portal in the lower part of the rotator interval, just over the subscapularis tendon and in line with the posterior portal; and an anterosuperior portal, placed at the upper edge of the rotator interval, almost perpendicular in direction to the anterior portal (Fig. 7.4).

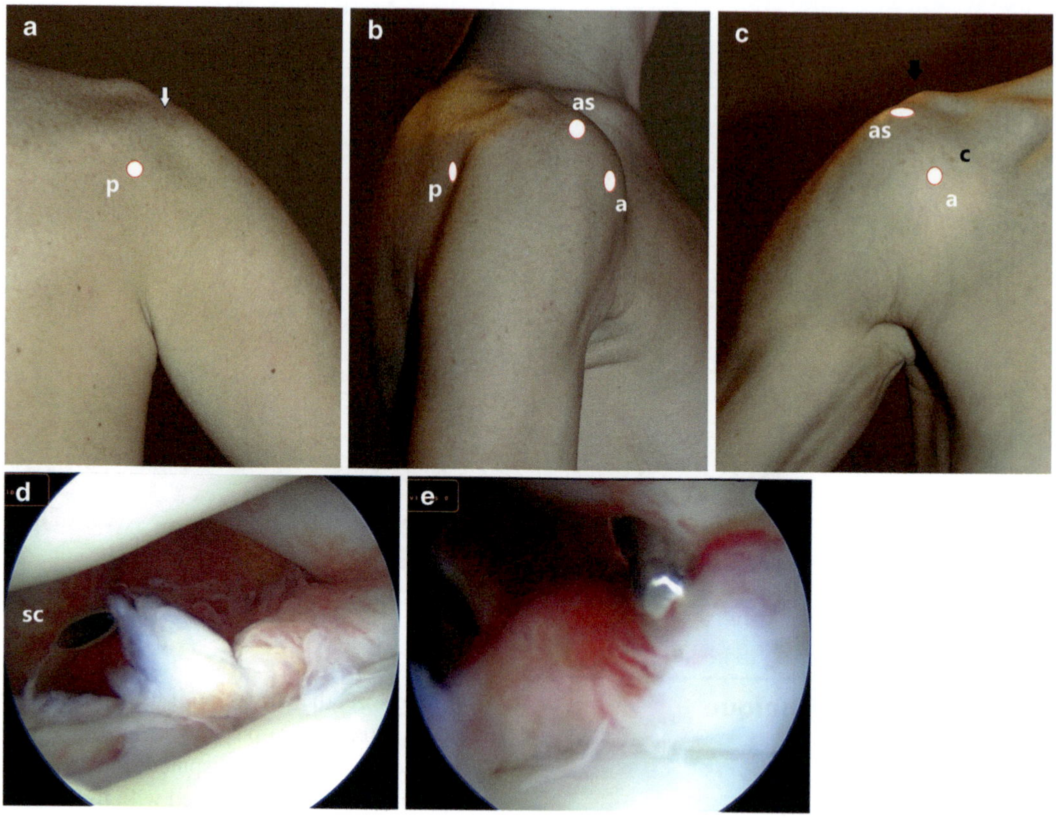

Fig. 7.4 The arthroscopic portals for an arthroscopic Bankart procedure presented in a posterior (**a**), lateral (**b**) and anterior (**c**) view of a model's shoulder and arthroscopic views through the posterior portal of the anterior (**d**) and anterosuperior portal positions (**e**). The posterior portal (p) is placed in an outside-inside fashion at the beginning of the procedure, a couple of cm distal and medial to the posterolateral edge of the acromion (white arrow), but the two other portals are placed into the joint with careful selection of the proper location under direct arthroscopic visualization, the anterior portal (a) starting lateral to the coracoid (c) just over the subscapularis tendon (sc) in line with the posterior portal, and the anterosuperior portal (as) starting just anterior to the anterolateral edge of the acromion (black arrow) and entering the superior edge of the rotator interval

- The use of an accessory 5 o'clock portal, placed through the subscapularis muscle, was recommended to access the lower anterior glenoid, but it is not really necessary with modern equipment.

7.4.3 Step-by-Step Description of the Procedure

1. Diagnostic arthroscopy and portal placement:
   - Initially a thorough evaluation of the glenohumeral joint should be performed, focusing specifically on identifying:
     – The pattern of the labral injury and its extension posteroinferiorly (to the posterior labrum) or superiorly (affecting the biceps insertion, a SLAP V lesion).
     – The presence of a relevant Hill-Sachs defect.
     – The amount of anteroinferior glenoid bone loss.
     – The competence of the anterior-inferior capsuloligamentous tissues with specific focus on addressing the possible presence of a HAGL lesion.

- The three above-mentioned portals should be defined and developed, placing a cannula in each of them. This allows for seamless translation of the optic to any of these, facilitating a more complete visualization of the joint.

2. Capsulolabral release
   - The antero-inferior labrum is better visualized from the superior portal. From this portal the characteristics of the labral injury can be carefully assessed, and the labral tissue can be separated, in conjunction with the periosteum, from the anterior glenoid surface (Fig. 7.5).
   - The detachment of the labrum from its displaced position is essential. A complete release is necessary to allow for adequate repositioning of the damaged labrum over the glenoid edge.
   - Detachment can be done with a combination of arthroscopic periostotomes and judicious use of the radiofrequency device, always taking care of maintaining labral circular continuity.
   - The detachment is better started in the most cephalad zone in which the labral tissue seems to be damaged. There, the healthy tissue is identified, and the detachment can progress caudally.
   - The most difficult part is always the most caudal part, and care should be taken to avoid progressing the detachment through the intact inferior labrum.
   - It is necessary to develop the plane between the anterior glenoid surface and the labrocapsular tissue way medially, reaching up to the fibres of the underlying subscapularis muscle.
   - Utmost care should be taken not to disrupt the circular continuity of the labrum.
   - When the release has been completed, the capsulolabral tissue should be mobilized with a grasper, confirming that it comes over the glenoid edge with ease.
3. Capsulolabral repair
   - The objective of this step is triple:
     - The labrum has to be replaced in its original position, shifting the damaged tissue laterally.
     - The capsular structures, attached to the labrum, have to be reattached to their original glenoid insertion; usually, the tissue has displaced distally, so some degree of proximal (cephalad) tissue shift is necessary.
     - The capsule and inferior glenohumeral humeral ligament have also suffered plastic deformation, and some degree of capsular plication is needed.
   - The optic can be transferred to the posterior portal. This allows a more precise assessment of the exact position of the anchors can be done.
   - The first anchor should be placed at the 4:30–5:00 position. More inferior placement of this anchor is unnecessary, as the capsule-labral tissue has to be displaced proximally, and a very distal anchor (5:30) won't facilitate this (Fig. 7.6).

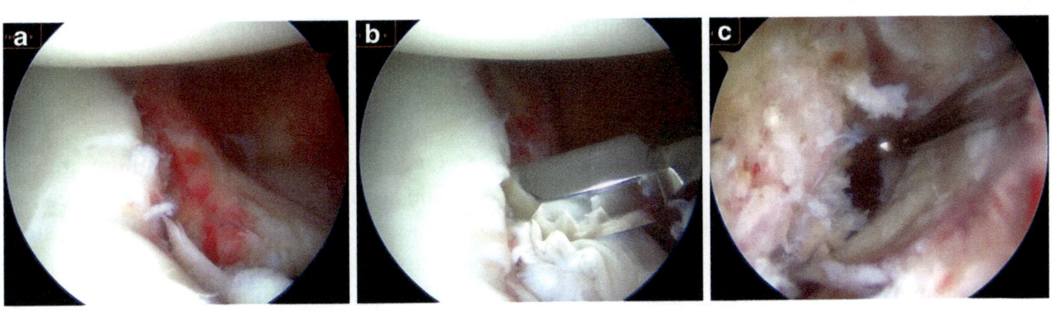

Fig. 7.5 Arthroscopic view from the anterosuperior portal of a left shoulder. The labral injury, in this case an ALPSA lesion, is seen (**a**). An arthroscopic periostotome is used, from cranial to caudal, to release the medialized capsulolabral tissue (**b**) until it is completely free from the anterior side of the glenoid (**c**)

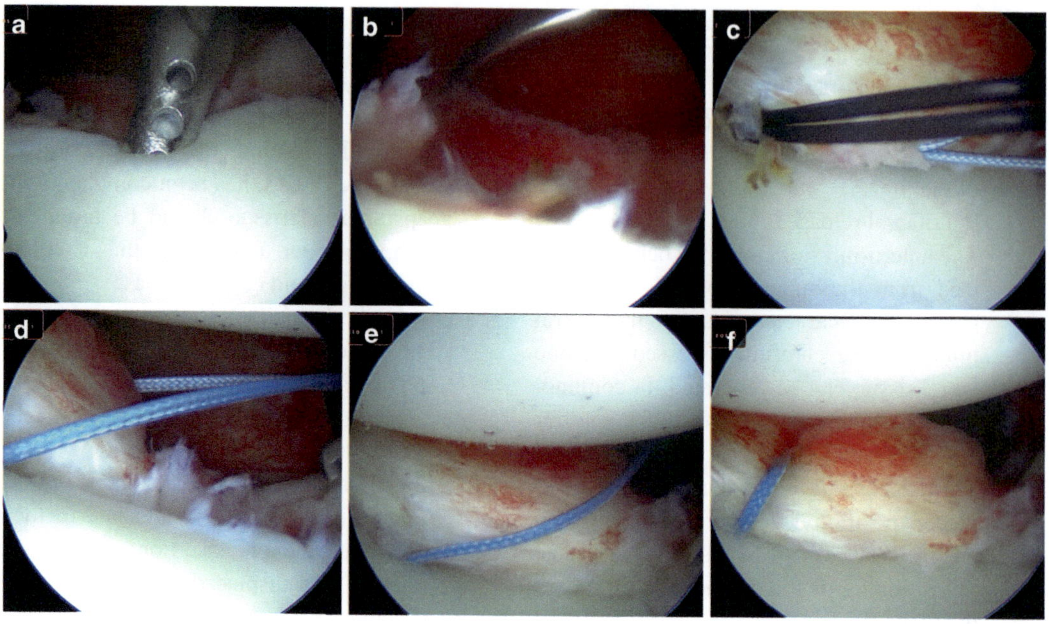

Fig. 7.6 Placement of the inferior-most anchor and suture. View from a posterior portal in a left shoulder. The all-suture anchor is placed at the 5:00 position, at the edge of the chondral surface (**a**). Then an indirect suture passer (**b**) is used to drive a passing suture through the labrum and capsule. Note that the piercing of the capsule and labrum are made more than 1 cm caudally to the anchor (**c**), almost at the 6:00 position. The suture from the anchors is driven through the labrum and capsule (**d**) and a grasper is used to apply traction to the labrum and capsule, placing it over the glenoid and causing a superior capsular shift (**e**); then the suture is tied over the anchor (**f**)

- The ideal position of the anchor relative to the anterior glenoid edge is disputed. Some authors recommend placing it 1–2 mm into the joint to obtain a good bumper effect with the repaired labrum, but, when doing that, some cartilage should be removed to assure good contact between the repaired labrum and the bone, which is needed for healing. The authors recommend a more conservative approach, placing all-suture anchors at the edge of the cartilage, making sure it is not medial to the glenoid edge but not into the cartilage.
- A single-use indirect suture passer is passed through the capsule, ideally 1 cm lateral to the labrum and 1 cm distal to the anchor. The sharp tip of the passer should contact the medial glenoid bone and slide laterally, making sure all labral tissue is captured.
- One of the suture limbs of the anchor is passed through the tissue.
- Knot-tying has to be done with care: one assistant will pick up the capsulolabral tissue with a grasper from the superior portal, then pull it laterally and proximally while the surgeon ties a sliding knot from the anterior portal, taking care to place the suture as distal as possible in the soft tissue. The knot should always be placed away from the joint, using the limb of the suture that goes through the tissue as the post.
- Sometimes both limbs of the suture can be passed through the tissue, allowing for a more superior and lateral capsulolabral shift.
- Once the first anchor and suture are tied and secure, the following anchors can be placed, repeating the same steps (Fig. 7.7).
- The optimal number of anchors depends on the extension of the labral lesion. In more limited injuries, three anchors might

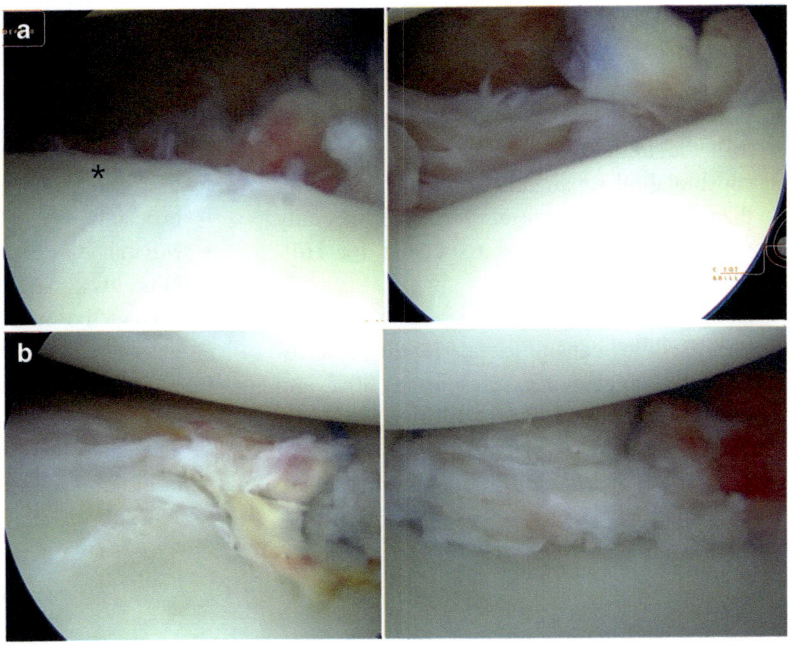

Fig. 7.7 The labral repair. View from a posterior portal in a left shoulder. Initial image of the labrum (**a**): there is severe medialization, especially in the caudal part, where it is not even visible (*). Final view after repair with 3 anchors (**b**): the labrum is restored over the glenoid and the tissue is shifted from medial to lateral and from caudal to cranial

be enough, but injuries that extend cranially might need more superior anchors, and injuries that extend posteroinferiorly might need placing anchors in the posterior glenoid.

- Although some authors recommend placing the anchors evenly along the anterior glenoid edge, it is often better to place the inferior anchors more tightly together than the superior anchors, as the inferior repair should and will sustain more forces when the patient gets back to sports.

7.5 Postoperative Protocol

- This procedure is best performed under general anesthesia with a previous interscalene nerve block performed with a long-acting anesthetic. This will allow for good early postoperative pain control.
- After surgery, the shoulder should be placed in a simple sling that needs to be maintained between 2 and 4 weeks (depending on surgeon preference) and non-narcotic oral analgesics should be able to control pain.
- Physical therapy can be structured in three separate phases:
  - The first "protection" phase extends for the first six postoperative weeks. During the initial 2 to 4 weeks, the arm should be kept in a sling and focus should be placed on pain control, isometric deltoid exercises, scapular balancing and wrist and elbow motion. After mobilization is allowed, gentle exercises focused on regaining passive flexion and abduction are authorized.
  - The second "active recuperation" phase should focus on regaining full active range of motion and usually last another 6 weeks.
  - In the third "return to sport" phase, the objective is regaining strength and restoring scapular kinematics. Return-to-sport times are at least 3 to 5 months.

7.6 Outcomes

- When used in subjects without significant risk factors for recurrence, midterm follow-up (5 years) recurrence rates are around 15% with very low complication rates [8].

- Return to sports rates are high with a capsulolabral repair, with rates over 80% in adolescent athletes [6].
- For subjects without relevant glenoid bone loss the midterm outcomes of arthroscopic capsulolabral repair are similar, if not better than those of the Latarjet procedure, specially when a remplissage is associated for Hill-Sachs defects [5].
- Long term outcomes (> 10 years) of arthroscopic capsulolabral repair deteriorate, with recurrence rates up to 30% and revision rates of 17%. Instability arthropathy is also a concern as it develops in 60% of subjects, 10% having moderate or severe arthropathy [7].

Take Home Messages

- The arthroscopic capsulolabral repair is a good procedure when performed on subjects with minimal glenoid bone defect and a Bankart lesion with good-quality capsule and labrum.
- A good capsulolabral detachment from the anterior glenoid is of paramount importance. The tissue should move freely.
- The capsulolabral tissue has to be reattached laterally and proximally. Furthermore, some degree of plication is most of the times necessary, as there is often some capsular plastic deformity.
- A well-performed capsulolabral repair can give you excellent results and is an anatomic procedure. If it fails, many well-established non-anatomic alternatives are available for your patient. This does not happen the other way around.

Pearls and Pitfalls:

- Always assess posterior instability during the physical exam. Some multidirectional and posterior instability patients first get a misguided anterior Bankart procedure.
- MRI is not a good tool to assess glenoid bone loss; use a CT scan, ideally comparing the affected and contralateral glenoids.
- Use three portals, place three cannulas. This will allow you to change views as needed and keep fluid extravasation to a minimum.
- The labrum needs to be assessed and released with the optic in the superior portal. Keeping your 30° scope in the posterior portal during all surgery is a good indicator of poor surgical technique.
- If, during the diagnostic arthroscopy, the labral lesions do not seem to be very important, special attention is to be given to identifying a HAGL lesion. This is an injury that can be easily overlooked in standard MRI studies.
- Look also to the inferior and posterior labrum; some labral tears will extend posteriorly and have to be dealt with.
- Superior involvement (an SLAP V lesion) is not a true SLAP tear; it is just the progression of the Bankart lesion. Anterior repair of the bicep's insertion is often more than enough; no posterior anchors are needed.
- There is no such thing as "too much capsulolabral detachment" as long as the circular continuity of the labrum is maintained. A good indicator that the dissection has been carried medially

(continued)

enough is the apparition of profuse bleeding, meaning that the instruments have reached the subscapularis muscle.

- While you do your knot-tying, make your assistant pick up the labral tissue and displace it proximally and laterally, this will bring the tissue into a better position.
- When you finish your procedure, have a look at the glenoid and humeral articular surface. Look for iatrogenic damage. A perfect capsulolabral repair is the objective, but chondral damage should also be avoided.

References

1. Bak K, Wiesler ER, Poehling GG. Consensus statement on shoulder instability. Arthroscopy. 2010;26(2):249–55. https://doi.org/10.1016/j.arthro.2009.06.022S0749-8063(09)00567-2.
2. Balg F, Boileau P. The instability severity index score. A simple pre-operative score to select patients for arthroscopic or open shoulder stabilisation. J Bone Joint Surg Br. 2007;89(11):1470–7. https://doi.org/10.1302/0301-620x.89b11.18962.
3. Bankart AS. Recurrent or habitual dislocation of the shoulder-joint. Br Med J. 1923;2(3285):1132–3. https://doi.org/10.1136/bmj.2.3285.1132.
4. Burkhart SS, De Beer JF. Traumatic glenohumeral bone defects and their relationship to failure of arthroscopic Bankart repairs: significance of the inverted-pear glenoid and the humeral engaging Hill-Sachs lesion. Arthroscopy. 2000;16(7):677–94.
5. Haroun HK, Sobhy MH, Abdelrahman AA. Arthroscopic Bankart repair with remplissage versus Latarjet procedure for management of engaging Hill-Sachs lesions with subcritical glenoid bone loss in traumatic anterior shoulder instability: a systematic review and meta-analysis. J Shoulder Elb Surg. 2020;29(10):2163–74. https://doi.org/10.1016/j.jse.2020.04.032.
6. Kasik CS, Rosen MR, Saper MG, Zondervan RL. High rate of return to sport in adolescent athletes following anterior shoulder stabilisation: a systematic review. J ISAKOS. 2019;4(1):33–40. https://doi.org/10.1136/jisakos-2018-000224.
7. Murphy AI, Hurley ET, Hurley DJ, Pauzenberger L, Mullett H. Long-term outcomes of the arthroscopic Bankart repair: a systematic review of studies at 10-year follow-up. J Shoulder Elb Surg. 2019;28(11):2084–9. https://doi.org/10.1016/j.jse.2019.04.057.
8. Ruiz Iban MA, Asenjo Gismero CV, Moros Marco S, Ruiz Diaz R, Del Olmo HT, Del Monte BG, Garcia Navlet M, Avila Lafuente JL, Diaz Heredia J. Instability severity index score values below 7 do not predict recurrence after arthroscopic Bankart repair. Knee Surg Sports Traumatol Arthrosc. 2019;27(12):7. https://doi.org/10.1007/s00167-019-05471-w.
9. Sugaya H, Kon Y, Tsuchiya A. Arthroscopic repair of glenoid fractures using suture anchors. Arthroscopy. 2005;21(5):635. https://doi.org/10.1016/j.arthro.2005.02.006.

The "Labral Bridge" Technique

8

R. C. Ostermann

Key Points

- The Labral Bridge is an arthroscopic anatomic knotless technique for capsulolabral Bankart repair that utilizes a 1.5 mm suture tape that is running alongside the newly created capsulolabral bump in a running mattress stitch configuration between the anchors.
- By placing all suture material medial to the capsulolabral bump, instead of letting it run across the bump, potential irritation of the cartilage is completely avoided.
- The technique provides better coverage of the native labral footprint and avoids spot welds of fixation due to a more uniform pressure distribution. It also seems to optimize blood supply to the labral tissue by avoiding constricting horizontal fixation of the labrum at the level of each anchor.
- The technique can also be used for a posterior capsulolabral repair.

Supplementary Information The online version contains supplementary material available at https://doi.org/10.1007/978-3-662-73064-5_8.

R. C. Ostermann (✉)
Competence Center for Sports and Joint Injuries, Die Praxis, Vienna, Austria
e-mail: ostermann@diepraxis-wien.at

8.1 Background

- Arthroscopic Bankart repairs are nowadays widely considered the "gold standard" surgical treatment for anterior shoulder instability without significant glenoidal or humeral bone loss following recurrent anterior shoulder dislocations.
- The "classic" arthroscopic Bankart repair technique consists of multiple suture anchors that are placed along the anterior glenoid rim from the 5:30 to 3 o'clock position to achieve a firm and stable fixation of the detached capsulolabral complex at its anatomic origin [1, 2].
- A simultaneous capsulolabral tissue shift from south to north is an essential and integral part of the procedure to reduce the capsule volume and to re-tension the attenuated inferior glenohumeral ligament complex.
- A variety of different anchor designs and materials have been utilized; therefore, knotless anchors are nowadays widely used for arthroscopic Bankart repairs, since they provide a fast and secure way of fixation with reliable long-term outcomes without the risk of potential knot impingement [3].
- The clinical success of an arthroscopic Bankart repair is mainly determined by the rate of recurrent instability. It should be pointed out that in the majority of outcome studies on this topic, not only a true recurrent

L. Kovačič et al. (eds.), *Surgical Techniques for Anterior Shoulder Instability*, https://doi.org/10.1007/978-3-662-73064-5_8

dislocation but also a positive apprehension test is considered a recurrence and thus a failure.
- Recurrence rates of arthroscopic Bankart repairs have been reported between 7% and 41% in the current literature but can also be as high as 89% in high-risk patients such as contact athletes [4–8].
- If evidence-based surgical indications and techniques are applied, the recurrence rate can drop to 7.8% even in this high-risk group [9].
- The literature of the last two decades is conflicting if arthroscopic or open Bankart repairs lead to better outcomes and lower recurrence rates. The only level I study to date, comparing recurrence rates of open and arthroscopic Bankart repairs, reported twice the recurrence rate for arthroscopic repairs [10]. A possible explanation for this finding could be a less sufficient reduction of the capsule volume, besides a potentially insufficient anatomic reconstruction of the capsulolabral complex with arthroscopic techniques.
- During the last decade, a variety of refined arthroscopic Bankart repair techniques have been reported in the literature in an attempt to potentially close the gap to the open technique and promote superior results with lower recurrence rates.
- The "Labral Bridge" is one of these techniques that has been presented in its original version in late 2014 and has since then been modified twice [11]. The technique utilizes a synthetic tape that is secured between the anchors in a type of running mattress stitch configuration in order to provide a more uniform pressure distribution of the entire labrum and to cover the native labral footprint to a greater extent than a traditional technique, where the labrum is only secured in "spot welds" at each anchor. Furthermore, the technique aims to minimize the potential contact of suture material with the cartilage of the humeral head. Figure 8.1 shows a schematic drawing of the suture configuration of a modified Labral Bridge Technique.

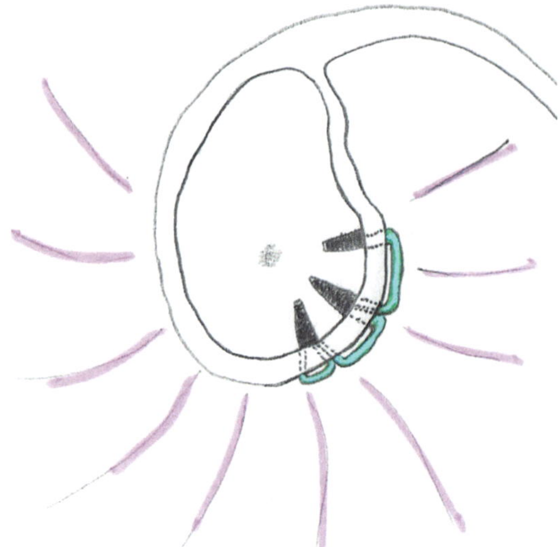

Fig. 8.1 Schematic drawing of the Labral Bridge stitch configuration. Turquoise lines showing the Labral Tape

8.2 Indications

8.2.1 Main

- In principle, the Labral Bridge Technique can be used in any case of recurrent anterior shoulder instability without significant glenoidal or humeral bone loss. However, there is ongoing debate about what amount of glenoidal bone loss should be considered "significant" in terms of changing the treatment strategy from a soft-tissue procedure to a bony augmentation technique. Instead of using a numeric cutoff value of critical glenoidal bone loss at the bare spot level, a critical range of 10–15% bone loss is nowadays considered as "significant."
- However, there is evidence that bone loss of more than 13.5% may lead to deterioration of clinical outcome score results [12]. As for the critical amount of humeral bone loss or Hill-Sachs lesion size, the On/Off track concept introduced by Di Giacomo et al. in 2014 is widely accepted as the currently most practical way to estimate significance and catego-

rize these lesions as critical for engagement or not [13].
- Personally, I consider cases of shoulder instability where there is close to significant glenoidal bone loss, and cases in patients who have a higher risk of redislocation, such as young male overhead or contact athletes, as a main indication for the Labral Bridge technique, because it aims to restore the capsulolabral complex more anatomically than traditional techniques.

8.2.2 Contraindication

- Cases of glenoidal bone loss of more than 15% at the bare spot level, and off-track Hill-Sachs lesions, that are not additionally addressed, can be seen as a clear contraindication.

8.2.3 Controversial

- Revision Bankart repairs without significant glenoidal or humeral bone loss can be seen as a controversial indication for the Labral Bridge technique as, regardless of the technique, the revision of a soft tissue repair with another Bankart repair is seen as controversial on its own.
- However, one has to keep in mind that before finally ruling out a revision Bankart repair, a thorough evaluation of the primary surgery is necessary in order to determine whether evidence-based technical criteria have been followed or not.
- That said, I would recommend the Labral Bridge technique as a worthy option if one considers a revision Bankart repair.

8.3 Goals of Surgical Procedure

- The main goal of any capsulolabral soft tissue repair is a secure fixation of the damaged capsulolabral complex to the glenoid rim in order to achieve healing to bone and to further retension the attenuated glenohumeral ligament complex, leading to a reduction of the capsule volume.
- The Labral Bridge technique aims to provide a secure fixation of the capsulolabral complex at its native footprint, utilizing a synthetic tape (LabralTape Arthrex Inc.) together with knotless suture anchors. The tape is placed in a running mattress stitch configuration between each suture anchor in order to provide an even pressure distribution alongside the whole construct and to cover the native labral footprint to a wider extent. At the same time, a potential irritation of the articular cartilage is avoided since no suture material at all is running over the newly created capsulolabral bump and the knotless nature of this technique.

8.4 Advantages

8.4.1 Biologic Advantages

- The main advantage of the Labral Bridge Technique is probably a potential biological healing benefit due to a number of technique-specific aspects.
- First, the LabralTape provides secure fixation of the labral tissue between each suture anchor, creating some kind of seal; this aims to provide a more uniform pressure distribution of the entire capsulolabral complex along the whole construct when compared to traditional techniques, where the labrum is secured only in "spot welds" at each suture anchor. However, since tissue-to-bone healing is what one wants to achieve when performing a soft tissue repair, one could expect that this is achieved to a superior grade if the tissue was attached to the bone over a larger total length. Preliminary results of an anatomic study show that the Labral Bridge technique is able to cover the native labral footprint to a significantly higher degree than a traditional knotted technique. Furthermore, this "seal" might also prevent synovial leakage between bone and capsulolabral tissue. This might be another

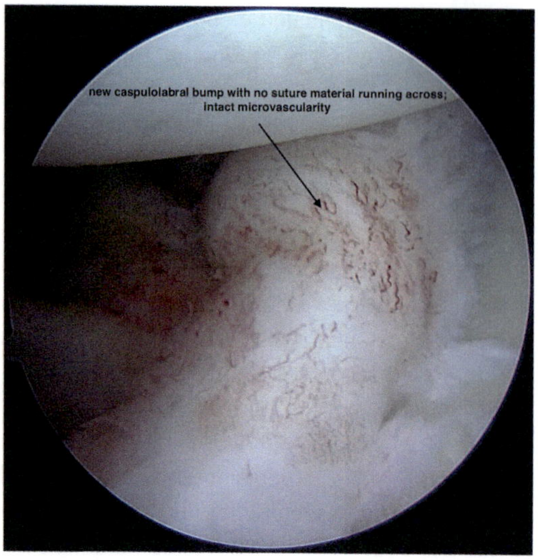

Fig. 8.2 Arthroscopic view from anterosuperior of the newly created capsulolabral bump with no suture material running across. The vascularity is still intact and does not seem to be compromised as one can still see the microvessels on the bump

possible advantage, as it has been shown that synovial leakage can potentially delay or disturb tissue-to-bone healing.

- Second, the technique potentially optimizes blood supply of the newly created labrum, since it avoids constricting horizontal sutures that run across the capsulolabral bump (Fig. 8.2), thus potentially preventing interruption of the blood supply to the labrum and capsule, as the vessels in this portion of the labrum tend to run in a more longitudinal (vertical) way [14].
- Third, since the LabralTape is running vertically between the anchors, no suture material is running across the newly created capsulolabral bump, thus, completely avoiding potential irritation of the articular cartilage.

8.4.2 Stability Advantages

- The second group of advantages can best be summarized as "stability advantages." The height of the native labrum and the concavity compression, or "suction cup effect," of the labrum are known to be important factors contributing to shoulder stability. Preliminary results of an anatomic study show that the labral height can be significantly better restored with the Labral Bridge Technique compared to a standard knotted technique. Besides, as no constricting sutures run across the newly created capsulolabral bump, one can assume that the "suction cup effect" might be less compromised compared to traditional techniques.

8.5 Disadvantages

- The main disadvantage is probably that the technique is technically demanding and therefore has a rather high learning curve. Thus, the use of cannulas to avoid potential problems with suture management and tissue bridges is highly recommended.
- Another potential disadvantage might be an inferior fixation strength and lower ultimate load to failure values compared to more traditional techniques. However, preliminary results of a biomechanical study show no significant difference regarding fixation strength and ultimate load to failure compared to a traditional knotted technique.
- Furthermore, published clinical results of the technique are still missing. However, unpublished preliminary results of a prospective clinical consecutive case series show a low failure rate of less than 6% at a minimum 2-year follow-up.

8.6 Surgical Technique

8.6.1 Equipment

- Device for getting the tissue stitches done (we prefer a 25° Suture Lasso, Arthrex Inc.)
- Suture grasper
- 2.9 mm biocomposite PushLock anchors (Arthrex Inc.) plus reamer and trochar
- 1.5 mm LabralTape (Arthrex Inc.)
- FiberLink #2 suture (Arthrex Inc.)
- TigerLink #2 suture (Arthrex Inc.)

- Gemini Cannula (Arthrex Inc.)
- Crystal clear Cannula (Arthrex Inc.)
- Cannulas are generally not a necessity but are highly recommended due to the complexity of the technique with a number of suture shuttling maneuvers!

8.6.2 Positioning & Portals

- The technique can be carried out in either the beach chair or the lateral decubitus position. Nevertheless, we strongly prefer the lateral decubitus position due to a subjective belief in a superior visualization and mobilization of the relevant anteroinferior structures. Besides, there is evidence in the literature that the lateral decubitus position seems to reduce the failure rate in arthroscopic soft tissue Bankart repair. Additionally, a double extension can only be carried out sufficiently in the lateral decubitus position.
- A standard posterior glenohumeral portal and an anterosuperior and anteroinferior glenohumeral portal are needed for the technique. The latter two portals are placed in an outside-in technique. A crystal-clear cannula is then placed in the anterosuperior portal and the Gemini Cannula in the anteroinferior portal.

8.6.3 Step-by-Step Prescription of the Procedure

1. Via the anterosuperior portal, a detachment of the scarred-down capsulolabral tissue from the anterior glenoid rim is carried out from the 2 to the 6 o'clock position (right shoulder). Care is taken to get a good tissue release to be able to achieve a sufficient south-north tissue shift for a profound reduction of capsule volume. The goal is proper tensioning of the anterior band of the inferior glenohumeral ligament (IGHL). This should be tested with a tissue grasper to make sure that the release is sufficient.
2. Once this is achieved, the bony bed at the anterior glenoid rim is prepared with a shaver, and a bleeding bony surface is created.
3. The first tissue stitch is carried out below the 5 o'clock position with a suture lasso via the anteroinferior portal, and a LabralTape is shuttled from the anteroinferior to the anterosuperior portal.
4. Close to the first stitch, a second tissue stitch is carried out with a suture lasso in the same fashion. This time a TigerLink is placed from the anteroinferior to the anterosuperior portal. The loop of the TigerLink must be placed in the anteroinferior portal.
5. Now one of the limbs of the LabralTape that is parked in the anteroinferior portal is loaded in the loop of the TigerLink together with the loop end of a FiberLink suture.
6. By pulling on the free end of the TigerLink in the anterosuperior portal, the free limb of the LabralTape and the loop end of the FiberLink are shuttled to the anterosuperior portal. This creates a mini mattress stitch with the LabralTape below the 5 o'clock position; the FiberLink is parked at this position, running from the anterosuperior to the anteroinferior portal through the capsulolabral tissue. Both limbs of the LabralTape are now in the anterosuperior portal.
7. Next, both LabralTape limbs are shuttled to the anteroinferior portal for anchor placement via that portal.
8. With an offset guide, a bone socket is drilled for a 2.9 biocomposite PushLock anchor through the anteroinferior portal at the 5 o'clock position directly on the glenoid rim. The limbs of the LabralTape are loaded in the anchor. Before anchor placement, one limb must be made longer than the other limb by pulling on it.
9. Then the first anchor is placed with sufficient tensioning of the LabralTape limbs to get a good tissue shift. After anchor placement, the shorter limb of the LabralTape is cut directly at the anchor, leaving the longer limb in place.
10. Now the remaining longer LabralTape limb is shuttled to the anterosuperior portal and

placed in the loop of the FiberLink suture that is parked there outside the cannula.

11. By pulling on the FiberLink end in the anteroinferior portal, the LabralTape limb is shuttled back through the tissue medially and into the anteroinferior portal.
12. The third tissue stitch is carried out with a suture lasso roughly 7–10 mm above the first anchor, approximately at the 4 o'clock position. The further medial this stitch is carried out, the higher the capsulolabral bump will be created.
13. The wire of the suture lasso is loaded with the TigerLink again, and the loop end of the TigerLink is shuttled out the anteroinferior portal.
14. Outside the cannula, the LabralTape limb and the loop end of a FiberLink are loaded in the loop end of the TigerLink, which is then shuttled out the anterosuperior portal. That way, the LabralTape limb creates a mattress stitch running from the first medial anchor through the tissue and lateral to the glenoid face again at the 4 o'clock position. The FiberLink is parked through the same tissue stitch with the loop end in the anterosuperior portal now and the free end in the anteroinferior portal.
15. Now the limb of the LabraTape needs to be shuttled back to the anteroinferior portal for anchor placement.
16. Via the anteroinferior portal, a bone socket for a 2.9 biocomposite PushLock anchor is drilled with an offset guide at the 4 o'clock position directly on the glenoid rim. The limb of the LabralTape is loaded in the anchor outside the anteroinferior portal, and then the anchor is placed via that portal. This step firmly secures the capsulolabral tissue from medial to the glenoid rim between the first anchor and the second anchor, creating a nice capsulolabral bump. We call this the first "bridge" between the anchors, which is now "closed."
17. After anchor placement, the limb of the LabralTape is shuttled to the anterosuperior portal again and loaded in the loop end of the FiberLink suture that is parked there, outside the cannula.
18. By pulling on the free end of the FiberLink suture in the anteroinferior portal, the LabralTape limb is shuttled back medially through the tissue and outside the anteroinferior portal again.
19. Now steps 12–17 can be repeated in the same way as before, and a third anchor can be placed at the 3 o'clock position on the glenoid rim. By placing the third anchor, the capsulolabral tissue is secured from medial to the glenoid rim between the second and the third anchor, and the second "bridge" is closed.

Normally three anchors and two tape "bridges" are sufficient. If needed, a fourth anchor can be placed, and a third "bridge" can thus be created.

To finalize the construct, the limb of the LabralTape is cut directly at the final anchor.

By looking at the final construct, you will find no suture material running across the newly created capsulolabral bump at all.

Pearls and Pitfalls

Pearls

- Creation of a sufficiently high labral bump at the chondrolabral junction due to the LabralTape mattress stitches
- No suture material potentially irritating the cartilage
- Uniform pressure distribution throughout the construct
- Better labral footprint coverage
- Blood supply to the capsulolabral tissue potentially optimized

Pitfalls

- Interlooping of the #2 FiberLink and the LabralTape limbs within the anteroinferior portal before placing the first anchor, creating high friction when shuttling back the FiberLink
- Placing the LabralTape mattress stitches too loosely
- Breakage of the Nitinol Wire loop from the SutureLasso

8.7 Postoperative Protocol

- The postoperative protocol usually is that of a standard Bankart repair. The patient is placed into a sling for 4–6 weeks, and passive ROM is allowed immediately. Assisted ROM is allowed from week 3 on, and active ROM from week 4 on. Elevation is restricted to 90° for the first 4 weeks for assisted and active ROM. External rotation above neutral is restricted for 6 weeks also for passive ROM.
- However, there are surgeons who prefer an early active rehabilitation after a Labral Bridge repair with good clinical outcomes. If early active rehabilitation is the goal, earlier unrestricted pain-led active mobilization is allowed, and sling immobilization is shortened.

8.8 Potential Complications

- As in standard arthroscopic Bankart repairs care must be taken to avoid any iatrogenic cartilage lesions.
- Another potential complication is anchor misplacement, either too far medial to the glenoid rim or too far onto the glenoid cartilage. However, suture management is crucial in a Labral Bridge repair, and twisting of the sutures inside the cannulas should be avoided.

Take Home Message

- The Labral Bridge is an arthroscopic knotless technique for a more anatomic reconstruction of the capsulolabral complex at the anterior or posterior glenoid rim.
- The technique creates a high capsulolabral bump and provides better labral footprint coverage.
- All suture material is placed away from the articular cartilage in a way to provide a uniform pressure distribution that potentially optimizes blood supply to the capsulolabral tissue.

References

1. Pope EJ, Ward JP, Rokito AS. Anterior shoulder instability – a history of arthroscopic treatment. Bull NYU Hosp Jt Dis. 2011;69(1):44–9. PubMed PMID: 21332438. Epub 2011/02/22. eng.
2. Cole BJ, Romeo AA. Arthroscopic shoulder stabilization with suture anchors: technique, technology, and pitfalls. Clin Orthop Relat Res. 2001;390:17–30. PubMed PMID: 11550863. Epub 2001/09/12. eng.
3. Ng DZ, Kumar VP. Arthroscopic Bankart repair using knot-tying versus knotless suture anchors: is there a difference? Arthroscopy. 2014;30(4):422–7. PubMed PMID: 24680302. Epub.
4. Porcellini G, Campi F, Pegreffi F, Castagna A, Paladini P. Predisposing factors for recurrent shoulder dislocation after arthroscopic treatment. J Bone Joint Surg Am. 2009;91(11):2537–42.
5. van der Linde JA, van Kampen DA, Terwee CB, Dijksman LM, Kleinjan G, Willems WJ. Long-term results after arthroscopic shoulder stabilization using suture anchors: an 8- to 10-year follow-up. Am J Sports Med. 2011;39(11):2396–403.
6. Adam M, Attia AK, Alhammoud A, et al. Arthroscopic Bankart repair for the acute anterior shoulder dislocation: systematic review and meta-analysis. Int Orthop. 2018;42:2413–22. https://doi.org/10.1007/s00264-018-4046-0.
7. Zimmermann SM, Scheyerer MJ, Farshad M, Catanzaro S, Rahm S, Gerber C. Long-term restoration of anterior shoulder stability: a retrospective analysis of arthroscopic Bankart repair versus open Latarjet procedure. J Bone Joint Surg Am. 2016;98(23):1954–61. https://doi.org/10.2106/JBJS.15.01398. PMID: 27926676.
8. Cho NS, Hwang JC, Rhee YG. Arthroscopic stabilization in anterior shoulder instability: collision athletes versus noncollision athletes. Arthroscopy. 2006;22(9):947–53.
9. Leroux TS, Saltzman BM, Meyer M, et al. The influence of evidence-based surgical indications and techniques on failure rates after arthroscopic shoulder stabilization in the contact or collision athlete with anterior shoulder instability. Am J Sports Med. 2017;45(5):1218–25. https://doi.org/10.1177/0363546516663716.
10. Mohtadi NG, Chan DS. A randomized clinical trial comparing open and arthroscopic stabilization for recurrent traumatic anterior shoulder instability: two-year follow-up with disease-specific quality-of-life outcomes. J Bone Joint Surg Am. 2014;96(5):353–60.
11. Ostermann RC, Hofbauer M, Platzer P, Moen TC. The "Labral Bridge": a novel technique for arthroscopic anatomic knotless Bankart repair. Arthrosc Tech. 2015;4(2):e91–5.
12. Shaha JS, Cook JB, Song DJ, et al. Redefining "critical" bone loss in shoulder instability: functional

outcomes worsen with "subcritical" bone loss. Am J Sports Med. 2015;43(7):1719–25. https://doi.org/10.1177/0363546515578250.

13. Di Giacomo G, Itoi E, Burkhart SS. Evolving concept of bipolar bone loss and the hill-Sachs lesion: from "engaging/non-engaging" lesion to "on-track/off-track" lesion. Arthroscopy. 2014;30(1):90–8, ISSN 0749-8063. https://doi.org/10.1016/j.arthro.2013.10.004.
14. Cooper DE, Arnoczky SP, O'Brien SJ, Warren RF, DiCarlo E, Allen AA. Anatomy, histology, and vascularity of the glenoid labrum. An anatomical study. J Bone Joint Surg Am. 1992;74(1):46–52. PMID: 1734013.

Biologic Labral Augmentation 9

Arianna Rizzo, Marco Adriani,
Maristella F. Saccomanno, and Giuseppe Milano

Key Points

- Failure rates of arthroscopic Bankart repair are still too high.
- The role of soft tissues is usually underestimated compared to bone defects.
- It has been shown that glenoid labral morphology plays a role in recurrent instability.
- Labral augmentation by using a collagen membrane aims to close the gap between an arthroscopic Bankart repair and bone block procedures.
- Labral augmentation aims to restore the anatomy when the main issue is the labral insufficiency.

A. Rizzo · M. Adriani
Department of Medical and Surgical Specialties, Radiological Sciences, and Public Health, University of Brescia, Brescia, Italy

M. F. Saccomanno (✉)
Department of Bone and Joint Surgery, Spedali Civili, Brescia, Italy

Department of Orthopedics, Fondazione Policlinico Univarsitario A Gemelli IRCSS, Rome, Italy

G. Milano
Department of Medical and Surgical Specialties, Radiological Sciences, and Public Health, University of Brescia, Brescia, Italy

Department of Bone and Joint Surgery, Spedali Civili, Brescia, Italy
e-mail: giuseppe.milano@unibs.it

9.1 Introduction

- Bankart repair showed an overall rate of recurrent instability of 31.2%, with 16.0% of patients having recurrent dislocations, and an overall revision rate of 17.0%. Evidence of instability arthropathy was found in 59.4% of patients [1].
- Labral morphology can influence the risk of re-dislocation after primary Bankart repair [2].
  - A glenoid labral injury is identified in almost all cases of acute or recurrent traumatic glenohumeral instability, but sometimes, especially in chronic instability, scarred and residual tissue look so poor that an anatomic capsulolabral restoration is almost unachievable.
  - Atraumatic instability is often associated with insufficient chondrolabral containment and a redundant capsule [3], which makes any attempt at capsulolabral reconstruction very difficult, surely raising up the failure rate after primary arthroscopic soft tissue stabilization [4].

9.2 Indications

The glenoid labral augmentation technique has been mainly designed to account for at least two common clinical scenarios:

L. Kovačič et al. (eds.), *Surgical Techniques for Anterior Shoulder Instability*,
https://doi.org/10.1007/978-3-662-73064-5_9

- Thinned or frayed glenoid labrum in traumatic recurrent glenohumeral instability with no or subcritical glenoid bone loss
- Hypoplastic labrum commonly encountered in atraumatic instability

9.2.1 Main Indications

- Intraoperative confirmation of insufficiency (severe thinning, hypoplasia, inconsistent scar tissue) of the glenoid labrum
- On-track lesions [5], including peripheral-track lesions [6, 7]

9.2.2 Controversial Indications

- Contact- or collision-sport athletes
- MDI: Reconstruction of the anterior and posterior labrum at the same time could be needed, thus requiring higher technical skills. Although the surgical technique has been described [8], no clinical studies have been conducted yet.

9.2.3 Contraindications

- Off-track lesion [5]
- Acute bony Bankart lesion

9.3 Relevant Physical Findings

Since the main indication is based on arthroscopic findings, there are no pathognomonic clinical features. From a clinical standpoint, all patients being evaluated for shoulder instability always undergo a complete history-taking and physical examination to aid in surgical decision-making.

Key points when evaluating patient history:

- Traumatic/atraumatic onset
- Position of the shoulder at the time of the initial dislocation
- Necessity for medically assisted reduction versus self-reduction
- Amount of time that has passed since the initial dislocation
- Frequency of dislocation episodes
- Functional impairment of daily-living activities
- Sport activity type and level
- Any previous treatment

A standard physical examination will then be performed:

- Assessment of passive and active range of motion
- Provocative tests for anterior instability: apprehension, relocation
- Provocative tests for posterior instability: Kim's test [9]
- Shoulder laxity: Add-ER >85° [10], Sulcus sign, Gagey test [11]
- Generalized hyperlaxity: Beighton score [12]

9.4 Relevant Imaging

Besides anteroposterior (AP) view and axillary x-rays, it is part of authors' standard diagnostic protocol to rule out critical humeral and glenoid bone loss by performing a computed tomography (CT) scan in all patients prior to surgery. The following features are estimated:

- *Glenoid bone loss*: based on the circle method and achieved on three-dimensional (3D) *en face* views of the glenoid by volume rendering technique (VRT) reconstruction [13–15];
- *Bipolar defects interaction*: a 3D osseous reconstruction is also performed to determine the Hill-Sachs interval and then to calculate if bone defects are on track or off track [5]. In case of on-track lesions, the "Hill–Sachs interval to glenoid track width ratio" (H/G ratio) [7] is always calculated to specifically identify peripheral track lesions.

9.5 Goals of Surgical Procedure

9.5.1 Advantages

- Anatomic technique
  - Restores an efficient capsulolabral containment (bumper effect)
  - Deepens glenoid cavity
  - Increasing the joint surface area
- Does not require a long learning curve

9.5.2 Disadvantages

- Costs related to the graft

9.6 Surgical Technique

9.6.1 Equipment

Besides standard equipment for a shoulder arthroscopy, the following specific instrumentation is used:

- Two cannulas: one operative (8 mm) and one for outflow (5.5 mm)
- Porcine dermal collagen matrix (DX Reinforcement Matrix, Arthrex Inc., Naples, FL, USA)
- Knotless PEEK suture anchors (2.9 mm PushLock Anchor, Arthrex)
- High-strength permanent braided sutures (FiberWire, Arthrex)
- Suture passing devices (SutureLasso, Arthrex)

9.6.2 Positioning and Portals

- *Anesthesia*: general
- *Position*: lateral decubitus with the arm distracted at 70° of abduction and 15° of forward flexion
- A marking pen is utilized to draw bony landmarks:
  - spine of the scapula
  - acromion
  - clavicle
  - coracoid process

A standard three-portal approach is performed.

- *Posterior portal*: standard viewing portal. In case of combined posterior labral tears, the scope is then switched to the anterior portal, and the posterior portal is used as an operative portal for anchor placement (otherwise, an additional 7 o'clock portal is added) and suture management.
- *Anterosuperior portal* placed with the outside-in technique. This portal is performed through the rotator interval. It is the authors' preference to use plastic cannulas for the entire duration of the procedure in order to avoid soft tissue damage or the creation of false routes during the passage of arthroscopic instruments. A 5.5-mm plastic cannula is usually placed in this portal.
- *Anterior mid-glenoid portal* placed with the outside-in technique. This portal is performed through the rotator interval, just above the subscapularis tendon. An 8-mm plastic cannula is then positioned. This portal is used for the passage of arthroscopic instruments, anchor placement and suture management.

9.6.3 Step-by-Step Description of the Procedure

Step-by-step procedure for anterior labral augmentation is now described, as this is the most common scenario. The same technique is also applicable for the posterior labrum in case of combined posterior labral deficiency.

- *Diagnostic arthroscopy*: performed systematically. It is important to assess for pathology commonly encountered in patients affected by glenohumeral instability: labral tears (anterior and/or posterior Bankart lesions, Perthes lesion, ALPSA lesion, Kim lesion, SLAP tears), HAGL or RHAGL lesion, capsule condition (tearing, thinning, or redundancy), glenoid and humeral head bone loss. Mobilization of the anteroinferior capsulolabral complex is then attempted by using a chisel dissector. At this point, if a glenoid labrum deficiency is encountered, a labral augmentation should be considered (Fig. 9.1).

- *Measurements*: after mobilization of the anteroinferior capsulolabral complex and abrasion of the anterior glenoid neck, a probe is used to measure the length of the labral lesion (from inferior to superior). This measure is used for the preparation of the scaffold (Fig. 9.2).
- *Graft preparation*: A porcine dermal collagen matrix (DX Reinforcement Matrix, Arthrex) is sized according to the measured length of the labral lesion and 2 cm in width. The membrane is then rolled up to obtain a cylindrical scaffold 5 mm thick and sutured in a continuous fashion with a 2.0 high-strength nonabsorbable braided suture (FiberWire, Arthrex). Each end of the scaffold is then armed with one #2 absorbable monofilament traction suture (Fig. 9.3).
- *Graft passage and fixation*: a suture hook is introduced from the anterior mid-glenoid cannula and passed through the capsulolabral junction at the most inferior aspect of the injured capsule (approximately at the 6-to-5 o'clock position for a right shoulder). The shuttle of the suture hook is retrieved out of the anterosuperior cannula, and one limb of the distal traction suture of the scaffold is loaded over the eyelet of the shuttle and retrieved out of the anterior mid-glenoid cannula after passing through the capsulolabral junction in a retrograde way. The other limb of the same traction suture is retrieved from the anterior mid-glenoid cannula, and the scaffold is introduced into the joint from the anterosu-

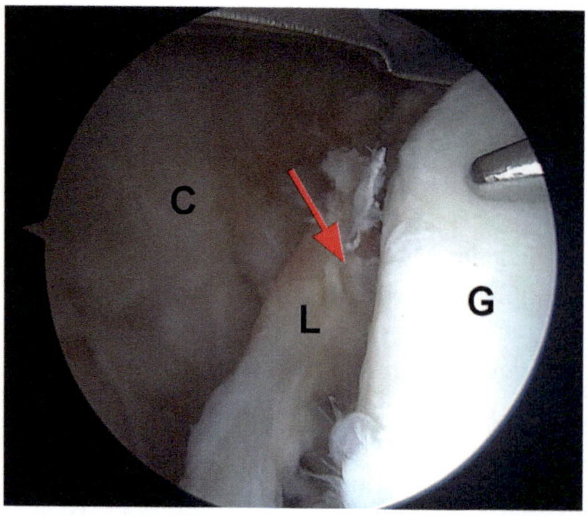

Fig. 9.1 Right shoulder. Scope in the antero-superior portal. Anterior glenoid labrum (arrow) is attenuated and scarred medially on the glenoid neck (C capsule, L labrum, G glenoid)

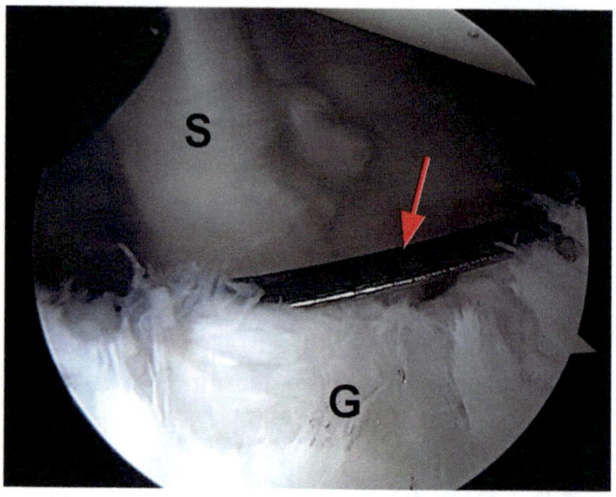

Fig. 9.2 Right shoulder. Scope in the posterior portal. A flexible probe (arrow) is used to measure the length of the labral lesion (from inferior to superior) (S subscapularis, G glenoid)

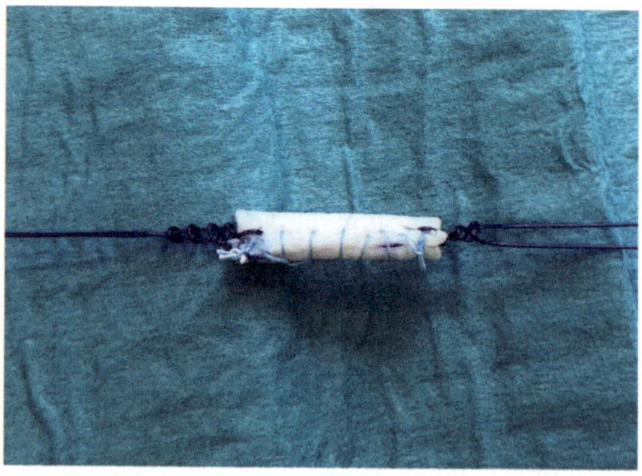

Fig. 9.3 A porcine dermal collagen matrix (DX Reinforcement Matrix; Arthrex Inc., Naples, FL) is sized according to the measured length. The membrane is rolled-up to obtain a cylindrical scaffold and sutured in a continuous fashion with a 2.0 absorbable braided suture. Each end of the scaffold is then armed with one #2 absorbable monofilament traction suture

perior cannula by pulling the inferior traction suture while maintaining a slight tension on the proximal traction suture. The scaffold is then placed over the anterior glenoid rim and fixed at its distal end to the capsule by knot tying of the distal traction suture (Fig. 9.4).

- *Capsulolabral repair*: performed in an inferior-to-superior direction by passing #2 FiberWire through the capsule and under the residual labrum and the scaffold in a simple configuration. Sutures are fixed to the anterior glenoid rim with 3–4 knotless suture anchors (2.9 PEEK Pushlock, Arthrex) placed over the articular margin of the anterior glenoid by including the capsule, the labrum and the scaffold (Fig. 9.5). Finally, the proximal traction suture is fixed to the most superior aspect of the stable capsulolabral tissue.

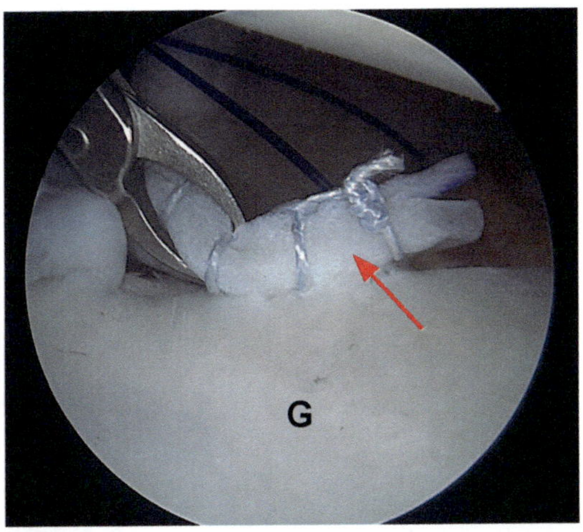

Fig. 9.4 Right shoulder. Scope in the posterior portal. The scaffold (arrow) is placed over the anterior glenoid rim by pulling the inferior traction suture (G glenoid)

9.6.4 Top Technical Recommendations from the Expert

- As described above, the scaffold is inserted into the joint through the antero-superior portal. Before scaffold introduction, remove the 5.5 mm cannula and place an 8 mm flexible cannula by using a switching stick to avoid a new route. The scaffold is quite stiff and thick, so the passage through a 5.5 mm cannula could require an unnecessarily high pulling strength.

Pearls and Pitfalls

- Lateral decubitus allows easy access to the entire glenoid, labrum, and capsule.
- Flexible cannulas can be used instead of plastic cannulas from the beginning of the procedure, thus avoiding any further switch.
- A flexible probe allows more precise measurements.
- Do not wet the graft before transferring it into the joint.
- A slight tension should be maintained on the proximal traction suture of the scaffold during tissue fixation.
- Accurate measurement of the labral tear is important: a short graft could be not enough; a long graft could be difficult to menage.

Fig. 9.5 Right shoulder. (**a**) Scope in the posterior portal. Final result: knotless suture anchors are used to fix the graft (arrow). (**b**) Scope in the antero-superior portal. Deepening of glenoid concavity as well as the bumper effect are appreciable (G glenoid)

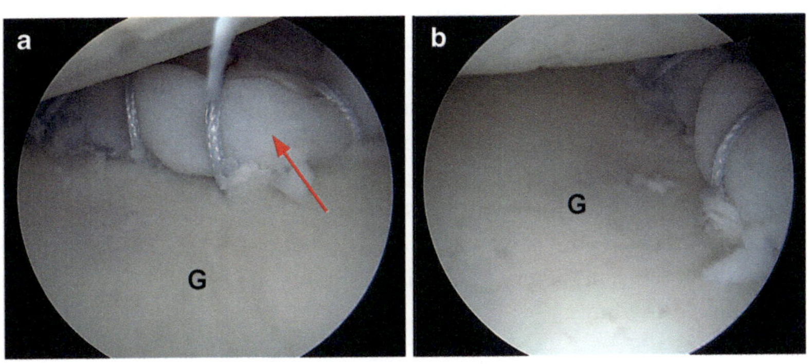

9.7 Postoperative Protocol

- Sling: 4 weeks after surgery
- Rehabilitation program:
  - Stage 1 (4–8 weeks after surgery): massotherapy and lysis of scar adhesions, passive mobilization for range of motion recovery
  - Stage 2 (9–12 weeks after surgery): closed kinetic chain exercises to strengthen the rotator cuff, the subscapularis, the biceps, the deltoid, the pectoralis major and the scapular stabilizers
  - Stage 3 (13–16 weeks after surgery): open kinetic chain exercises, proprioceptive and plyometric exercises, and postural rehabilitation of the kinetic chain (lumbo-pelvic, thoracolumbar and scapulothoracic muscles).
- Return to sports activities and heavy manual work is allowed 6 months after surgery.

9.8 Outcomes

Glenoid labral augmentation is one of the innovative surgical strategies to address the "grey zone" of glenohumeral instability: when an arthroscopic Bankart repair is not enough, and a bone augmentation procedure is too much.

Several techniques have been recently described aiming for the same purpose:

- *Arthroscopic Bankart-Plus procedure* [16]: described to fix small to intermediate glenoid bone defects by using an allogeneic demineralized spongy bone matrix between the glenoid neck and the labrum, in addition to the conventional capsulolabral repair
- *Arthroscopic subscapularis augmentation (ASA) technique* [17]: a tenodesis of the upper third of the subscapularis tendon in addition to a Bankart repair. The authors reported good functional results not only after treating recurrent anterior instability with capsular inconsistency and subcritical glenoid bone loss, but also after revision surgery of failed prior stabilization procedures.
- *The "between glenohumeral ligaments and subscapularis muscle stabilization" (BLS) technique* [18]: an anterior extracapsular stabilization, which relies on augmentation of the damaged anterior soft tissues by a part of the subscapularis muscle
- *Dynamic anterior shoulder stabilization (DAS)* [19, 20]: transposition of the long head of the biceps tendon within a subscapularis split to the anterior glenoid margin.

None of the above-described soft tissue procedures can be considered anatomic. Labral augmentation by using a biologic scaffold is a viable and safe option to address labral deficiency. Restoring the normal anatomy is the main advantage of the procedure, with a low risk of ROM restrictions and degenerative changes of the glenohumeral joint, often reported with non-anatomic procedures [21]. In the authors, experience, labral augmentation provided very good restoration of joint stability (recurrence rate at 2 years: 5%) and good integration of the graft with the glenoid and with the surrounding tissue (Fig. 9.6) (*unpublished data).*

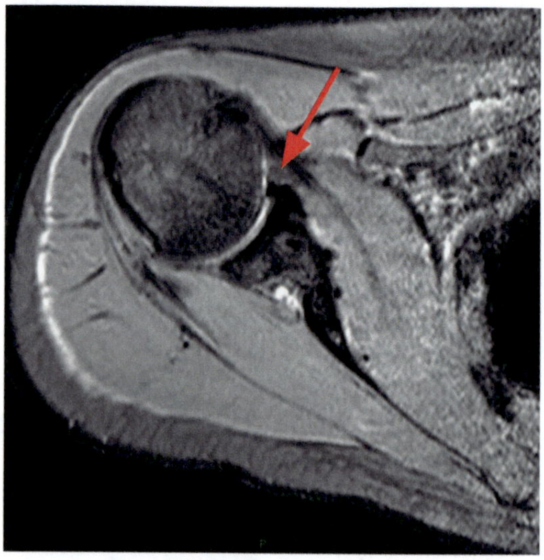

Fig. 9.6 Postoperative MRI at 6-month follow-up. Good integration of the graft (arrow) with the glenoid and with the surrounding tissue can be seen

9.9 Potential Complications

No specific intraoperative or postoperative complications related to the scaffold itself or to the surgical technique have been encountered up to now.

Take Home Messages

- Soft tissues matter!
- Anatomy should always be the goal of any surgical procedure performed in young people.
- Labral augmentation by using a collagen membrane is easy to perform and can effectively restore the anatomy when the main issue is the labral insufficiency.

References

1. Murphy AI, Hurley ET, Hurley DJ, Pauzenberger L, Mullett H. Long-term outcomes of the arthroscopic Bankart repair: a systematic review of studies at 10-year follow-up. J Shoulder Elb Surg. 2019;28:2084–9.
2. Vaswani R, Gasbarro G, Como C, Golan E, Fourman M, Wilmot A, Borrero C, Vyas D, Lin A. Labral morphology and number of preoperative dislocations are associated with recurrent instability after arthroscopic Bankart repair. Arthroscopy. 2019;36:993–9.
3. Doehrmann R, Frush TJ. Posterior shoulder instability. In: StatPearls. Treasure Island: StatPearls Publishing; 2021.
4. Longo UG, Rizzello G, Loppini M, Locher J, Buchmann S, Maffulli N, Denaro V. Multidirectional instability of the shoulder: a systematic review. Arthroscopy. 2015;31:2431–43.
5. Di Giacomo G, Itoi E, Burkhart SS. Evolving concept of bipolar bone loss and the Hill-Sachs lesion: from "engaging/non-engaging" lesion to "on-track/off-track" lesion. Arthroscopy. 2014;30:90–8.
6. Yamamoto N, Shinagawa K, Hatta T, Itoi E. Peripheral-track and central-Track Hill-Sachs lesions: a new concept of assessing an on-track lesion. Am J Sports Med. 2020;48:33–8.
7. Yang T-C, Chen K-H, Chiang E-R, Chang M-C, Ma H-L. Using the "Hill-Sachs interval to glenoid track width ratio" for prediction of recurrent instability after arthroscopic Bankart repair. Orthop Traumatol Surg Res. 2018;104:797–801.
8. Gervasi E, Sebastiani E, Spicuzza A. Multidirectional shoulder instability: arthroscopic labral augmentation. Arthrosc Tech. 2017;6:e219–25.
9. Kim S-H, Park J-S, Jeong W-K, Shin S-K. The Kim test: a novel test for posteroinferior labral lesion of the shoulder–a comparison to the jerk test. Am J Sports Med. 2005;33:1188–92.
10. Boileau P, Villalba M, Héry J-Y, Balg F, Ahrens P, Neyton L. Risk factors for recurrence of shoulder instability after arthroscopic Bankart repair. J Bone Joint Surg Am. 2006;88:1755–63.
11. Gagey OJ, Gagey N. The hyperabduction test. J Bone Joint Surg Br. 2001;83:69–74.
12. Beighton P, Horan F. Orthopaedic aspects of the Ehlers-Danlos syndrome. J Bone Joint Surg Br. 1969;51:444–53.
13. Magarelli N, Milano G, Baudi P, Santagada DA, Righi P, Spina V, Leone A, Amelia R, Fabbriciani C, Bonomo L. Comparison between 2D and 3D computed tomography evaluation of glenoid bone defect in unilateral anterior Gleno-humeral instability. Radiol Med (Torino). 2012;117:102–11.
14. Magarelli N, Milano G, Sergio P, Santagada DA, Fabbriciani C, Bonomo L. Intra-observer and interobserver reliability of the "Pico" computed tomography method for quantification of glenoid bone defect in anterior shoulder instability. Skeletal Radiol. 2009;38:1071–5.
15. Milano G, Saccomanno MF, Magarelli N, Bonomo L. Analysis of agreement between computed tomography measurements of glenoid bone defects in anterior shoulder instability with and without comparison with the contralateral shoulder. Am J Sports Med. 2015;43:2918–26.
16. Moroder P, Böhm E, Scheibel M. The arthroscopic Bankart-Plus procedure for treatment of anterior shoulder instability with small to intermediate glenoid defects. Arthrosc Tech. 2018;7:e379–84.
17. Maiotti M, Russo R, Zanini A, Schröter S, Massoni C, Bianchedi D. Arthroscopic Bankart repair and subscapularis augmentation: an alternative technique treating anterior shoulder instability with bone loss. J Shoulder Elb Surg. 2016;25:898–906.
18. Brzóska R, Laprus H, Michniowski P, Solecki W, Klon W, Błasiak A. Novel and effective arthroscopic extracapsular stabilization technique for anterior shoulder instability-BLS. Knee Surg Sports Traumatol Arthrosc. 2019;27:3897–904.
19. Collin P, Lädermann A. Dynamic anterior stabilization using the long head of the biceps for Anteroinferior Glenohumeral instability. Arthrosc Tech. 2018;7:e39–44.
20. Mehl J, Otto A, Imhoff FB, Murphy M, Dyrna F, Obopilwe E, Cote M, Lädermann A, Collin P, Beitzel K, Mazzocca AD. Dynamic anterior shoulder stabilization with the long head of the biceps tendon: a biomechanical study. Am J Sports Med. 2019;47:1441–50.
21. Waterman BR, Kilcoyne KG, Parada SA, Eichinger JK. Prevention and management of post-instability glenohumeral arthropathy. World J Orthop. 2017;8:229–41.

Hill-Sachs and Remplissage

10

Gonzalo Samitier and Gustavo Vinagre

Key Points

- Physical examination of a patient's unstable shoulder should be done bilaterally.
- Surgical treatment of anterior shoulder instability and each complementary procedure should be an "a la carte" decision-making process.
- The Hill-Sachs lesion should be considered in conjunction with the glenoid bone defect using the on-track/off-track concept.
- The remplissage technique is a tenodesis of the infraspinatus over the Hill-Sachs lesion (posterolateral humeral head bone loss secondary to the impact during dislocation).
- An arthroscopic remplissage procedure should be considered to be added to an arthroscopic Bankart repair in cases of medium to large engaging Hill-Sachs ('off-track') defects—even in first-time traumatic dislocations.
- The remplissage procedure can potentially decrease the external rotation so that it should be carefully indicated in competitive thrower athletes who need extreme external rotation range of motion.

10.1 Introduction

- Traumatic anterior shoulder instability is a common condition in sports injuries with a high risk of recurrence in young and active patients [1].
- Recurrence risk factors include young age, number of episodes, capsular laxity, glenoid bone loss, large Hill-Sachs defects, type, competitive sports, and reduced time to return to sports/competition after shoulder dislocation.
- Hill-Sachs injury is a posterolateral impaction fracture of the humeral head, which results from the anterior glenoid rim impacting the humeral head during anterior/inferior dislocation [2, 3]. This happens in 65–71% of initial

Supplementary Information The online version contains supplementary material available at https://doi.org/10.1007/978-3-662-73064-5_10.

G. Samitier (✉)
Centro Médico Quironsalud Aribau, Barcelona, Spain
e-mail: contacto@samitiersports.com

G. Vinagre
Department of Orthopaedic Surgery, Aspetar Orthopaedic and Sports Medicine Hospital, Doha, Qatar
e-mail: gustavovinagre@gustavovinagre.com

L. Kovačič et al. (eds.), *Surgical Techniques for Anterior Shoulder Instability*,
https://doi.org/10.1007/978-3-662-73064-5_10

glenohumeral dislocations [2, 4–6] and 93–100% of patients with recurrent dislocations [4, 7, 8]. It can cause recurrent locking, catching, and re-dislocations events.

- A combination of a glenoid defect and a Hill-Sachs defect is entitled "bipolar bone loss."
- Subsequent dislocations and subluxations can increase the size of the Hill-Sachs and increase the risk of recurrence, even after primary Bankart repair [9–11].
- An engaging Hill-Sachs ('off-track') is an injury that comes out of the glenoid coverage and engages with the anterior rim of the glenoid, causing a dislocation (Fig. 10.1).
- A remplissage is a soft-tissue nonanatomic surgical technique that consists of the fixation of the infraspinatus tendon and posterior capsule (capsulotenodesis) to the abraded surface of the Hill-Sachs lesion. The remplissage does "fill" the Hill-Sachs lesion with capsular and posterior cuff tissue so that it can no longer engage, transforming an engaging Hill-Sachs ('off-track') into a non-engaging Hill-Sachs ('on-track') injury [12, 13]. It also prevents anterior humeral head translation.
- The remplissage procedure converts an intra-articular Hill-Sachs into an extra-articular defect.
- Arthroscopic remplissage is usually a complementary and combined procedure along with an arthroscopic Bankart repair.

10.2 Indications for Remplissage

- Different factors play a role in the surgical decision-making process of the treatment of the anterior shoulder instability: age, the number of dislocations, symptoms, type of activity/sports, level of sports competition, the position of the athlete (overhead/thrower vs. non-overhead/non-thrower), type of lesion (soft-tissue vs. bony lesion), and time of sports season.
- Complementary surgical treatment of Hill-Sachs injury should also consider different aspects such as the size, location, and symptoms of the lesion.
- The procedure of arthroscopic remplissage is a concomitant procedure along with arthroscopic Bankart repair that has been used to improve shoulder stability in cases in which the humerus engages with the glenoid ('off-track' lesion) [14] with glenoid bone loss less than 25% ("subcritical" bone loss) and the humeral head involvement (Hill-Sachs) is moderate to large (higher than 25%) [13].

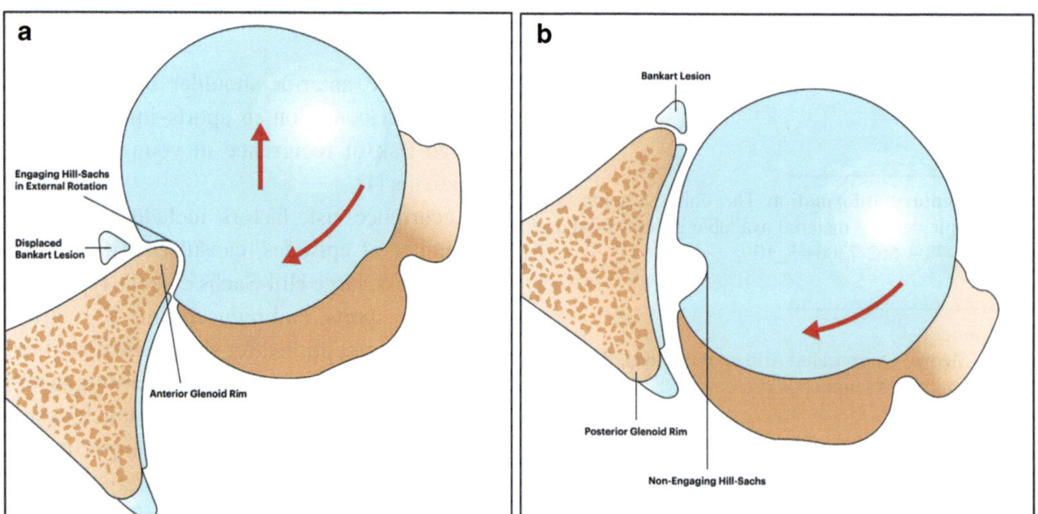

Fig. 10.1 (**a**) Engaging Hill-Sachs. (**b**) Non-engaging Hill-Sachs

Table 10.1 Treatment algorithm for Hill-Sachs (HS) injuries [13]

Glenoid bone loss <25% ("subcritical")	Non-engaging HS 'on-track': *arthroscopic Bankart repair*
	Engaging HS 'off-track': *Arthroscopic Bankart repair + remplissage*
Glenoid bone loss ≥25% ("critical")	Non-engaging HS 'on-track': *Latarjet*
	Engaging HS 'off-track': *Latarjet +/− Remplissage or humeral head grafts*

- Remplissage complementary procedure may compromise glenohumeral range of motion (ROM) external rotation [14–16]. Therefore, should be cautiously indicated in overhead/thrower athletes who need extreme external rotation movements.
- Further surgical indications for the treatment of Hill-Sachs injuries in shoulder instability are detailed in (Table 10.1).

10.3 Relevant Physical Findings

- A clinical and diagnostic examination should start with a detailed history.
- It is crucial to know individual factors (age, gender, type of sports, hand dominance) and to understand the history of shoulder instability, inquiring about the details on the first dislocation event (age, mechanism of injury, shoulder and arm position that led to dislocation, and treatment), the number of subsequent dislocations or subluxations, and how easily the shoulder dislocates and reduces.
- Differential diagnosis should focus on traumatic (TUBS) versus atraumatic (AMBRI) shoulder instability.
- It is also key to know the actual symptoms of the patient: if there is glenoid bone loss or an engaging Hill-Sachs defect, the patient may describe a sensation of "catching" or "the shoulder falls out." These symptoms should be corroborated with a physical exam.
- Physical examination of a patient's unstable shoulder should start with an inspection to rule out an obvious deformity, open wound, scapular dyskinesis, and limited range of motion.
- Palpation of the shoulder is intended to localize any tender spots or crepitus.
- Both active and passive ranges of motion (ROM) should be determined and registered.
- Also, assessment of the muscular status (check for atrophy in the deltoid and supraspinatus fossa), rotator cuff strength (especially in patients over the age of 40), and ligamentous laxity tests should also be made to complement and support the differential diagnosis.
- A complete neurovascular exam is mandatory, especially in the acute shoulder dislocation, to evaluate the presence of any sensory-motor impairment—before and after any reduction maneuver attempt.
- The apprehension test is an essential tool to be made in the outpatient setting: the patient is supine, and the arm is passively abducted and externally rotated, both to 90°. The test is positive if the patient feels discomfort or pain. The examiner can push posterior the humeral head by applying a direct force to the shoulder—the so-called Jobe relocation test—and the patient will feel a relief from the pain [17]. A positive surprise test is when the examiner suddenly removes the hand after a relocation test, and the patient re-experiences the symptoms.
- Stability of the glenohumeral joint should also be evaluated by the anterior and posterior drawer tests (positive if the humerus has an increased translation compared to the contralateral shoulder); the sulcus sign (depression that occurs after the inferior traction of the arm); the Gagey hyperabduction test (assessment of the laxity of the inferior glenohumeral ligament); the jerk test; and the load-and-shift test (positive if the humeral head can be shifted anteriorly off the glenoid). These tests can be done either supine or sitting upright.

10.4 Relevant Imaging

- Shoulder instability overall radiological evaluation should include routine X-rays in three views: true Grashey AP view, West Point Axillary view, and trans-scapular Y view or lateral Subacromial (Outlet) view.
- West Point Axillary view is the best projection for bony Bankart evaluation.
- Axial view and Stryker (Notch) view are the best projections for Hill-Sachs evaluation.
- Glenoid profile (Bernageau) can evaluate both: Bankart and Hill-Sachs injuries.
- A CT scan should be performed when bone loss is suspected for quantification and calculation of the glenoid and humerus bone loss (glenoid track and Hill-Sachs interval).
- CT arthrogram and 3D CT scan are complementary tools to assess glenoid bone defects and/or Hill-Sachs lesions.
- Magnetic resonance imaging (MRI) or arthro-MRI can be used to evaluate the size and extent of Bankart lesions and screen for any associated lesions (e.g., SLAP lesions, rotator cuff tears).

10.5 Goals of Surgical Procedure

- An arthroscopic Hill-Sachs remplissage is a combined procedure that transforms intra-articular engaging Hill-Sachs ('off-track') into an extra-articular non-engaging Hill-Sachs ('on-track') defect.
- The goal of this surgical procedure is to improve shoulder stability and reduce the chance of re-dislocation and symptoms.

10.6 Surgical Technique

- An upper limb regional anesthetic block is performed, and general anesthesia is administered with endotracheal tube intubation.
- The procedure can be performed in lateral decubitus or in a beach chair position. In our group, we use lateral decubitus with the arm abducted at 70° and 5–7 kg of traction.
- The bony landmarks and portals of the shoulder can be outlined with a sterile marker.
- Standard posterior and anterosuperior portals are performed, and an additional accessory posterolateral portal centered over the Hill-Sachs is created, enabling preparation and insertion of suture anchors into the defect. The authors recommend inserting cannulas in all the portals to facilitate suture passage; 8 mm cannulas are used in the anteroinferior and posterior portals. Meanwhile, a 7 mm cannula is usually enough at the anterosuperior portal, as this is mostly a visualization portal.
- An arthroscopic diagnostic systematic evaluation of the shoulder is initially performed to understand the extent of the injuries.
- First, the humeral head Hill-Sachs defect is prepared; an arthroscopic remplissage is performed with two anchors using the posterior cannula and recovering sutures through the capsule; the final remplissage suturing tightening should not be performed until the Bankart is completed.
- Our preference for remplissage is using knotless anchors with interconnected sutures that are linked out of the posterior capsule on the posterior cannula.
- In case of the presence of a posterior Bankart, a repair should be done with proper labrum repair—before closing the Hill-Sachs remplissage.
- The anterior Bankart glenoid preparation and insertion of the anchors and labrum sutures should then be passed through the anterior labrum.
- Completion of the anterior Bankart labral suture tightening repair should be performed at this point.
- As the final step, remplissage sutures are tied to close and fill the Hill-Sachs humeral defect (Table 10.2).

Table 10.2 Pearls and pitfalls of arthroscopic remplissage surgical technique

Pearls	Pitfalls
Examine under anesthesia to identify the directions and degree of humeral translation relative to the glenoid In the remplissage technique, the procedures of anchor implanting and suture passing (without tying the sutures) must be completed before the anterior Bankart repair. Final tightening of the Hill-Sachs remplissage should be performed after anterior Bankart repair For Bankart repair the authors recommend using tensionable knotless anchors (3.0 mm knotless SutureTak®) or sutures with a closed loop in the end (Fiberlink®) and knotless anchors (Pushlock®) For remplissage, an interconnected knotless technique can be used (Video 10.1) in an attempt to improve biomechanical strength and compression of the infraspinatus [18] After anchor fixation on the humeral Hill-Sachs defect, the cannula should be slowly pulled back off the capsule for capsule re-penetration and suture retrieval with the help of a suture manipulator grasper.	Posterior Bankart repair should be performed before tightening the remplissage sutures Avoid over-tightening the remplissage in a position of excessive internal or external rotation In case of traction use, release it before remplissage suture tightening

10.7 Postoperative Protocol

- Postoperative rehabilitation protocol should be individualized for each patient/athlete according to the type of surgery.
- Early phases should include a sling for 3 weeks for soft tissue protection, control of inflammation, and healing.
- Passive ROM with daily pendulum exercises is recommended from the beginning to avoid shoulder stiffness. Hand, wrist, and elbow active exercises are also encouraged to start immediately.
- From the third week, active-assisted ROM is gradually increased, and isotonic and gentle closed-chain exercises are started, along with progressive strengthening and joint neuromuscular control.
- Abduction and external rotation beyond neutral are avoided until 6 weeks.
- The sling is usually discontinued at four postoperative weeks, and full ROM is allowed after 6 weeks.
- Final rehabilitation phases should aim for sports-specific movements and tests.
- Return-to-sports is expected from 4 to 6 months (4-month period on average) [19].

10.8 Outcomes

- For primary anterior shoulder dislocation, early surgical stabilization has a better outcome and lower recurrent instability rate compared to nonoperative treatment, especially for younger and active individuals [20].
- According to Friedman et al. [21] systematic review, in cases of glenoid bone loss less than 30% or non-engaging ('on-track') Hill-Sachs, open Bankart repair was successful in 100% of patients (no recurrences). If the glenoid bone loss is greater than 30% or engaging Hill-Sachs ('off-track'), open Bankart repair yielded 57.1% of recurrences.
- According to Balg and Boileau [22, 23], bone loss (both at the glenoid or at the humeral side), patient age under 20 years at the time of surgery, contact sports or overhead activity, and shoulder hyperlaxity are risk factors for recurrence after arthroscopic Bankart repair.
- These authors developed the "instability severity index score" (ISIS score), a numerical scoring system that takes into account the previously named risk factors and determines which patient would be better treated by an arthroscopic (Bankart repair) vs. open proce-

dure (i.e., Latarjet) [22]. If there is an ISIS >3 they suggest augmenting a Bankart repair with a remplissage (engaging Hill-Sachs), Latarjet (anteroinferior glenoid bone loss), or Trillat (no glenoid or humeral bone loss) procedure [9].

- In a cadaveric study by Elkinson et al. [23], Hill-Sachs lesions sized at 15% and 30% were treated with a combination of Bankart repair with remplissage. They found that when treated with Bankart alone, none of the 15% Hill-Sachs lesions engaged and dislocated, whereas all of the 30% lesions did. However, the dislocation rate of the 30% Hill-Sachs lesions was significantly reduced if remplissage was added in conjunction with Bankart repair. So that remplissage is most effective in the setting of minimal glenoid bone loss and moderate to large engaging Hill-Sachs defects.
- One anchor may fill large defects and transform critical lesions into noncritical, nonengaging defects. However, two anchors are often needed. Despite that, it seems that there is no difference between using one or two anchors [24].
- According to several studies [24–28], at least partial healing of the remplissage is shown in 100% of patients, with >74% of patients demonstrating healing of >75% of the footprint by MRI or CT arthrogram. It is difficult to calculate the exact percentage of healing using MRI due to artifacts from the anchors [28], but by adding contrast to a CT, the assessment of healing is improved [25].

10.9 Potential Complications

- One of the most frequent complications after conservative or surgical treatment of shoulder instability is a failure of stabilization and subsequent recurrent shoulder dislocations and/or apprehension. This can be due to the failure to correct the pathology, failure of healing, or poor patient compliance.
- Potential complications related to the treatment of shoulder instability can be neurovascular problems, infection, postoperative degenerative changes, hardware failure, and patient expectations mismatch.
- Specific possible complications of arthroscopic remplissage have been described, such as posterosuperior shoulder pain, partial infraspinatus tears, tendinopathy or fatty infiltration, and loss of shoulder motion, particularly in external rotation [28, 29].

10.10 Video

- Remplissage arthroscopic technique with tips and pearls is detailed in (Video 10.1).

Take Home Message

- Large engaging Hill-Sachs deformity, if not properly managed, may compromise a Bankart repair and lead to recurrent instability.
- Preoperative and intraoperative assessments of humeral head defects are mandatory for patients with shoulder instability.
- Remplissage should be considered to be added into Bankart repair in cases of bipolar "subcritical" glenoid bone loss and engaging Hill-Sachs defects (particularly moderate-large humeral head defects)—to decrease postoperative recurrent instability and re-dislocation rate.
- Recurrence, external rotation loss, and posterior shoulder pain are the most frequent complications observed following remplissage.
- All potential causes of failure or complications must be fully evaluated and understood to properly address a solution/treatment.

References

1. Rowe CR. Prognosis in dislocations of the shoulder. J Bone Joint Surg Am. 1956;38-A(5):957–77.
2. Calandra JJ, Baker CL, Uribe J. The incidence of Hill-Sachs lesions in initial anterior shoulder dislocations. Arthroscopy. 1989;5(4):254–7.
3. Spatschil A, et al. Posttraumatic anterior-inferior instability of the shoulder: arthroscopic findings and clinical correlations. Arch Orthop Trauma Surg. 2006;126(4):217–22.
4. Yiannakopoulos CK, Mataragas E, Antonogiannakis E. A comparison of the spectrum of intra-articular lesions in acute and chronic anterior shoulder instability. Arthroscopy. 2007;23(9):985–90.
5. Longo UG, et al. Shoulder injuries in soccer players. Clin Cases Miner Bone Metab. 2012;9(3):138–41.
6. Longo UG, et al. Video analysis of the mechanisms of shoulder dislocation in four elite rugby players. J Orthop Sci. 2011;16(4):389–97.
7. Lynch JR, et al. Treatment of osseous defects associated with anterior shoulder instability. J Shoulder Elb Surg. 2009;18(2):317–28.
8. Maffulli N, et al. Sport injuries: a review of outcomes. Br Med Bull. 2011;97:47–80.
9. Boileau P, Villalba M, Hery JY, Balg F, Ahrens P, Neyton L. Risk factors for recurrence of shoulder instability after arthroscopic Bankart repair. J Bone Joint Surg Am. 2006;88(8):1755–63.
10. Rowe CR, Zarins B, Ciullo JV. Recurrent anterior dislocation of the shoulder after surgical repair. Apparent causes of failure and treatment. J Bone Joint Surg Am. 1984;66(2):159–68.
11. Burkhart SS, De Beer JF. Traumatic glenohumeral bone defects and their relationship to failure of arthroscopic Bankart repairs: significance of the inverted-pear glenoid and the humeral engaging Hill-Sachs lesion. Arthroscopy. 2000;16(7):677–94.
12. Di Giacomo G, Itoi E, Burkhart SS. Evolving concept of bipolar bone loss and the Hill-Sachs lesion: from "engaging/non-engaging" lesion to "on-track/off-track" lesion. Arthroscopy. 2014;30:90–8.
13. Park MJ, Tjoumakaris FP, Garcia G, Patel A, Kelly JD IV. Arthroscopic remplissage with bankart repair for the treatment of glenohumeral instability with hill-sachs defects. Arthroscopy. 2011;27:1187–94.
14. Purchase RJ, Wolf EM, Hobgood ER, Pollock ME, Smalley CC. Hill-Sachs "remplissage": an arthroscopic solution for the engaging Hill-Sachs lesion. Arthroscopy. 2008;24:723–6.
15. Romeo AA, Provencher MT. Shoulder instability: a comprehensive approach. Philadelphia: Saunders; 2012.
16. Young DC, Rockwood CA Jr. Complications of a failed Bristow procedure and their management. J Bone Joint Surg Am. 1991;73:969–81.
17. Jobe FW, Kvitne RS, Giangarra CE. Shoulder pain in the overhand or throwing athlete. The relationship of anterior instability and rotator cuff impingement. Orthop Rev. 1989;18(9):963–75.
18. Funakoshi T, Hartzler R, Stewien E, Burkhart S. Remplissage using interconnected knotless anchors: superior biomechanical properties to a knotted technique? Arthroscopy. 2018;34:2954–9.
19. Jaggi A, Lambert S. Rehabilitation for shoulder instability. Br J Sports Med. 2010;44(5):333–40.
20. Brophy RH, Marx RG. The treatment of traumatic anterior instability of the shoulder: nonoperative and surgical treatment. Arthroscopy. 2009;25(3):298–304.
21. Friedman LG, Griesser MJ, Miniaci AA, Jones MH. Recurrent instability after revision anterior shoulder stabilization surgery. Arthroscopy. 2014;30(3):372–81.
22. Balg F, Boileau P. The instability severity index score. A simple pre-operative score to select patients for arthroscopic or open shoulder stabilisation. J Bone Joint Surg Br. 2007;89(11):1470–7.
23. Elkinson I, et al. The effect of the remplissage procedure on shoulder stability and range of motion: an in vitro biomechanical assessment. J Bone Joint Surg Am. 2012;94(11):1003–12.
24. Franceschi F, Papalia R, Rizzello G, Franceschetti E, Del Buono A, Panasci M, et al. Remplissage repair—new frontiers in the prevention of recurrent shoulder instability: a 2-year follow-up comparative study. Am J Sports Med. 2012;40(11):2462–9.
25. Boileau P, O'Shea K, Vargas P, Pinedo M, Old J, Zumstein M. Anatomical and functional results after arthroscopic Hill-Sachs remplissage. J Bone Joint Surg. 2012;94(7):618–26.
26. Park MJ, Garcia G, Malhotra A, Major N, Tjoumakaris FP, Kelly JD. The evaluation of arthroscopic remplissage by high-resolution magnetic resonance imaging. Am J Sports Med. 2012;40(10):2331–6.
27. Zhu YM, Lu Y, Zhang J, Shen JW, Jiang CY. Arthroscopic Bankart repair combined with remplissage technique for the treatment of anterior shoulder instability with engaging Hill-Sachs lesion: a report of 49 cases with a minimum 2-year follow-up. Am J Sports Med. 2011;39(8):1640–7.
28. Nourissat G, Kilinc AS, Werther JR, Doursounian L. A prospective, comparative, radiological, and clinical study of the influence of the remplissage procedure on shoulder range of motion after stabilization by arthroscopic Bankart repair. Am J Sports Med. 2011;39(10):2147–52.
29. Deutsch AA, Kroll DG. Decreased range of motion following arthroscopic remplissage. Orthopedics. 2008;31(5):492.

Anterior Shoulder Instability Treatment with BLS Technique

11

Roman Brzóska and Hubert Laprus

Key Points

- Arthroscopic Bankart repair in the treatment of shoulder instability is associated with a high prevalence of instability recurrence.
- The extracapsular stabilization of the glenohumeral joint with enhancement of anterior wall soft tissues could be an alternative and more efficient procedure, especially in cases of anterior glenoid bone loss or anterior wall insufficiency. Following this point of view, a novel anterior extracapsular stabilization technique—"Between glenohumeral Ligaments and Subscapularis tendon" (BLS)—was introduced.
- Effectiveness of BLS technique was studied retrospectively by assessing patients with anterior shoulder instability who underwent surgical treatment with the novel arthroscopic BLS technique.
- At final assessment, 86% of patients were categorized as having a positive outcome, with full restoration of joint stability.
- Recurrence of shoulder instability was observed in 14 (14%) patients including 6 (6%) cases following major trauma.
- The frequency of failure was higher in patients with a more severe glenoid bone loss (GBL) and with a greater baseline range of ER.
- There was no statistically relevant limitation of external or internal rotation.
- The BLS technique has been shown to be an effective way of treating anterior shoulder instability in patients without significant glenoid bone loss. It was also shown that this technique does not decrease shoulder range of motion.

Supplementary Information The online version contains supplementary material available at https://doi.org/10.1007/978-3-662-73064-5_11.

R. Brzóska · H. Laprus (✉)
St Luke's Hospital, Bielsko-Biala, Poland

11.1 Introduction

- Treatment of anterior shoulder instability is currently a subject of debate. Several different operative techniques, with varying effectiveness, have been proposed, and there is yet no consensus on which technique provides the best outcome.
- For many years, open or arthroscopic Bankart repair procedure was the proposed treatment for every case [1, 4]. Unfortunately, studies showed that approximately one third of patients had instability

L. Kovačič et al. (eds.), *Surgical Techniques for Anterior Shoulder Instability*,
https://doi.org/10.1007/978-3-662-73064-5_11

recurrence after arthroscopic Bankart repair and among patients younger than 21 years, the risk of failure was shown to be even higher, with a reported failure rate of more than 50% [4, 5, 7].

- In the pursuit of a surgical technique that could prevent recurrent anterior shoulder instability, the authors developed a new arthroscopic technique, which could be seen as a modification of the classic Bankart procedure [2, 3].
- This non-anatomic technique relies on augmentation of the damaged anterior wall soft tissues by a part of the subscapularis muscle and was named "between glenohumeral ligaments and subscapularis muscle stabilization" (BLS).
- This technique enables restoration of the original capsulolabral footprint while protecting the articular surface by extracapsular knots placement, thus, reducing the risk of future articular damage by abrasion.

11.2 Surgical Technique

11.2.1 Positioning and Portals

- For performance of the BLS procedure, the patient is placed in the beach chair position under general anesthesia following an interscalene block.
- The standard posterior portal is created.
- Two additional portals: anterolateral and anterior are created.

11.2.2 Step-by-Step Description of the Procedure

- During the initial arthroscopic examination, a Hill-Sachs lesion should be identified.
- In case of arthroscopically confirmed engaging Hill-Sachs lesion [9], remplissage standard technique is performed [8].
- Viewing through the posterior portal, the glenoid labrum pouch (GLP) and ligament subscapularis pouch (LSP) are marked with electrothermal cautery inserted through the anterolateral portal (Fig. 11.1).
- The GLP is prepared first in the standard fashion, using a rasp to approximately the 6-o'clock position.
- The LSP is then marked through the direct anterior portal, viewing through the anterolateral portal (Fig. 11.1). To create this space, the capsule must be separated from the overlying subscapularis, and this delicate dissection is carried out medially and inferiorly until the subscapularis muscle fibers are visualized.
- Care must be taken to orient the electrothermal cautery toward the subscapularis and away from the anterior capsule, which might otherwise become injured.

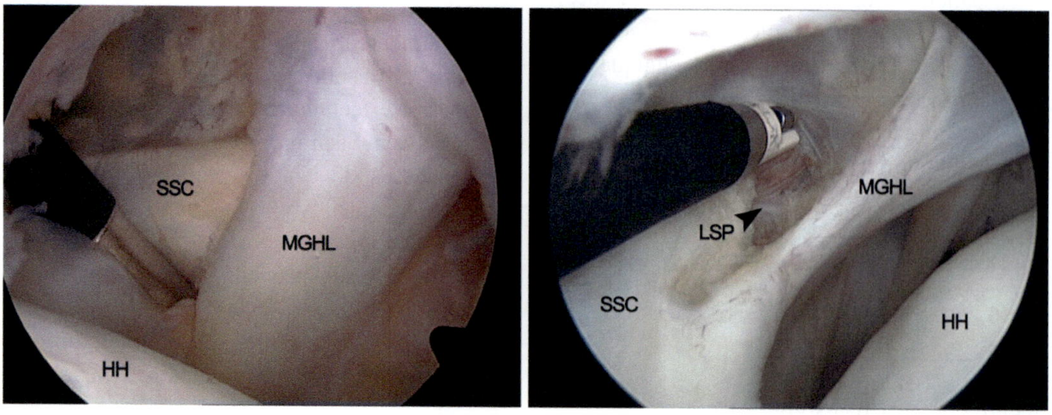

Fig. 11.1 Arthroscopic view of makred glenoid labrum pouch (GLP) and ligament subscapularis pouch (LSP) and arhtoscopic view of LSP through the anterolateral portal

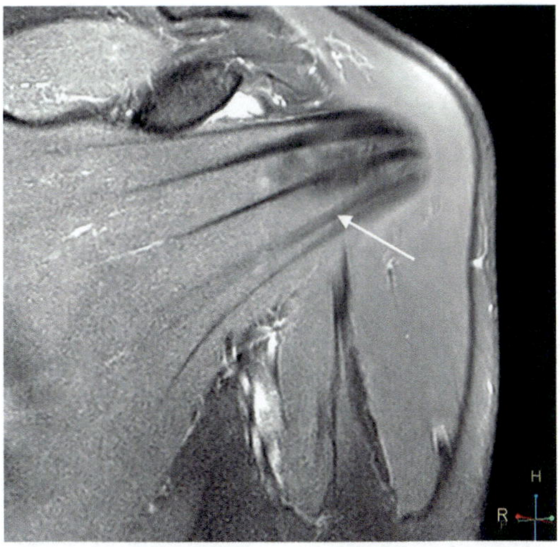

Fig. 11.2 Subscapularis muscle tendinous cords in MRI imaging- white arrow indicates proper cord used for anterior wall augmentation

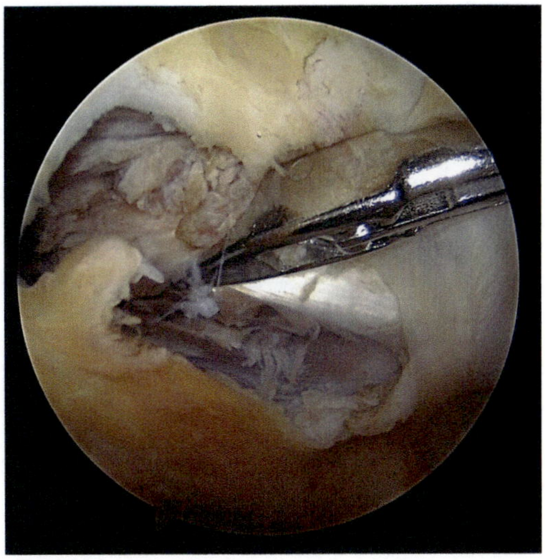

Fig. 11.3 Lower cord of subscapularis muscle used in anterior wall augmentation

- Because the anterior capsular tissues are usually deficient, a lower third or fourth tendinous cord of subscapularis muscle is separated with a grasper in order to augment the repair without affecting motion (Figs. 11.2 and 11.3).
- A double-loaded suture anchor is inserted into the glenoid rim at the 5:30. The threads from the anchor must pass through the center of the labrum, anterior capsule, and glenohumeral ligaments, and finally attach a silver cord of the subscapularis tendon to augment the repaired anterior stabilizers.
- Using the grasper through the posterior portal to pull up the anterior wall complex and hold it in position, a second double-loaded suture anchor is placed at 4 o'clock, and 2 additional mattress sutures are placed.
- The previously dissected third or fourth tendinous cord of the subscapularis muscle has to be surrounded and stitched by threads from the lowest anchor (Figs. 11.4 and 11.5).

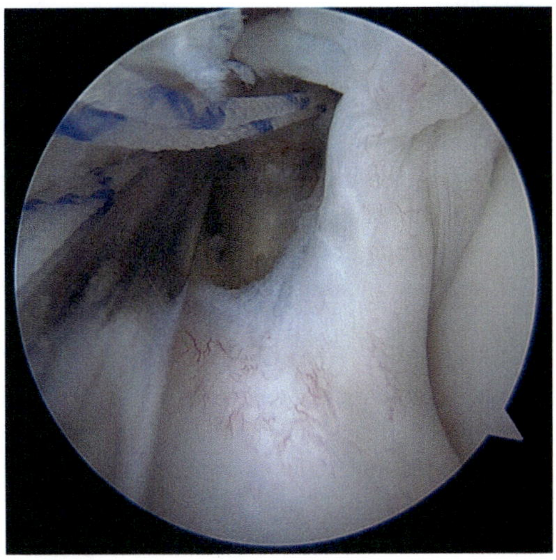

Fig. 11.4 Cord of subscapularis muscle used for anterior wall augmentation

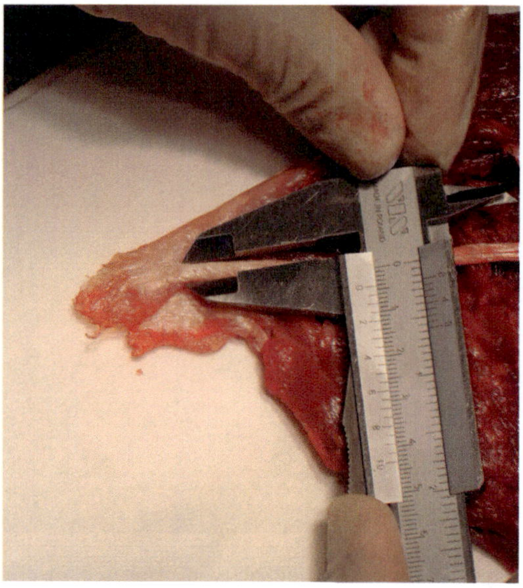

Fig. 11.5 Cadaveric view of subscapularis muscle tendinous cord

- It should be underlined that thread passing through the tendon and knot tying should be performed with the shoulder in external rotation, which is crucial so that after the suturing this part of the subscapularis muscle, there is no restriction in the external rotation.
- If necessary another anchor is placed like in the standard arthro-Bankart procedure (Fig. 11.6).
- After suture tying, tendinous cord dissected previously from subscapularis muscle is parallel to the lower glenohumeral ligament, thus strengthening the anterior capsulo-ligamentous complex.
- The use of mattress sutures helps to position the suture material away from the articular surface, and the knots used to control the LSP are truly extracapsular, lying between the capsule and subscapularis (Fig. 11.7).

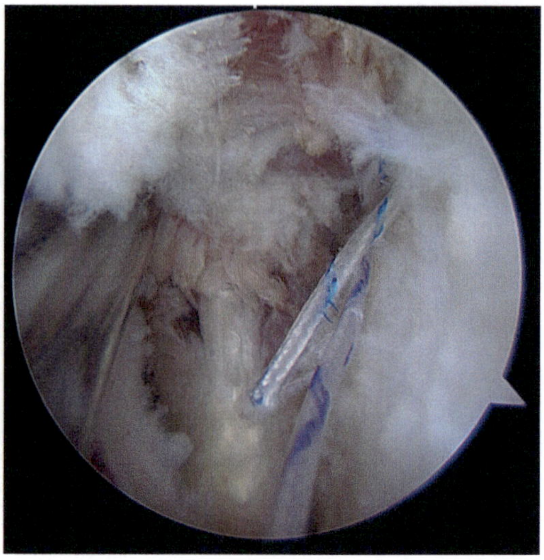

Fig. 11.6 BLS technique before knot tying

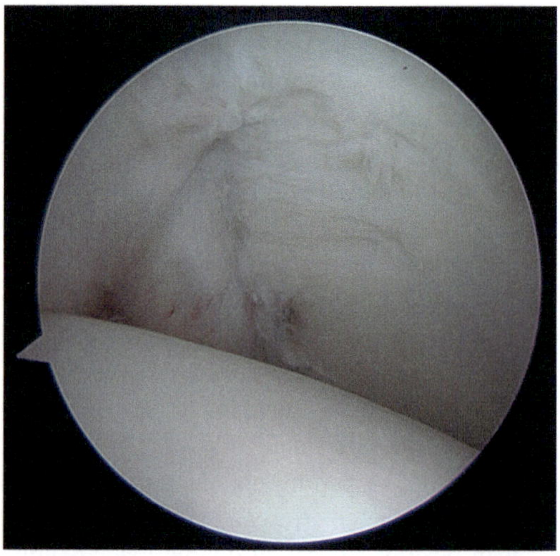

Fig. 11.7 Final intraarticular view after BLS technique

Pearls and Pitfalls

Portals	Location	Pearl	Pitfalls
Antero-lateral (for visualization)	Above bicipital groove	Allows frontal visualization of the glenoid	Be aware not to damage transverse humeral ligament
Antero-inferior portal (5 o'clock portal)	Location lateral to coracoid process tip, about 3 cm below the coracoid process tip	Using antero-lateral portal to visualization dissection continued after conjoint tendon visualization Grabbing tendinous cord of subscapularis muscle and antero-inferior capsule	Avoiding sharp dissection and deep incision due to the axillary or musculocutaneous nerve injury
Superior	About 1cm in front of the AC joint, laterally to the coracoid process. Necessity of partial dissection of CA lig	Possibility to separate soft tissue from the glenoid and visualize glenoid neck	To avoid bleeding from the branches of thoracoacromial artery use radiofrequency device (RD)

11.3 Outcomes

- The authors studied a cohort of 150 patients who underwent arthroscopic BLS surgery during the study period 2008–2016. Fifty patients were lost to follow-up, leaving 100 patients for final analysis in the present study.
- The study cohort consisted of 74 men and 26 women with a mean age of 27.5 years [SD 10.3] at the time of surgery. The dominant shoulder was affected in 62 cases. The mean follow-up was 82.9 months [SD 29.4].
- The Constant Score increased statistically significant from mean 82.89 [SD 9.1], preoperatively, to mean 88.2 [SD 10.3] ($p < 0.001$) at final follow-up.
- The corresponding numbers for the Walch-Duplay Score were a mean 5of 2.0 [SD 11.1] preoperatively and mean 81.1 [SD 19.0] ($p < 0.001$) at final follow-up.
- At final follow-up, there was no statistically significant difference in shoulder ER [n.s] or IR [n.s] compared with the preoperative range of motion.
- Analysis of outcomes between the different GBL-groups (Table 11.1) did not show any statistically significant differences in the Constant score [n.s], Walch-Duplay score [n.s], shoulder ER [n.s] or shoulder IR [n.s].

Table 11.1 Variables of GBL groups

Baseline variables of the patients GBL	
Variable	Number of patients
Glenoid bone loss group	
Group 1 (0–5%)	34
Group 2 (6–10%)	32
Group 3 (11–15%)	24
Group 4 (>15%)	10

- Patients whose affected shoulder was the non-dominant arm improved more in the Walch-Duplay score compared with patients whose dominant arm was affected, mean 34.8 points [SD 14.9] and 25.4 points [SD 19.2] ($p = 0.01$), respectively.
- At final assessment, 86 patients (86%) were categorized as having a positive outcome, with full restoration of joint stability. These patients did not experience any dislocation or subluxation episodes during the follow-up period and had a negative apprehension test at final clinical examination or did not report apprehension in questionnaire.
- Failure of the treatment was observed in 14 patients (14%). In six cases, the reason for recurrence of anterior dislocation was a major trauma during sport activity. Patients with recurrent dislocation were younger compared to patients without recurrent dislocation: mean age 23.9 years [SD 6.7] compared with

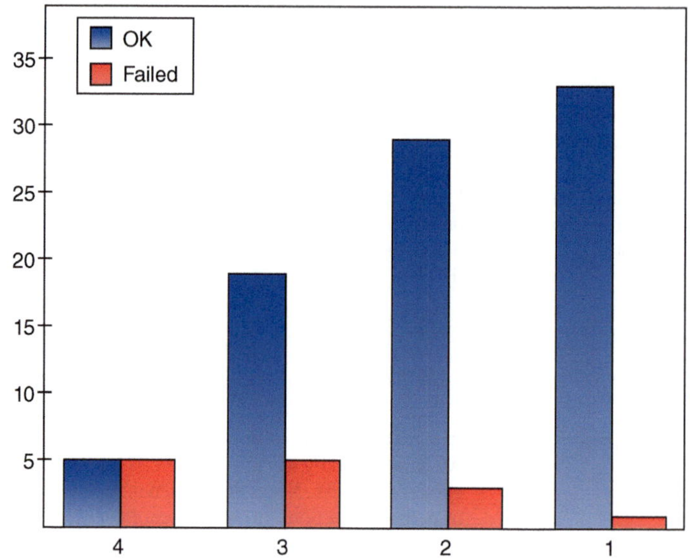

Fig. 11.8 Failure distribution according to size of GBL

a mean age 28.1 years [SD 10.7]; however, this age differences was not statistically significant (n.s).

- The frequency of failure was higher in patients with a more severe GBL [$p = 0.001$]. In GBL group 1, only one case of recurrence was observed, and the reason for re-dislocation was major trauma. In GBL group 2, there were three cases of failure, including two after trauma. In GBL group 3, five cases of failure were observed, including one posttraumatic case. In GBL group 4, there were five instability recurrences, including two cases of post-traumatic patients.
- Failure distribution according to the size of GBL is presented in Fig. 11.8. Patients who failed also had a greater baseline range of ER compared with patients with a positive outcome [mean 87.1° vs 76.8°, $p = 0.02$].
- No severe complications, like postoperative infection or persistent pain were observed.

11.4 Recommendations from the Expert

- The most important finding of the study on the BLS technique was that this technique was shown to provide a good clinical outcome with high shoulder stability and functional improvement, without decreasing shoulder range of motion.
- After a mean follow-up of 82.9 months, 86% of the patients who underwent surgery with the BLS technique regained satisfactory shoulder stability.
- Among the 14 failures observed in the present study, six were the consequence of high-energy trauma during sport activity. Thus, the BLS technique presented high effectiveness as an arthroscopic anterior instability treatment technique.
- Another important finding was that no patient developed postoperative mobility limitation or infection, which indicates a high safety of this technique.
- Complications after traditional arthroscopic Bankart repair have been reported to occur in 21–68% of cases and typically involve significant labral damage and cartilage destruction, partially due to suture knot placement too close to the articular surface [2, 5, 8, 10–12]. The BLS method described in the present study relies on placing the sutures and the knots that are harmful to cartilage outside the joint and, instead, placing them in the space between the medial glenohumeral ligament (MGHL) and subscapularis muscle. Thus,

similarly to the open Bankart technique, all suture materials are placed outside the joint, and the risk of cartilage and labrum abrasion is reduced.

- The improvement in constant score showed that satisfactory patient-reported outcome could be expected 2–9 years postoperatively.
- Future study comparing preoperative and postoperative radiographs in long-time follow-up is necessary to prove that extracapsular suture placing reduce the risk of osteoarthritis after Bankart repair.
- Several modified Bankart techniques have been described previously. For instance, Maiotti et al. [13] reported satisfactory results after an arthroscopic Bankart repair augmented by subscapularis muscle tenodesis, even in cases of chronic anterior shoulder instability, with GBL less than 25% and capsular joint deficiency [13]. However, Maiotti et al. also reported a significant reduction of shoulder joint ER, which is an inevitable complication of whole subscapularis muscle tenodesis. Recently, a new technique of dynamic anterior stabilization (DAS) with the long head of the biceps tendon was proposed [14] to close the gap between clean indications for Bankart and Latarjet techniques.
- The BLS technique is advantageous since it results in a significant increase in anterior joint stabilization while not limiting ER.
- Assessment of GBL and its effect on outcome is important. According to Owens' recommendations [6] concerning GBL measurement, the authors of this study divided the GBL into 4 groups based on a MRI examination to avoid the harmful CT radiation in preoperative diagnosis, especially after considering the young age of patients (Table 11.1).
- Patients with GBL >15% or with an intraoperatively observed "flat-line" shaped front wall of the glenoid were considered to have the largest defect. The term "flat-line" refers to the bony loss of the anteromedial glenoid, resulting in the lack of the anterior curvature, thereby creating a straight vertical cut-off line. It is possible that this type of glenoid damage predisposes to recurrent dislocations to a similar extent as the "inverted pear" described by Burkhart [15] and can be a severe risk factor for treatment failure.
- There was a statistically significant correlation between the GBL level and a higher frequency of treatment failure. Consideration the size of the GBL in particular groups, patients with recurrent instability had a median GBL group of 3 (11–15%), while patients with a positive outcome had a median GBL group of 2 (6–10%).
- Burkhart et al. and other studies investigating the effect of the GBL size reported that a GBL size of 21–25% predisposes recurrence of anterior shoulder instability [15–17]. However, a later study by Shaha et al. suggested a GBL of 13.5% to be sufficient to predispose recurrent instability [18]. This is in line with authors' data which shows a higher recurrence rate of shoulder instability among patients with a GBL of 11% or more [2].
- It should be underlined that there is still lack of gold standard for GBL calculating method and recent study showed that many differences in GBL calculating came from differences in its assessment [19].

Take Home Messages

- The BLS technique has been shown to be an effective method for anterior shoulder instability in patients without significant glenoid bone loss.
- Technique provides significant improvement in shoulder function without reducing shoulder range of motion.

References

1. Bankart AS. Recurrent or habitual dislocation of the shoulder. BMJ. 1923;2:1132–3.
2. Brzoska R, Blasiak A, Hldaki W, Streit JJ, Toussaint B, Solecki W. Arthroscopic Bankart repair using extracapsular suture between the Glenohumeral

ligaments and subscapularis tendon (BLS technique): a technical note. Tech Should Surg. 2012;13:86–9.
3. Brzóska R, Laprus H, Michniowski P et al. Knee Surg Sports Traumatol Arthrosc. 2019. https://doi.org/10.1007/s00167-019-05496-1.
4. Fabbriciani C, Milano G, Demontis A, Fadda S, Ziranu F, Mulas PD. Arthroscopic versus open treatment of Bankart lesion of the shoulder: a prospective randomized study. Arthroscopy. 2004;20:456–62.
5. Flinkkilä T, Knape R, Sirniö K, Ohtonen P, Leppilahti J. Long-term results of arthroscopic Bankart repair: minimum 10 years of follow-up. Knee Surg Sports Traumatol Arthrosc. 2018;26:94–9.
6. Owens BD, Burns TC, Campbell SE, et al. Simple method of glenoid bone loss calculation using ipsilateral magnetic resonance imaging. Am J Sports Med. 2013;41:622–4.
7. Privitera DM, Bisson LJ, Marzo JM. Minimum 10-year follow-up of arthroscopic intra-articular Bankart repair using bioabsorbable tacks. Am J Sports Med. 2012;40:100–7.
8. Purchase RJ, Wolf EM, Hobgood ER, Pollock ME, Smalley CC. Hill-sachs "remplissage": an arthroscopic solution for the engaging Hill-sachs lesion. Arthroscopy. 2008;24:723–6.
9. Yamamoto N, Itoi E, Abe H, Minagawa H, Seki N, Shimada Y, Okada K. Contact between the glenoid and the humeral head in abduction, external rotation, and horizontal extension: a new concept of glenoid track. J Shoulder Elb Surg. 2007;16:649–56.
10. Franceschi F, Papalia R, Del Buono A, Vasta S, Maffulli N, Denaro V. Glenohumeral osteoarthritis after arthroscopic Bankart repair for anterior instability. Am J Sports Med. 2011;39:1653–9.
11. Kavaja L, Pajarinen J, Sinisaari I, Savolainen V, Björkenheim J-M, Haapamäki V, et al. Arthrosis of glenohumeral joint after arthroscopic Bankart repair: a long-term follow-up of 13 years. J Shoulder Elb Surg. 2012;21:350–5.
12. Kowalsky MS, et al. Evaluation of suture abrasion against rotator cuff tendon and proximal Humerus bone. Arthroscopy. 2008;24(3):329–34.
13. Maiotti M, Massoni C, Russo R, Schroter S, Zanini A, Bianchedi D. Arthroscopic subscapularis augmentation of Bankart repair in chronic anterior shoulder instability with bone loss less than 25% and capsular deficiency: clinical multicenter study. Arthroscopy. 2017;33:902–9.
14. Mehl J, Otto A, Imhoff FB, Murphy M, Dyrna F, Obopilwe E, Cote M, Lädermann A, Collin P, Beitzel K, Mazzocca AD. Dynamic anterior shoulder stabilization with the long head of the biceps tendon: a biomechanical study. Am J Sports Med. 2019;47(6):1441–50. https://doi.org/10.1177/0363546519833990. Epub 2019 Apr 9. PMID: 30964697.
15. Burkhart SS, De Beer JF. Traumatic glenohumeral bone defects and their relationship to failure of arthroscopic Bankart repairs: significance of the inverted-pear glenoid and the humeral engaging Hill-Sachs lesion. Arthroscopy. 2000;16:677–94.
16. Griffith JF, Antonio GE, Tong CW, Ming CK. Anterior shoulder dislocation: quantification of glenoid bone loss with CT. Am J Roentgenol. 2003;180:1423–30.
17. Griffith JF, Antonio GE, Yung PS, et al. Prevalence, pattern, and spectrum of glenoid bone loss in anterior shoulder dislocation: CT analysis of 218 patients. Am J Roentgenol. 2008;190:1247–54.
18. Shaha JS, Cook JB, Song DJ, Rowles DJ, Bottoni CR, Shaha SH, Tokish JM. Redefining "critical" bone loss in shoulder instability: functional outcomes worsen with "subcritical" bone loss. Am J Sports Med. 2015;43:1719–25.
19. Verweij LPE, Schuit AA, Kerkhoffs GMMJ, Blankevoort L, van den Bekerom MPJ, van Deurzen DFP. Accuracy of currently available methods in quantifying anterior glenoid bone loss: controversy regarding gold standard-a systematic review. Arthroscopy. 2020;36(8):2295–2313.e1. https://doi.org/10.1016/j.arthro.2020.04.012. Epub 2020 Apr 21. PMID: 32330485.

12 Arthroscopic Subscapularis Augmentation (ASA) Technique

Emmanouil Brilakis
and Emmanouil Antonogiannakis

Key Points

- The long-term results of the classic arthroscopic Bankart repair are not satisfactory.
- In order to decrease recurrences, augmentation of the classic arthroscopic Bankart repair with additional soft tissue procedures has been proposed and seems to significantly improve the recurrence rate of anterior instability.
- Arthroscopic subscapularis augmentation (ASA) is one of these additive arthroscopic soft-tissue procedures for anterior shoulder instability.
- The concept is to use the subscapularis tendon to recentralize the humeral head by push it posteriorly during the external rotation of the arm.
- The main advantage of this procedure is that can be considered an easy, safe and effective procedure. Easy, because it is a feasible and reproducible technique with low learning curve since the surgical skills required are equal to those of performing a simple arthroscopic Bankart repair.
- The standard postoperative protocol followed in instability cases is also applied in the postoperative period.
- The surgical technique and its outcomes are described in this chapter as well as to technical considerations, pearls and pitfalls.

12.1 Introduction/Background

- The restoration of the normal anatomy is the goal of surgical management. Therefore, the restoration of the anterior torn labrum to its anatomic attachment and the re-establishment of the appropriate tension of the glenohumeral ligaments and capsule is the primary goal of every instability surgery.
- The long-term results of the classic arthroscopic Bankart repair are not satisfactory. A recurrence rate of 30% after ten years of follow-up has been reported, with 52% occurring within the first two years postoperatively [1].

Supplementary Information The online version contains supplementary material available at https://doi.org/10.1007/978-3-662-73064-5_12.

E. Brilakis (✉) · E. Antonogiannakis
3rd Orthopaedic Department, Hygeia General Hospital, Athens, Greece

L. Kovačič et al. (eds.), *Surgical Techniques for Anterior Shoulder Instability*,
https://doi.org/10.1007/978-3-662-73064-5_12

- In order to decrease the recurrence rate, augmentation of the classic arthroscopic Bankart repair with additional soft tissue procedures has been proposed. This addition seems to significantly improve the recurrence rate of anterior instability [2].
- Arthroscopic subscapularis augmentation (ASA) is one of these additive arthroscopic soft-tissue procedures for anterior shoulder instability. The Hill-Sachs Remplissage (Chap. 10), the BLS technique (Chap. 11) and the dynamic anterior stabilization (DAS) with the long head of biceps tendon (Chap. 13) are also options for augmenting the classic Bankart repair.
- The role of the subscapularis muscle and tendon in the pathogenesis and management of anterior dislocation of the shoulder has been highlighted since the early '70s [3]. Moreover, the most successful open operations used during the pre-arthroscopic era had in common the shortening of the subscapularis muscle. The arthroscopic augmentation of the classic Bankart repair with the subscapularis tendon was initially described in 2013 [4].

12.2 Indications

- This procedure is rarely performed as a standalone operation. It is mainly an additive procedure to the classic arthroscopic Bankart repair. Since this is primarily an augmenting procedure, surgeons should give particular attention to the indications of the primary procedure (soft tissue or bony procedure).
  - Its main indication is chronic anterior shoulder instability with bone loss of less than 25% and capsular deficiency [5]. The threshold of 25% of bone loss has been used traditionally for anterior instability since the initial publication in 2000 [6]. Over time, this threshold for performing soft-tissue or bony procedures is decreasing. We use the so-called subcritical bone loss [7], which is 13.5% and has a decreasing trend. In our department, the threshold for performing soft-tissue procedures is 10%. If the bone defect is larger, we use bony procedures. However, more clinical studies are needed to confirm this observation.
  - A second indication is the treatment of anterior shoulder instability in collision and contact sports athletes associated with GBL (<15%) and hyperlaxity [8].
  - A third indication of ASA is to augment an arthroscopic Eden-Hybinette or other bone grafting procedures (apart from Latarjet), especially in cases with insufficiency of the anterior soft tissue wall of the shoulder [9]. This combination could be an alternative equivalent to the arthroscopic or open Latarjet procedures [10]. However, this comparison needs to be studied and validated.
- Another possible and controversial indication is using this tenodesis in lax patients with anterior labrum and capsular deficiency without a Bankart lesion. In those cases, this technique can offer plication of the anterior inferior capsular tissue and decrease the volume of the anterior capsule. However, this indication also needs to be studied and validated.
- Contraindication for performing ASA is the chronic anterior shoulder instability due to structural failure of the subscapularis muscle and the anterior capsule because of the insufficiency of the subscapularis tendon. Several failed instability correction surgeries can cause this rare clinical situation.

12.3 Relevant Physical Findings

- First-time dislocators present after a single acute event and typically report a recent history of high-energy trauma or collision impact causing the dislocation.
- The patient's age, the degree of trauma (high- or low-energy impact mechanisms), and the sporting activity (type of sport and level of participation) are important information from the medical record.

- Particular attention should be given during the clinical examination to detect possible generalized hyperlaxity. The Beighton score is mainly used for classifying the patient's laxity.
- In chronic cases, patients typically present when limitations begin to significantly impact daily or sporting activities.
- Clinicians should get a detailed medical record with the data mentioned above. In addition, attention should be paid for low-energy, recurrent subluxation cases or instability episodes during sleep that may indicate significant bone loss. Previous failed instability surgeries should also be recorded.

12.4 Relevant Imaging

- Magnetic resonance (MR) imaging is highly sensitive for evaluating anterior shoulder instability because of its ability to detect soft tissue injuries.
- 3D CT scan is an important diagnostic tool for the osseous evaluation of Bankart and Hill-Sachs lesions. In particular, this modality is highly sensitive in assessing the size of the bone loss and the location of the bony defect.
- The data acquired from these two imaging modalities can properly indicate which patients are suitable for either arthroscopic soft tissue repair or bony reconstruction.

12.5 Goals of Surgical Procedure

- The main goal of every surgical procedure for shoulder instability is to produce a stable shoulder and prevent recurrence.
- A secondary goal is to avoid apprehension when the arm is in abduction and external rotation.
- ASA allows the recentralization of the humeral head, pushing it posteriorly and acting opposite to that of the Remplissage technique, creating a lift-up effect on the anterior part of the inferior capsule (Fig. 12.1). The procedure achieves closure of the axillary pouch and increases the contact between the glenoid (or the bone graft), the subscapularis muscle/tendon, and the residual capsule.
- The effect of this tenodesis could be comparable to that of the conjoint tendon in the Latarjet procedure.
- The subscapularis tenodesis to the glenoid apply stress to the anterior capsuloligamentous structures and the coracohumeral ligament. Through the tissue's connections, this stress is transmitted to the rotator interval. The tension of the rotator interval's tissue restrains the anterior translation when the glenohumeral joint is in internal or external rotation at lower levels of abduction [11].

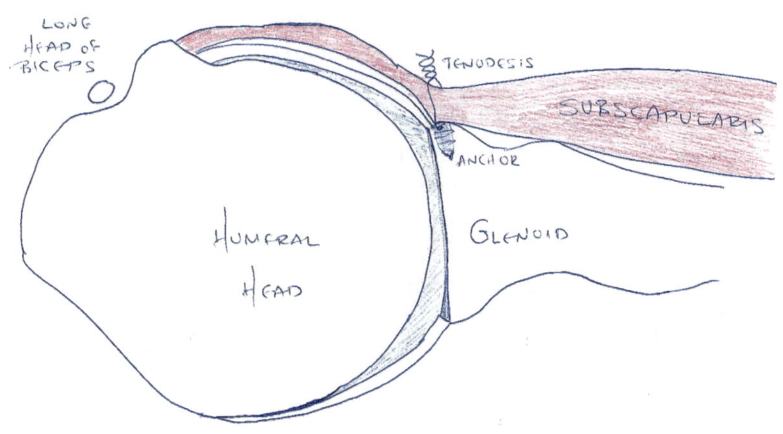

Fig. 12.1 Sketch of the ASA

12.6 Advantages and Disadvantages

- The main advantage of this procedure is that it can be considered an easy, safe, and effective procedure.
- It is easy because it is a feasible and reproducible technique with a low learning curve. The surgical skills required are equivalent to those needed for performing a simple arthroscopic Bankart repair.
- It is safe because the risk of nerve damage is equal to a simple Bankart repair and because of its low complication rate.
- It is effective because it reduces the recurrence rate of the primary procedure performed (classic arthroscopic Bankart repair or Arthroscopic Eden-Hybinette).
- One additional advantage is the ease of revision in case of recurrence.
- The main disadvantage of this procedure is that the long-term outcomes are still unknown since this is a relatively new technique. When instability cases are concerned, a minimum of 10 years of follow-up is required to properly evaluate a new technique.

12.7 Surgical Technique

12.7.1 Equipment

- Standard arthroscopic equipment with no special instrumentation is required for performing this technique. Strong orthopedic sutures are required for the tenodesis. These sutures are constructed of a multi-strand, long-chain ultra-high molecular weight polyethylene (UHMWPE) core with a braided jacket of polyester and UHMWPE that gives superior strength, soft feel, and abrasion resistance. Tapes can also be used for the tenodesis. Standard soft tissue or knotless anchors are also needed for fixing the subscapularis tendon to the anterior glenoid rim.

12.7.2 Positioning and Portals

- Anesthesia may be general or under interscalene block, with supplemental local anesthetic as necessary. Patient positioning and preparation are the same as with standard arthroscopy. The patient can be placed in a beach chair or lateral decubitus position depending on the surgeon's preference. The traditional posterior, anterior, and anterosuperior portals are used. Special care is given to place the anterior portal just over the superior border of the subscapularis tendon to obtain a straightforward approach for passing instruments through the subscapularis tendon.
- The authors' preference is positioning the patient in lateral decubitus with arm traction of 3 kg under general anesthesia with supplemental glenohumeral joint anesthetic injection.

12.7.3 Step-by-Step Description of the Procedure

- A diagnostic examination of the glenohumeral joint is initially carried out to confirm the presence of the Bankart lesion, measure any glenoid bone defect, evaluate the tissue quality of the anterior capsule, confirm and calculate the size of the Hill-Sachs lesion, and detect any other concomitant pathology.
- The dynamic evaluation completes the diagnostic part of the arthroscopy. With the traction removed, the arm is abducted and externally rotated to detect whether the Hill-Sachs lesion engages the anterior glenoid rim.
- Subsequently, viewing from the anterosuperior portal, the anterior labrum-capsule complex is mobilized, and a Bankart repair is performed in a standard fashion. The authors prefer to use a double-loaded soft anchor inserted in the glenoid rim at 5 or 7 o'clock (for the right or left shoulder, respectively). Additional anchors are implanted as required

(usually 2 or 3 double-loaded anchors in total). The sutures are passed through the anterior labrum and the capsule, and are tied. However, any type of anchor (metal, bio-composite, absorbable, or knotless) can be used as well, according to the surgeon's preference.

- In cases managed by bony procedures, the authors prefer to perform an arthroscopic Eden-Hybinette using an autologous bone graft from the iliac crest and fixate it with four buttons (two anteriorly and two posteriorly) [12].
- In very lax cases with large and medially engaging Hill-Sachs lesions, the authors combine ASA with Remplissage [13].
- After completing the techniques mentioned above according to the indications and the surgical plan, the subscapularis tenodesis is performed in the following fashion.
  - Viewing from the posterior portal, one all-suture anchor is inserted into the anterior glenoid rim between 2 and 3 o'clock.
  - The traction of the arm is released, and only the assistant holds the arm in 0° of abduction and maximum external rotation.
  - The subscapularis tendon is penetrated at least 5 mm inferior to its superior border at the glenoid level, and one suture limp is grasped and looped. The loop is exported from the anterior portal.
  - The suture limp of the loop and the unpassed suture limp are brought to the same portal also, posteriorly to the subscapularis belly. With a loop and two limps from the anterior portal, the surgeon performs a Nice knot [14], which combines a doubled suture with a sliding knot and provides a robust fixation.
  - Alternatively, a suture limp is passed from the subscapularis belly at the same level, and it is tied with the unpassed limp of a soft anchor implanted into the anterior glenoid rim, as mentioned earlier.
  - Another possible way is to use a tape passed through the subscapularis tendon as a loop at the same level. The free limps of the tape are passed through the loop and secured to the anterior glenoid rim with a knotless anchor.
  - Finally, the centralization and the stability of the humeral head with the glenoid is checked under arthroscopy from the anterosuperior portal (Fig. 12.2), bringing the arm in full abduction and external rotation. The assistant brings the arm at 90° of abduction and maximum external rotation, checking that it can reach this position without any disengagement of the anchor or loosening of the knot.
  - A standard closure of the arthroscopy portals is performed with a 3-0, Nylon suture.

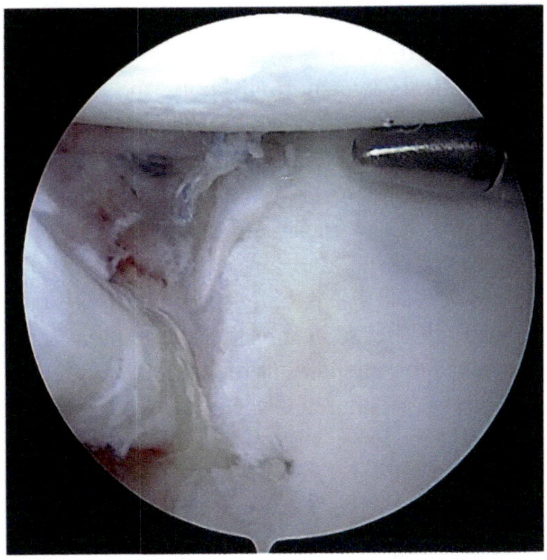

Fig. 12.2 The final outcome of the subscapularis tenodesis as this is revealed from the anterosuperior portal

12.8 Technical Recommendations

- Viewing from the posterior portal and working from the anterior portal is recommended.
- The position of the anterior portal just over the superior border of the subscapularis tendon is recommended to obtain a straightforward approach for the passing instruments through the subscapularis tendon.
- When the tenodesis is performed, the traction of the arm is released, and only the assistant

holds the arm in 0° abduction and maximum external rotation.

- In patients with normal laxity, the anchor is inserted at 3 o'clock, while in hyper-lax patients, the anchor is inserted at 2 o'clock.
- The subscapularis tendon is penetrated at least 5 mm inferior to its superior border to have enough tissue and prevent cutting by the suture itself. The passing should be done at the glenoid level to ensure that the tendon is not pushed too medially or too laterally.
- The use of sutures is recommended. The use of tapes is also a valid selection.
- The use of the Nice knot is recommended for maximizing the stabilizing force of the tenodesis.
- Always check the shoulder ROM after the tenodesis under arthroscopic observation to ensure that the subscapularis tendon is not overtightened. The anchor that has been inserted has not disengaged when the arm is brought in the end-range of its motion.

Pearls

- The position of the anterior portal should be just over the superior border of the subscapularis tendon in order to obtain an easy approach for the passing instruments through the subscapularis tendon.
- The traction of the arm should be released during the tenodesis and only the assistant holds the arm in 0° abduction and maximum external rotation (this is referred to lateral decubitus positioning).
- In patients with normal laxity the anchor is inserted at 3 o'clock, while in hyperlax patients, the anchor is inserted at 2 o'clock.
- The subscapularis tendon should be penetrated at least 5 mm inferior to its superior border in order to have enough tissue and decrease the possible cutting by the suture itself.
- Always, check under arthroscopy the shoulder ROM with the arm in 90° of abduction and maximum external rotation in the end of the procedure.

Pitfalls

- Positioning of the tenodesis too superior to the glenoid may decrease the external rotation.
- The penetration of the suture through the tendon too laterally may decrease the external rotation.
- Disengagement of the anchor in the anterior glenoid rim.

12.9 Postoperative Protocol

- The operated arm is kept in a sling for the first six weeks, but the patient is allowed to remove the sling for passive exercises or to perform daily activities.
- The ROM is restricted to the front of the body (90° of forward flexion, internal rotation towards the belly, and no more than 10° of external rotation).
- Active-assisted exercises are started during the third postoperative week, increasing the ROM gradually and progressing to active exercises based on the patient's progress.
- After the restoration of the ROM (at least 160° of FF, 70° of ER, and IR to the L1), strengthening exercises are started.
- Overhead activities and contact sports are allowed after 6–9 months following surgery, depending on patient rehabilitation progress and the level of participation.
- In athletes, sport-specific activities are permitted after the 3rd month and return to sport is allowed when the ROM, the strength and the agility of the arm is >90% of the contralateral side.

12.10 Outcomes

- The outcome of the ASA—arthroscopic subscapularis augmentation of Bankart repair—in chronic anterior shoulder instability with bone loss less than 25% and capsular deficiency, as they have published in a clinical multicenter study, is excellent:

- The recurrence rate is equal to 2.7% with a mean follow-up of 3 years (40.5 months). The functional results are excellent and statistically significant. The Rowe score increased from 57.4 preoperatively to 95.3 postoperatively, and the ASES score increased from 66.5 to 96.5.
- The mean deficit of external rotation is 8° with the arm at the side of the trunk and 4° with the arm in 90° of abduction.
- No limitation in everyday activities has been reported. At the same time, a mild restriction of the pre-injury level of sporting activity occurs in 16.3% and a moderate limitation in 7.2% of the patients treated with this technique, probably due to the restriction of external rotation [5].
- In athletes with evidence of shoulder hyperlaxity, the recurrence rate is 3.9%. External rotation deficit is 15° with the arm in adduction and 10° in abduction after a mean follow-up of 2.5 years (30.5 months) [8].
- Finally, a recurrence rate of 11% is expected in patients with recurrent anterior instability associated with critical bone loss and hyperlaxity. No persistent anterior apprehension or other complications have been noticed in this group of patients [9].
- In summarizing, according to the authors' experience, the outcome is excellent when the glenoid bone defect is less than 10%, and the postoperative deficit of external rotation is a rare clinical problem if the patient follows a proper rehabilitation program. The integration of the subscapularis and the healing on the anterior rim of the glenoid is very solid as this can be revealed in a second look arthroscopy (Fig. 12.3).

12.11 Potential Complications

- No early or late postoperative complications have been referred to in published studies.
- A deficit of external rotation has been noticed. However, this is not a clinically or statistically significant deficit in the vast majority of the patients.
- The risk of nerve damage is minimal and comparable to the respective of a simple Bankart repair.

Take Home Message

- The ASA is an additional procedure used to augment the classic Bankart repair, and it cannot be used as a standalone operation.
- This is an option for decreasing the recurrence rate of the classic Bankart repair.
- ASA allows the recentralization of the humeral head, using the subscapularis tendon to push it posteriorly during external rotation of the arm.
- It is a safe alternative to other additive procedures like Remplissage, DAS, BLS, etc.
- The midterm recurrence rate is 2.7%.
- There is probably an external rotation deficit, which is not clinically significant as far as the patient's everyday and sporting activities are concerned.
- Long-term results are needed in order to confirm the encouraging mid-term results.

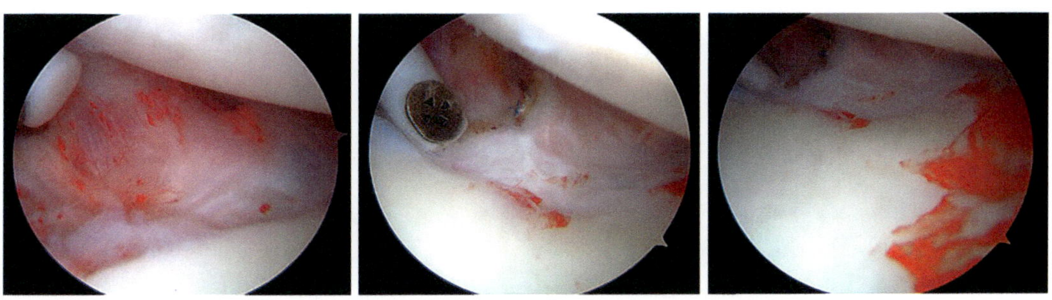

Fig. 12.3 Second look arthroscopy showing the healing of the subscapularis on the anterior rim of the glenoid

References

1. Flinkkilä T, Knape R, Sirniö K, Ohtonen P, Leppilahti J. Long-term results of arthroscopic Bankart repair: minimum 10 years of follow-up. Knee Surg Sports Traumatol Arthrosc. 2018;26(1):94–9. https://doi.org/10.1007/s00167-017-4504-z.
2. Trellopoulos A, Brilakis E, Antonogiannakis E. Alternative and additive arthroscopic soft-tissue procedures for anterior shoulder instability. Subscapularis tenodesis, remplissage, and more. Obere Extremität. 2021;16:8–15. https://doi.org/10.1007/s11678-021-00634-z.
3. Symeonides PP. The significance of the subscapularis muscle in the pathogenesis of recurrent anterior dislocation of the shoulder. J Bone Joint Surg Br. 1972;54(3):476–83.
4. Maiotti M, Massoni C. Arthroscopic augmentation with subscapularis tendon in anterior shoulder instability with capsulolabral deficiency. Arthrosc Tech. 2013;2(3):e303–10. https://doi.org/10.1016/j.eats.2013.04.005.
5. Maiotti M, Massoni C, Russo R, Schroter S, Zanini A, Bianchedi D. Arthroscopic subscapularis augmentation of Bankart repair in chronic anterior shoulder instability with bone loss less than 25% and capsular deficiency: clinical multicenter study. Arthroscopy. 2017;33(5):902–9. https://doi.org/10.1016/j.arthro.2016.09.008.
6. Burkhart SS, De Beer JF. Traumatic glenohumeral bone defects and their relationship to failure of arthroscopic Bankart repairs: significance of the inverted-pear glenoid and the humeral engaging Hill-Sachs lesion. Arthroscopy. 2000;16(7):677–94. https://doi.org/10.1053/jars.2000.17715.
7. Shaha JS, Cook JB, Song DJ, et al. Redefining "critical" bone loss in shoulder instability: functional outcomes worsen with "subcritical" bone loss. Am J Sports Med. 2015;43(7):1719–25. https://doi.org/10.1177/0363546515578250.
8. Maiotti M, Russo R, Zanini A, Castricini R, Castellarin G, Schröter S, Massoni C, Savoie FH. Bankart repair with subscapularis augmentation in athletes with shoulder Hyperlaxity [published online ahead of print, 2021 Feb 10]. Arthroscopy. 2021;S0749-8063(21):00126–2. https://doi.org/10.1016/j.arthro.2021.01.062.
9. Russo R, Maiotti M, Cozzolino A, Della Rotonda G, Guastafierro A, Massoni C, Viglione S. Arthroscopic iliac crest bone allograft combined with subscapularis upper-third Tenodesis shows a low recurrence rate in the treatment of recurrent anterior shoulder instability associated with critical bone loss. Arthroscopy. 2021;37(3):824–33. https://doi.org/10.1016/j.arthro.2020.11.037.
10. Russo R, Maiotti M, Taverna E, Rao C. Arthroscopic bone graft procedure combined with arthroscopic subscapularis augmentation for recurrent anterior instability with glenoid bone defect. Arthrosc Tech. 2018;7(6):e623–32. https://doi.org/10.1016/j.eats.2018.02.009.
11. Lee TQ, Black AD, Tibone JE, McMahon PJ. Release of the coracoacromial ligament can lead to glenohumeral laxity: a biomechanical study. J Shoulder Elb Surg. 2001;10(1):68–72. https://doi.org/10.1067/mse.2001.111138.
12. Avramidis G, Kokkineli S, Trellopoulos A, Tsiogka A, Natsika M, Brilakis E, Antonogiannakis E. Excellent clinical and radiological midterm outcomes for the Management of Recurrent Anterior Shoulder Instability by all-arthroscopic modified Eden-Hybinette procedure using iliac crest autograft and double-pair button fixation system: 3-year clinical case series with no loss to follow-up. Arthroscopy. 2021;37(3):795–803. https://doi.org/10.1016/j.arthro.2020.10.036.
13. Brilakis E, Avramidis G, Malahias MA, Stathellis A, Deligeorgis A, Chiotis I, Mataragas E, Chronopoulos E, Antonogiannakis E. Long-term outcome of arthroscopic remplissage in addition to the classic Bankart repair for the management of recurrent anterior shoulder instability with engaging Hill-Sachs lesions. Knee Surg Sports Traumatol Arthrosc. 2019;27(1):305–13. https://doi.org/10.1007/s00167-018-5261-3.
14. Boileau P, Alami G, Rumian A, Schwartz DG, Trojani C, Seidl AJ. The doubled-suture Nice knot. Orthopedics. 2017;40(2):e382–6. https://doi.org/10.3928/01477447-20161202-05.

13 Dynamic Anterior Stabilization (DAS): Stabilization with the Long Head of the Biceps Tendon

Clara de Campos Azevedo
and Ana Catarina Ângelo

Key Points

- In arthroscopic DAS, the LHB is transferred and fixed to the anterior glenoid.
- The LHB passing through the subscapularis tendon split stabilizes the glenohumeral joint by producing a hammock and sling effect that prevents anterior dislocation of the humeral head in patients with anterior glenohumeral instability.
- Clinical studies report good results ranging from 1- to 3-year minimum follow-up in recreational athletes with anterior glenohumeral instability with ≤20% anterior glenoid bone loss.

13.1 Introduction

- Dynamic anterior stabilization (DAS) using the long head of the biceps (LHB) tendon is a new arthroscopic technique that fills a treatment algorithm gap between soft-tissue and bony procedures for chronic anteroinferior glenohumeral instability with limited to subcritical glenoid bone loss (GBL).
- Biomechanical cadaveric studies have shown that in instability models with 10% and 20% GBL, the relative anterior glenohumeral translation is significantly lower after DAS than after isolated Bankart repair [1]; and in instability models with 13% GBL, DAS is significantly stronger than both the isolated Bankart repair by 16.3% and the conjoint tendon transfer procedure by 16.6% [2].
- Several technical notes, [3–11], one case report [12], and four cases series [13–16] have described different arthroscopic methods of transposing and fixing the LHB tendon to the anteroinferior glenoid rim.
- Substantial improvements in the Western Ontario Shoulder Instability Index [17] and Rowe score [18] from the preoperative to the 12-month postoperative follow-up, with successful healing of the transposed LHB, have been shown; patients returned to their recreational level of sporting activity, with no apprehension or instability, and were very satisfied with the procedure [12, 13]. Case series with a minimum follow-up of 3 years showed no recurrence of glenohumeral dislocation after DAS [16].
- The originally proposed indication for DAS is chronic anteroinferior glenohumeral instability with limited bone defects, associated with a supe-

Supplementary Information The online version contains supplementary material available at https://doi.org/10.1007/978-3-662-73064-5_13.

C. de Campos Azevedo (✉) · A. C. Ângelo
Hospital dos SAMS, Lisbon, Portugal

Joaquim Chaves Saúde, Lisbon, Portugal

L. Kovačič et al. (eds.), *Surgical Techniques for Anterior Shoulder Instability*,
https://doi.org/10.1007/978-3-662-73064-5_13

rior labral tear from anterior to posterior (SLAP) [3, 4], or in overhead athletes and throwers [3].

- However, indications for arthroscopic DAS are expanding, as more clinical and biomechanical studies are published.
- In the case report by Defroda et al. [19], an open DAS technique was described for a case of recurrent dislocation and musculocutaneous palsy, in which a revision of the previously performed Bankart repair to either the Latarjet or Bristow procedures was relatively contraindicated because of the increased risk of neurologic injury (musculocutaneous nerve) [20, 21].
- In this chapter, the all-arthroscopic technical variation of DAS that uses all-suture anchors and a double double-pulley intra-articular shuttling method to transpose the LHB tendon to the anteroinferior glenoid rim through the subscapularis tendon is presented [6, 12].

13.2 Surgical Rationale

- The main purpose of the transposition of the LHB tendon (Fig. 13.1) through the subscapularis tendon is to dynamically increase the stability of the glenohumeral joint through both a "hammock" (Fig. 13.2) and a "sling" (Fig. 13.3) effect throughout the range of motion [22].

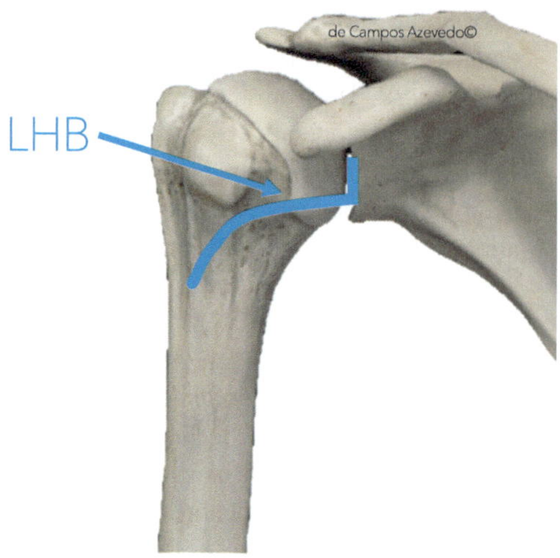

Fig. 13.1 Anterior view of a right shoulder after dynamic anterior stabilization with the long head of the biceps transposed to the anteroinferior glenoid rim. LHB long head of the biceps

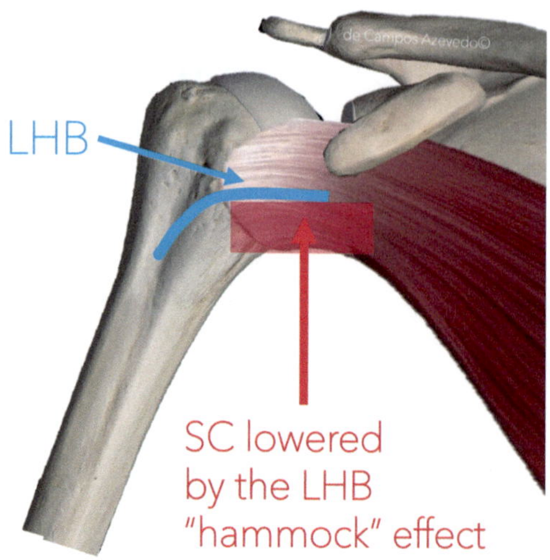

Fig. 13.2 Anterior view of a right shoulder after dynamic anterior stabilization. The "hammock effect" occurs in the lower ranges of abduction motion and consists of the lowering of the inferior part of the subscapularis muscle done by the LHB tendon, which represents a muscular effect by the subscapularis. LHB long head of the biceps, SC subscapularis tendon

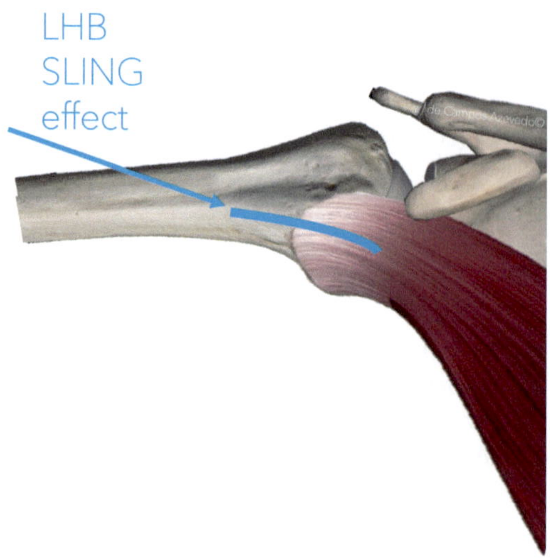

Fig. 13.3 Anterior view of a right shoulder after dynamic anterior stabilization. The "sling effect" occurs at higher ranges of abduction, when the LHB tendon is more horizontal and does not lower the inferior part of the subscapularis muscle anymore. Instead, the LHB forms a sling in front of the shoulder, providing anterior stability to the shoulder

13.3 Indications and Contraindications

- Recreational overhead athletes and throwers who have sustained 2 or more episodes of anteroinferior glenohumeral dislocations, presenting with shoulder pain and apprehension refractory to conservative treatment, are the ideal candidates for DAS.
- DAS may be indicated for chronic anteroinferior glenohumeral instability with limited (<13.5%) to subcritical (<25%) anteroinferior GBL and an engaging Hill-Sachs lesion, and/or a superior labrum anterior-posterior (SLAP) type I–III lesion.
- Additionally, DAS may be indicated for recurrent dislocation after failed Bankart repair and/or musculocutaneous palsy.
- DAS may be contraindicated for anteroinferior glenohumeral instability with 25% or more of GBL, or a tear of the LHB tendon.

13.4 Surgical Technique

- Arthroscopic DAS was first described in the studies by Collin and Lädermann, [3] and by Milenin and Toussaint [4], who performed the procedure with the patient in the semi- or beach-chair position, using 3 arthroscopic portals, and fixed the LHB to the anterior glenoid using either an inlay technique that utilizes one tenodesis screw, or an onlay technique that utilizes three push-in suture anchors, respectively.
- In this chapter, the preferred arthroscopic DAS technique described and used by de Campos Azevedo and Ângelo is detailed [6, 12].

13.5 Patient Positioning

- Patients undergo surgery under general anesthesia and in the beach-chair position.
- The shoulder is surgically draped for shoulder arthroscopic surgery.
- Shoulder passive ROM and the direction(s) of the instability are confirmed under general anesthesia.
- The forearm is placed in 3 kg forward traction at 70° of forward flexion and 10° of abduction and in neutral shoulder rotation.
- Alternatively, a mechanical arm positioner may be used to achieve equivalent shoulder position and traction during the procedure.

13.6 Portals

- DAS is performed through a 3-portal arthroscopic technique:
- a posterior (first) viewing portal is established 2 cm medial and 2 cm inferior to the posterolateral corner of the acromion (soft spot), aiming the 4-mm and 30-degrees arthroscope at the coracoid process;
- an anterior (second) portal is established from outside-in under direct vision using an 18-gauge needle directed to the union of the upper two-thirds with the lower third of the subscapularis tendon, lateral to the conjoint tendon, and a working cannula (a 5–6 × 85-mm cannula) with an outflow connection (attached to a closed-system arthroscopic pump) is placed through it;
- an anterolateral (third) portal is established from outside-in, distal to the anterolateral aspect of the acromion, using the needle directed laterally to the transverse humeral

ligament (THL), parallel and slightly distal to the superior border of the subscapularis.
- A 3.5 × 135-mm radiofrequency ablator probe is introduced through the anterolateral portal and is used to cut the THL laterally to the LHB tendon, thereby completely releasing the LHB tendon from the bicipital groove.

13.7 Subscapularis Tendon Split

- The subscapularis tendon split is performed using the switching stick and the radiofrequency ablator. The radiofrequency ablator may be used either through the anterior portal after placing the switching stick through the posterior portal to mark the level of the split at the middle third and using the anterolateral portal as a viewing portal with the arthroscope through it, or through the anterolateral portal after placing the switching stick through the anterior portal.
- After debridement using a 4 × 125-mm automated shaver, two 1.8-mm all- suture double-loaded anchors are implanted on the anteroinferior glenoid rim, through the subscapularis split, one at the 4 o'clock and the other at the 5 o'clock position (right shoulder), approximately 5 mm apart.
- All limbs of the sutures from the glenoid anchors are passed through the LHB tendon with the suture passer according to the following sequence: first, 2 different limbs of the sutures from the superior glenoid anchor are passed distal to the bicipital anchor on the labrum, and a surgeon's knot and 2 half-stitches are tied to be used as the first double-pulley knot; second, approximately 5 mm distal to this knot, 2 different limbs of the sutures from the inferior glenoid anchor are passed, and the second double-pulley knot is tied (Fig. 13.4).
- Using the ablator, the LHB is tenotomized distally to the bicipital anchor on the superior

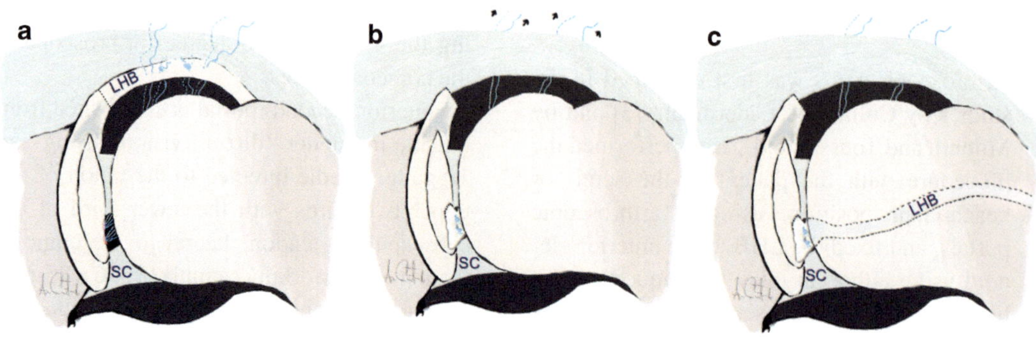

Fig. 13.4 Representation of the posterior portal arthroscopic view of the trans-subscapular transposition of the long head of the biceps using the double double-pulley on a right shoulder in the beach-chair position. (**a**) Two knots of the double pulley are tied after all suture limbs were passed through the long head of the biceps (LHB) tendon; (**b**) the remaining 4 opposing suture limbs are pulled and the LHB tendon reaches the anteroinferior glenoid rim after passing through the subscapularis tendon (SC) split; (**c**) the dashed line represents the final course of the LHB tendon through and anteriorly to the subscapularis tendon. The opposing 4 suture limbs will each be used to obtain an additional 2 knots to reinforce the fixation of the LHB to the glenoid rim. *(Free License (Number 5045451250785) was obtained from Wolters Kluwer Health, Inc. and JBJS Case Connector, for print and electronic publishing of figure 4 from the licensed content entitled "All-Suture Anchor Dynamic Anterior Stabilization Produced Successful Healing of the Biceps Tendon: A Report of 3 Cases", authored by Clara de Campos Azevedo and Ana Catarina Ângelo* [12]*)*

labrum and proximally to the first double-pulley knot (Fig. 13.5).

- The opposing limbs of the different sutures from the glenoid anchors are pulled while the 2 double-pulley knots are used to push the tenotomized LHB through the subscapularis tendon split.
- A suture retriever may be used to assist in guiding the LHB shuttling through the subscapularis tendon split.
- The suture limbs are tied once the LHB reaches the anteroinferior glenoid rim (Fig. 13.6).
- One 1.3-mm all-suture single-loaded anchor is implanted between the 4 and 5 o'clock positions, adjacent to the superior half of the transposed LHB tendon on the glenoid rim, and a simple knot is tied to plicate the remaining anteroinferior labrum or capsular tissue onto the glenoid rim.
- A stepwise approach to DAS and the pearls and pitfalls of the procedure are summarized in Table 13.1.

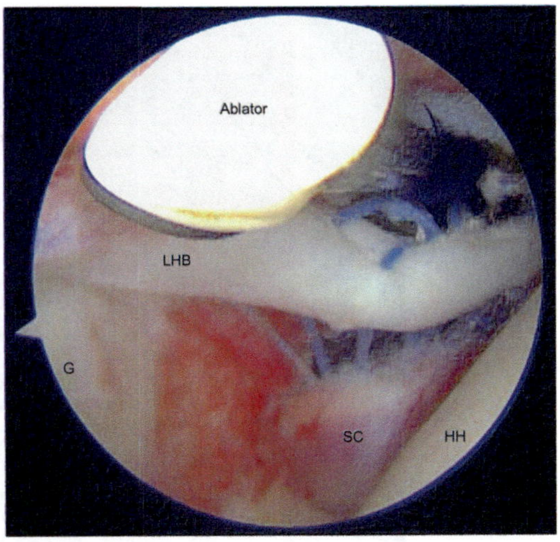

Fig. 13.5 Arthroscopic image of the right shoulder of patient 13 of the authors' case series. Posterior portal view. The ablator is placed over the long head of the biceps (LHB) to cut the LHB distally to the bicipital anchor on the superior labrum and proximally to the suture limbs of the double pulley. G Glenoid, HH humeral head, SC subscapularis tendon

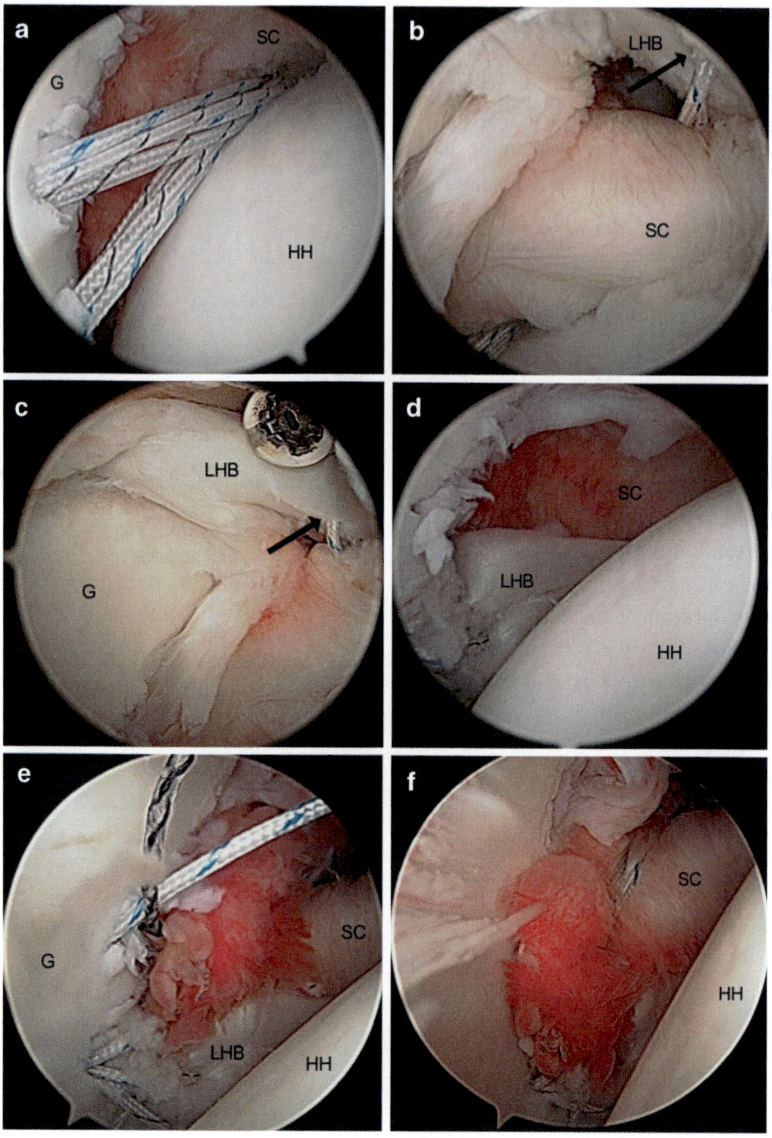

Fig. 13.6 Arthroscopic images of the right shoulder of patient 3 of the authors' case series. Posterior portal view. (**a**) Two double loaded all-suture anchors were implanted on the anteroinferior glenoid (G) rim; (**b**) all the suture limbs were passed through the subscapularis tendon (SC) and through the long head of the biceps (LHB, black arrow); (**c**) the ablator was used to perform the LHB tenotomy proximally to the most proximal suture fixation point on the LHB (black arrow); (**d**) the transposed LHB was fixed to the anteroinferior glenoid rim; (**e**) a suture passer is used to shuttle one suture limb of the all-suture anchor implanted superiorly to the transposed LHB tendon on the glenoid rim; (**f**) the superior anchor knot is tied with the capsular remnants partially covering the transposed LHB tendon. HH = humeral head. *(Free License (Number 5045451250785) was obtained from Wolters Kluwer Health, Inc. and JBJS Case Connector, for print and electronic publishing of figure 5 (renamed* Fig. 13.6 *in this chapter) from the licensed content entitled "All-Suture Anchor Dynamic Anterior Stabilization Produced Successful Healing of the Biceps Tendon: A Report of 3 Cases", authored by Clara de Campos Azevedo and Ana Catarina Ângelo* [12]*)*

Table 13.1 Stepwise approach to dynamic anterior stabilization after the first posterior viewing portal is placed through the soft spot[a]

Order	Surgical step	Rationale	Pearl	Pitfall
1	Anterior portal at the superior border of the lower third of the SC	Working portal, used to place the switching stick to help split the SC and to place the drilling guide for the glenoid anchors	Correct level of placement helps ensure that the transposed LHB tendon will be fixed at the ideal level, below the equator of the glenoid	Placing this portal too high risks either placing the anchors above the equator or kinking the suture limbs during shuttling the LHB tendon through the SC split
2	Cleaning the rotator interval	To ensure adequate visibility to perform the cutting of the THL, SC split, and LHB tendon shuttling steps	Enables an extra-articular view of the THL while the shoulder is in forward flexion and enables changing the arthroscope from the posterior to the anterolateral portal afterwards to have a perfect view both of the THL and of the SC split while the switching stick is placed through the posterior portal to help with the split	Inadequate cleaning may lead to poor visibility during the THL cutting and SC split steps and lead to difficult suture management during the shuttling step and to an increased risk of damage to the SC insertion and axillary nerve
3	Anterolateral portal distal to the level of the superior border of the SC	Working portal used during the THL cutting step, and viewing portal used during the SC split step	Ensures adequate distal access to the THL and visibility during the SC split and LHB tendon shuttling steps	Placing this portal too high risks either not adequately releasing the THL or poor visibility during the SC split
4	Cutting the THL lateral to the LHB tendon	To completely release the LHB tendon from the bicipital groove	After the LHB tendon subluxates medially, it becomes easier to pass the sutures from the anterior portal using the suture passer; complete release avoids kinking or catching of the LHB tendon at the bicipital groove after the transposition through the SC is performed	Cutting the THL medially risks damage to the SC insertion; incomplete LHB release may cause painful kinking
5	Passing the sutures through the LHB tendon using a low-profile suture passer and tying two double-pulley knots	To ensure the LHB tendon is fixed securely to the anteroinferior glenoid	The nitinol needle of the suture passer is not aggressive to the LHB tendon; suture management is easier if the LHB is intraarticularly shuttled while pulling the opposing suture limbs and pushing each double-pulley knot simultaneously	Avoid using bulky suture piercers to pass sutures through the LHB because the LHB may be damaged and tear longitudinally

[a]*LHB* long head of the biceps, *SC* subscapularis tendon, *THL* transverse humeral ligament

13.8 Postoperative Rehabilitation Protocol

- For the first 3 weeks, patients wear a sling and are instructed to remove it several times a day to perform passive forward flexion shoulder and elbow exercises. Shoulder exercises are limited to the range of 0°–90° of forward flexion, and external-internal rotation exercises with the arm at the side from internal rotation to the neutral position. Full range of flexion-extension passive exercises of the elbow are allowed. The purpose of the passive ROM exercises is to avoid postoperative adhesions of the transposed long head of the biceps to the subscapularis tendon while avoiding compromising the first stages of tendon-to-bone healing of the LHB tendon to the glenoid rim.
- From weeks 3 to 6, shoulder and elbow ROM exercises progress from passive to active-assisted, non-resistant exercises. Use of the sling is subsequently diminished, and patients undergo a shoulder rehabilitation protocol with progressive active non-resistant ROM exercises. Shoulder external and internal rotation exercises with the arm at the side progress gently from internal to external rotation exercises beyond the neutral position.
- Until 6 weeks postoperatively, active resistant elbow exercises are not allowed. The purpose is to continue to protect the tendon-to-bone healing of the LHB tendon to the anteroinferior glenoid rim during the first 6 weeks.
- From weeks 6 to 8, active resistant exercises of the elbow progress from 1 to 2 kg.
- After week 8, active resistant elbow exercises progress according to the patients' tolerance to pain, but active resistant abduction in external rotation exercises are avoided until 3 months postoperatively.
- After 6 months, a full return to their previous level of sports activity is progressively allowed.

13.9 Discussion

- Arthroscopic DAS using the transposed LHB tendon fixed to the anteroinferior glenoid rim using all-suture anchors offers the combined theoretical advantages of the decreased shoulder morbidity of the minimally invasive arthroscopic technique that uses an in situ autograft and avoids the donor site morbidity of harvesting the iliac bone or of other distant types of grafts, with several other advantages in comparison with either isolated Bankart repair, or bony and coracoid transfer procedures.
- First, DAS utilizes soft suture anchors to fix the LHB to the glenoid, thereby avoiding hardware-related complications and decreasing the risk of implant-related postoperative complications in comparison with bony and coracoid transfer procedures.
- Second, DAS avoids traction to the musculocutaneous nerve because the LHB is transposed instead of the conjoint tendon; therefore, there is decreased risk of injury to the musculocutaneous nerve in comparison with the coracoid transfer procedures.
- Third, arthroscopic DAS utilizes typical arthroscopic instrumentation, and does not require specific arthroscopic guides, while arthroscopic bony or coracoid transfer procedures usually do; therefore, DAS decreases the need for bulky instrumentation sets, and adds an option to the surgeon's treatment armamentarium when faced intra-operatively with increased bony loss and engaging Hill-Sachs lesions in preoperatively apparent on-track bipolar lesions.
- Fourth, at postoperative time zero, DAS has been shown to increase glenohumeral stability in subcritical GBL and humeral head bone loss models in comparison with either an isolated Bankart repair [1] or conjoint tendon transfer procedures [2].

- Fifth, the LHB tendon combines the increased biologic healing potential and the decreased immunologic reaction potential of an autograft in comparison with either soft- or bony-allografts or xenografts.
- Sixth, in patients with concomitant SLAP type I–III lesions, DAS provides a "fill two needs with one deed" treatment option, simultaneously addressing the SLAP lesion and the anteroinferior glenohumeral instability in an "all-in-one procedure."
- Finally, DAS may avoid the risk of scapular dyskinesis and respective potential nefarious long-term consequences, because only the LHB tendon is transposed, whereas after coracoid and conjoint tendon transfer procedures, the risk of scapular dyskinesis is increased. The Latarjet procedure has been shown to permanently disturb the physiological scapular kinesis because the pectoralis minor is detached, and the vector and the working length of the coracobrachialis and the short head of the biceps are changed [23].
- However, clinical studies on the long-term outcomes of arthroscopic DAS are lacking, and this procedure requires significant surgical skills [4], and may be time-consuming even for experienced shoulder surgeons, particularly in the first few cases, with an average operative time of 87 min (range, 79–101 min) [12].
- Furthermore, postoperative rehabilitation is restrictive, which may limit the indication of DAS to recreational athletes.
- Nevertheless, this procedure is a new treatment alternative that may avoid the complications of extending the Bankart repair, Hill-Sachs remplissage, or bone block procedures beyond their ideal indications.

13.10 Summary

Arthroscopic DAS using the LHB tendon is a minimally invasive technique that fills a treatment algorithm gap between soft-tissue and bony procedures for chronic anteroinferior glenohumeral instability with limited to subcritical anteroinferior GBL (≤25%) and an engaging Hill-Sachs lesion, and/or a SLAP type I–III lesion, in recreational overhead athletes or throwers. The rationale behind DAS is that the LHB dynamically increases the stability of the glenohumeral joint through both an "hammock" and a "sling" effect. Good short-term clinical outcomes have been reported, but studies reporting the long-term clinical outcomes are lacking.

Pearls and Pitfalls

- Adequate arthroscopic portal placement improves visualization during the most critical phases of arthroscopic DAS; the pitfall of placing the viewing portal too low should be avoided.
- Usage of the first 90° of range of forward flexion of the shoulder improves the visualization of the bicipital groove while viewing with the arthroscope placed in the posterior portal.
- All-suture anchors double-loaded with sutures allow for the use of a double double-pulley technique to shuttle the LHB through the subscapularis split.
- Cutting the THL only after having passed each of the eight limbs of the sutures through the LHB facilitates the approach to the LHB when the suture passer is used through the anterior portal.
- The inferior capsule should be plicated in addition to performing the DAS in severely hypertax patients to avoid recurrence by inferior dislocation of the humeral head under the transferred LHB.

Take Home Message

- DAS using the LHB is a safe and viable option for the treatment of anterior glenohumeral instability with ≤20% of anterior glenoid bone loss.

Permissions Free License (Number 5045451250785) was obtained on April 10, 2021, from Wolters Kluwer Health, Inc., and JBJS Case Connector, for print and electronic publishing of figures/tables/illustrations from the licensed content entitled "All-Suture Anchor Dynamic Anterior Stabilization Produced Successful Healing of the Biceps Tendon: A Report of 3 Cases," authored by Clara de Campos Azevedo and Ana Catarina Ângelo.

References

1. Mehl J, Otto A, Imhoff FB, Murphy M, Dyrna F, Obopilwe E, et al. Dynamic anterior shoulder stabilization with the long head of the biceps tendon: a biomechanical study. Am J Sports Med. 2019;47(6):1441–50.
2. Bokshan SL, Gil JA, DeFroda SF, Badida R, Crisco JJ, Owens BD. Biomechanical comparison of the long head of the biceps tendon versus conjoint tendon transfer in a bone loss shoulder instability model. Orthop J Sports Med. 2019;7(11):2325967119883549.
3. Collin P, Ladermann A. Dynamic anterior stabilization using the long head of the biceps for Anteroinferior Glenohumeral instability. Arthrosc Tech. 2018;7(1):e39–44.
4. Milenin O, Toussaint B. Labral repair augmentation by labroplasty and simultaneous trans-subscapular transposition of the long head of the biceps. Arthrosc Tech. 2019;8(5):e507–e12.
5. Ibrahim M, Narbona P, Denard PJ, Arrigoni P, Collin P, Ladermann A. A reproducible technique for creation of the subscapularis Split during dynamic anterior stabilization for shoulder instability. Arthrosc Tech. 2020;9(9):e1433–e8.
6. de Campos Azevedo CI, Ângelo AC. Dynamic anterior stabilization of the shoulder: Onlay biceps transfer to the anterior glenoid using the double double-pulley technique. Arthrosc Tech. 2023;12(7):e1097–e106.
7. Popescu IA, Neculau DC, Simion C, Popescu D. Modified dynamic anterior stabilization (DAS) and Hill-Sachs Remplissage for the treatment of recurrent anterior shoulder dislocation. Arthrosc Tech. 2022;11(2):e147–e52.
8. Garcia JC Jr, Belchior RJ, Mello MBD, Cardoso AM Jr. The long head of the biceps Bristow-Bankart procedure for anterior shoulder instability. Arthrosc Tech. 2019;8(10):e1185–e91.
9. Nair AV, Mohan PK, Jangale A, Kuntwad V, Kumar MP, Goud N, et al. Dynamic anterior stabilization using transosseous bone tunnel technique with the adjustable loop length cortical button incorporating high-strength suture augmentation for recurrent shoulder instability. Arthrosc Tech. 2022;11(11):e1929–e35.
10. Tang J, Zhao J. Arthroscopic transfer of the long head of the biceps Brachii for anterior shoulder instability. Arthrosc Tech. 2017;6(5):e1911–e7.
11. Garcia JC, Mendes RB, Muzy PC, de Paiva Raffaelli M, Dumans e Mello MB. Dynamic anterior stabilization of the shoulder with adjustable-loop device. Arthrosc Tech. 2022;12:e39.
12. de Campos Azevedo C, Ângelo AC. All-suture anchor dynamic anterior stabilization produced successful healing of the biceps tendon: a report of 3 cases. JBJS Case Connect. 2021;11(1):e20.00149.
13. de Campos Azevedo CI, Ângelo AC. Onlay dynamic anterior stabilization with biceps transfer for the treatment of anterior glenohumeral instability produces good clinical outcomes and successful healing at a minimum 1 year of follow-up. Arthrosc Sports Med Rehabil. 2023;5:e445.
14. Collin P, Nabergoj M, Denard PJ, Wang S, Bothorel H, Ladermann A. Arthroscopic biceps transfer to the glenoid with Bankart repair grants satisfactory 2-year results for recurrent anteroinferior glenohumeral instability in subcritical bone loss. Arthroscopy. 2022;38(6):1766–71.
15. Garcia JC, Yukie Nakano Schincariol C, Mendes RB, Muzy PC. Dynamic anterior stabilization of the shoulder using buttons. JSES International. 2024;8(6):1169–74.
16. Wu C, Xu J, Fang Z, Chen J, Ye Z, Wang L, et al. Arthroscopic dynamic anterior stabilization using either long head of the biceps or conjoined tendon transfer for anterior shoulder instability results in a similarly low recurrence rate. Arthroscopy. 2023;39:1618.
17. Kirkley A, Griffin S, McLintock H, Ng L. The development and evaluation of a disease-specific quality of life measurement tool for shoulder instability. The Western Ontario Shoulder Instability Index (WOSI). Am J Sports Med. 1998;26(6):764–72.
18. Rowe CR, Patel D, Southmayd WW. The Bankart procedure: a long-term end-result study. J Bone Joint Surg Am. 1978;60(1):1–16.
19. DeFroda SF, Gil JA, Owens BD. Recurrent shoulder stabilization with open bankart repair and long head biceps transfer. J Orthop. 2018;15(2):401–3.
20. Hendy BA, Padegimas EM, Kane L, Harper T, Abboud JA, Lazarus MD, et al. Early postoperative complications after Latarjet procedure: a single-institution experience over 10 years. J Shoulder Elbow Surg. 2020;30:e300–8.
21. Bokshan SL, DeFroda SF, Owens BD. Comparison of 30-day morbidity and mortality after arthroscopic Bankart, open Bankart, and Latarjet-Bristow procedures: a review of 2864 cases. Orthop J Sports Med. 2017;5(7):2325967117713163.

22. Goetti P, Denard PJ, Collin P, Ibrahim M, Hoffmeyer P, Lädermann A. Shoulder biomechanics in normal and selected pathological conditions. EFORT Open Rev. 2020;5(8):508–18.
23. Carbone S, Moroder P, Runer A, Resch H, Gumina S, Hertel R. Scapular dyskinesis after Latarjet procedure. J Shoulder Elb Surg. 2016;25(3):422–7.

Open Latarjet

14

V. Housset, A. Kamel, V. Martinel, and G. Nourissat

Key Points

- The Latarjet procedure is recommended for patients presenting with humeral and/or glenoid bone loss, practicing professional activities or sports at risk of recurrence, without any proof of the superiority between the arthroscopic and the open techniques.
- During the open Latarjet procedure, the capsular management has an important place, in particular by preventing glenohumeral arthritis that may follow this surgery.
- The optimal capsular management technique to use is still under debate.
- The chapter presents the open Latarjet procedure with the association of a vertical capsular shift to treat patients with an important risk of anterior shoulder instability recurrence.

14.1 Introduction

- The Latarjet procedure is currently the gold standard surgical option for patients with recurrent anterior shoulder instability associated with a major risk of recurrence, according notably to the ISIS score [1].
- The presence of bony lesions at the glenoid rim or the humeral head represents an indication for the Latarjet procedure, as underlined by the on−/off-track assessment of the glenoid track concept [2].
- The revision rate with good patient selection and surgical technique is from 1% to 3% [3], and the overall complication rate is evaluated at 15% [4]. It has also been shown to have good result in the treatment of first anterior dislocation for well-indicated patients to prevent the recurrence of anterior instability [5].
- The main objectives of this procedure are to augment and reconstruct the anterior glenoid

Supplementary Information The online version contains supplementary material available at https://doi.org/10.1007/978-3-662-73064-5_14.

V. Housset (✉) · G. Nourissat
Clinique des Maussins, Paris, France

A. Kamel
Hôpital Intercommunal de Villeneuve-Saint-Georges, Villeneuve-Saint-Georges, France

V. Martinel
Clinique de l'Ormeau – Site Pyrénées – ELSAN, Tarbes, France

L. Kovačič et al. (eds.), *Surgical Techniques for Anterior Shoulder Instability*,
https://doi.org/10.1007/978-3-662-73064-5_14

rim and to use the concept of "triple-locking" as demonstrated by Patte [6]. The augmentation of the glenoid surface area with the addition of the "bony effect" is associated with the dynamic "sling-effect" obtained after the anatomic modification of the inferior part of the subscapularis and the conjoint tendon, which achieves a dynamic blocking function on the humeral head in the abduction and external rotation arm position. Eventually, the capsulolabral complex can be repaired directly to the bone or using the stump of the coracoacromial ligament.

- Neer and Foster first described the open capsular shift with a "T" juxta- humeral capsulotomy to treat anteroinferior shoulder instability due to a redundant and overstretched capsule [7]. Altchek et al. then described the glenoid-based T-capsulotomy to allow the treatment of Bankart lesions with transosseous capsulolabral repair [8].
- The addition of a horizontal superior capsular shift to the bone block Latarjet procedure has been shown to have a good efficiency in the decrease of both recurrent dislocation and subluxation [9].
- The limitation of the external rotation remains the most argued limitation concerning the effect of the capsular repair. If the added capsular repair does not result in a significant improvement in terms of stability, cadaveric study seems to show that it may have an effect of restricting external rotation compared with the Latarjet procedure without capsular repair [10].
- Many surgical techniques have been described concerning the management of the capsular tissue during the open Latarjet procedure, with different shaped capsulotomies and different types of flaps [11, 12]. It may also include a capsulolabral repair [13], and augmentation techniques using the coracohumeral ligament or the long head of the biceps have also been described [14, 15].
- The objective is to present a stepwise to approach of the open Latarjet for the treatment of recurrent anterior instability associated with a capsular shift for the management of the capsule.

Table 14.1 Main indications and contraindications of this procedure

Indications	Contraindications
Recurrent anterior shoulder instability (more than 2 episodes) Bony lesions: Hill-Sachs lesion on plain x-ray, "off-track" hill-Sachs lesion, critical glenoid bone loss and "subcritical" bone loss, or bony Bankart for patients at risk Collision sport (especially in competition) Occupation at risk in case of recurrence for the patient or other.	Voluntary shoulder dislocation Isolated posterior instability Multidirectional shoulder instability Uncontrolled epilepsy for less than 6 months Rotator cuff tears in elderly patients (indication for a rotator cuff repair) Unique episode in a non-sportive patient without lesion at imaging (a conservative treatment is recommended)

14.2 Indication

- We systematically perform this procedure when an open Latarjet procedure is indicated:
  - Recurrent shoulder instability with patients having an ISI score of 3 or above.
  - Previous failed arthroscopic stabilization procedure.
  - Hill-Sachs lesion identified on plain X-ray and "Off-track" Hill-Sachs lesion.
  - A subcritical glenoid bone loss for patient at risk (patient practicing a collision sports or at-risk professions).
- Mains indications and contraindications are given in Table 14.1.

14.3 Relevant Physical Findings

- Clinical evaluation must start with an investigation of the patient's instability history: age at the first dislocation and mechanism of injury, residual apprehension, level of sport participation, especially the involvement in contact sports, occupation, and nerve injury. A voluntary component must be evaluated and contraindicates surgery.
- The most important physical findings are:
  - Bilateral passive and active range of motion is performed first to evaluate the presence of a limitation or a shoulder hyperlaxity

(external rotation with the elbow at the side >85°).
- An anterior drawer test is performed to confirm the direction of the dislocation, and differential diagnostics must be eliminated:
  - A posterior drawer test to eliminate a posterior instability.
  - A painful Kim test may be explained by a posterior labral tear in the context of an unstable painful shoulder.
  - A positive hyperabduction test and the presence of a sulcus sign must be evaluated to eliminate multidirectional shoulder instability.
  - The Beighton score, especially for young patients, must be calculated to search for generalized ligamentous hyperlaxity.
- The search for a positive apprehension test in a seated or supine position, with the patient's arm positioned in abduction and external rotation.
- The relocation test in a patient in supine position, with a diminution of the apprehension, can help in the diagnosis, despite the fact that this test was initially described for the posterior superior conflict.
- A neurological deficit of the axillary nerve must be research.
- In older patients, especially over 40 years old, a rotator cuff assessment with special attention to the presence or absence of lag signs is mandatory.

14.4 Relevant Imaging

- X-rays are the first exam and are mandatory before any surgical treatment. Plain X-rays with three rotations and an axillary view are recommended. An X-ray showing the dislocated shoulder allows a certainty diagnosis. These exams can identify associated lesions such as glenoid or humeral bone loss or fracture.
- Second-intention imaging is necessary to search for associated lesions; it will help surgeons in the decision of the most appropriate treatment as well:
  - A CT scan can be performed to better assess bony lesions and more precisely quantify them.
  - Arthro-CT scan can be useful for the evaluation of cartilage, capsular tissue, and ligamentous lesions such as Bankart and bony-Bankart lesions, Hill-Sachs lesion, and rotator cuff tears.
  - The use of 3D-CT is the most accurate exam to evaluate bone loss of the glenoid and at the humeral head.
  - MRI is recommended for older patients (over 40 years old) to evaluate the presence of lesion of the rotator cuff lesions but is also informative for glenohumeral ligaments and other soft tissue lesions such as ALPSA, GLAD, HAGL, or Perthes lesions.

14.5 Goal of Surgical Procedure

- The main goals of this procedure are to improve shoulder function in these patients by stabilizing the joint and preventing recurrent instability of the shoulder through to the restoration of a glenoid bone defect and/or prevention of Hill-Sachs lesion engagement, especially when the arm is in an abducted and externally rotated position.
- The final objective is to enhance the quality of life of the patients by allowing them to return to their occupation and previous sport activities, if possible at the same level.

14.6 Surgical Technique

14.6.1 Equipment

- A classic surgical table and basic surgical instruments, notably osteotomes, Gelpi and Fukuda retractors, and a motorized saw, are enough to perform this procedure.
- Two screws of 3.5 mm are needed for the fixation of the coracoid process, and two all-suture anchors of less than 2 mm are needed for the capsular shift.

14.6.2 Patient Positioning and Surgical Approach

- The patient is positioned in the supine position with the whole upper limb included in the surgical field to allow rotational movements during the surgery.
- A head positioner device is used.
- General anesthesia is administered after a preoperative anesthetic interscalene block.
- A deltopectoral approach is used.

14.6.3 Step-by-Step Description of the Procedure

- Skin incision starts 1.5 cm above the apex of the coracoid, with a length of 5–7 cm.
- A lateral and medial dissection of the coracoid process is performed to expose both the coracoacromial ligament and the pectoralis minor tendon insertion.
- The coracoacromial ligament is sectioned with the arm positioned in external rotation, with specific caution regarding the coracoacromial artery to minimize bleeding.
- The pectoralis minor tendon is released with the arm maintained in neutral rotation.
- A Hohmann retractor is positioned above the elbow of the coracoid for good visualization.
- A first incomplete osteotomy of the inferior and medial part of the coracoid process with a curved osteotome is performed to prevent the risk of scapular fracture during the later osteotomy. The Hohmann retractor is then replaced with the osteotome to perform the final osteotomy of the coracoid at the desired position.
- Electrocautery of the bone section is performed to minimize the bleeding.
- The coracoid process is then fully mobilized, and the adherences on the conjoint tendon are released.
- Cortical bone of the inferior aspect of the coracoid process is removed and leveled using the oscillating saw.
- A square point is used to prepare the two future screw holes. A minimum distance of 7 mm is maintained between the two drilled holes in the coracoid, and the distance between holes from the lateral side of the coracoid can be measured to anticipate the best positioning of the drilled holes at the anterior glenoid rim.
- Using a Kolbel self-retaining retractor, the coracoid process is positioned medially to avoid over-tensioning of the musculocutaneous nerve.
- The subscapularis muscle is exposed and is horizontally splited at the junction between the distal third and the two upper thirds, with the arm maintained in external rotation.
- Metzenbaum scissors are used to dissect the muscle fibers to expose the anterior glenohumeral capsule.
- A horizontal capsulotomy is performed at the center of the anterior capsule, with special caution not to damage the underlying cartilage of the humeral head (Fig. 14.1).
- A glenoid "T"-based capsulotomy is then performed on the anterior glenoid rim for the release of the capsule.
- Two threads are passed superiorly and inferiorly at the medial side of the inferior flap and are separated by 1 cm.
- The anterior aspect of the scapular neck is exposed, with the square point used as a Steinmann pin to retract the superior muscle body of the separated subscapularis muscle. A Hohmann retractor is positioned at the inferior part of the glenoid rim.
- The anterior cortical bone of the glenoid rim is removed using the osteotome.
- The distal hole at the glenoid rim is performed first. It is marked and drilled at the desired position, with a possible visual control of the mediolateral distance to favorize the flush positioning of the coracoid.
- The distal single-loaded suture anchors (SUTUREFIX ULTRA, 1.7 mm, Smith & Nephew) is then positioned at the inferior part of the anterior glenoid rim, with a specific attention not to cross the inferior drilled hole for the distal screw (Fig. 14.2).
- A guide wire is positioned in the distal drilled hole, and the distal drilled hole of the coracoid bone block can be positioned on the guide wire.

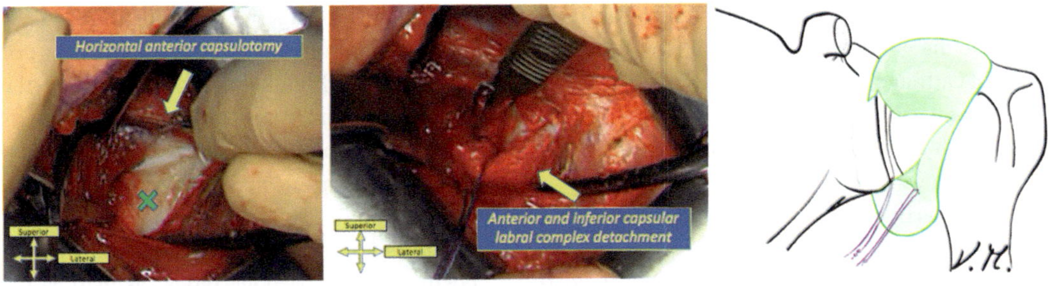

Fig. 14.1 Anterior horizontal capsulotomy (green cross, on the left) and inferior release from the anterior scapular neck performed to prepare the anterior capsulorrhaphy after the coracoid bone block fixation

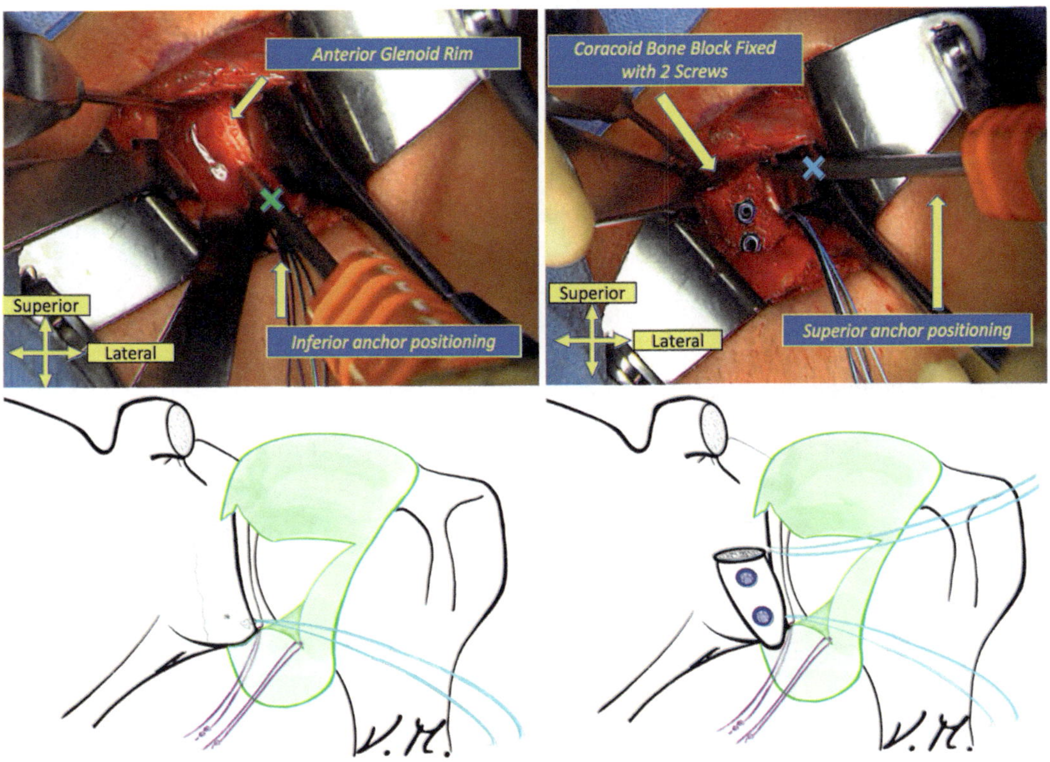

Fig. 14.2 First and second anchors positioning to perform the open capsular shift-Latarjet procedure on a left shoulder. On the left, the first glenoid anchor (green cross) is positioned before the bone block fixation. On the right, the second glenoid anchor positioning after the bone block fixation is shown (blue cross)

- The distal screw is then tightened carefully while the good positioning relative to the glenoid cartilage is controlled by hands.
- The anterior scapular neck is then drilled through the superior drilled hole of the coracoid process while the good positioning is still controlled to be flush with the anterior glenoid rim.
- A second single-loaded suture anchor is positioned medially and superiorly to the bone block and just anteriorly to the glenoid cartilage.
- The thread passed superiorly through the capsule then serves as a shuttle relay with the thread of the superior glenoid anchor (Fig. 14.3).
- The inferior-to-superior capsular shift is realized by fixing the medial and superior part of the capsular flap at the superior part of the anterior glenoid rim. The same technique is repeated with the inferior thread passed through the capsule and the thread of the inferior anchor.
- At the end of the procedure, the extra-articular positioning of the bone block, as well as the good closing and tensioning of the capsule, are controlled (Fig. 14.4).
- Top technical recommendations are given in Table 14.2.

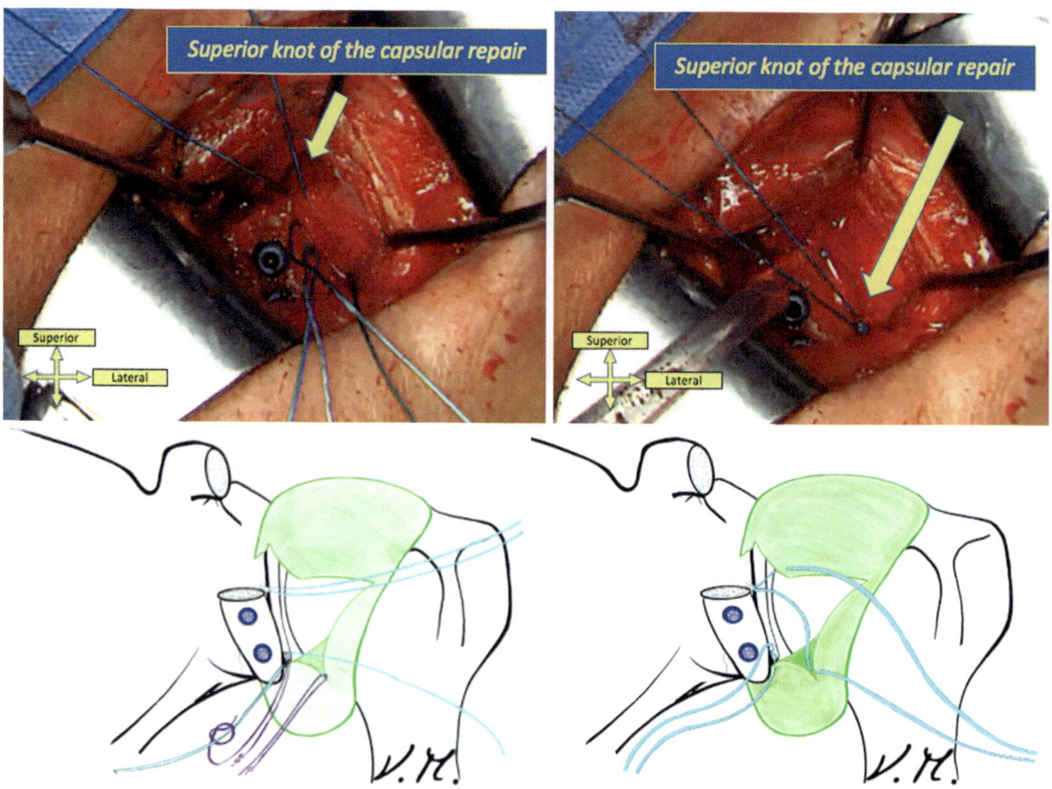

Fig. 14.3 The *shuttle relay* procedure for passing the threads of the anchors through the capsular tissue is shown in both drawn figures below

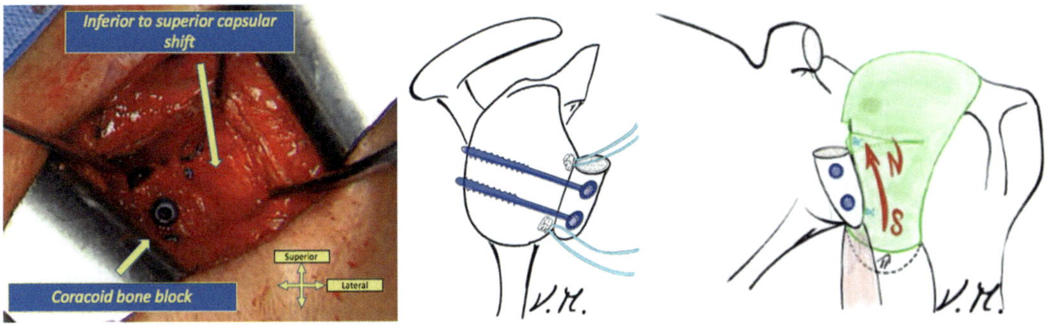

Fig. 14.4 Final aspect of the capsular repair of the anterior capsule at the end of the open Latarjet procedure

Table 14.2 Top technical recommendations

Use of two double-loaded suture anchors to perform the capsulorrhaphy
Order of anchors and screw positioning
1. Positioning of the inferior anchor at the 5 o'clock position
2. Miking the inferior screw hole after a measurement of its good location with a rule if necessary
3. Positioning of the superior screw of the Latarjet fixation
4. Position of the superior anchor for the capsulorrhaphy
A special caution must be made not to position the screws for the bone block fixation in the same direction as the double-loaded glenoid rim anchors
We recommend the use of surgical threads of different colors and performing a knot on their extra-articular to facilitate the recognition of each part of the passed threads

14.7 Postoperative Protocol

- Postoperative care includes a strict internal rotation positioning of the arm for 2 days, and the patient needs to visit a physiotherapist on the third day.
- Follow up includes a radiological and clinical control at the third and the sixth weeks.
- A 3D scan can be performed in the third month postoperatively to ensure the flush positioning of the bone block transfer, the absence of mis-positioning of the screws and the glenoid anchors. A second 3D CT scan can be performed at 1 year postoperatively to control good healing of the coracoid and the absence of osteolysis of the bone block.
- Mains steps of the postoperative protocol are detailed in Table 14.3.

Pearls and Pitfalls

Pearls	Pitfalls
Realization of a first inferior and medial osteotomy of the coracoid process to prevent any risk of scapular fracture Using all-suture anchors to minimize glenoid bone loss First closing of the medial passing threads with the superior glenoid anchors to obtain the best tensioning of the capsular repair without risk of capsular tear Minimizing bone block resorption by avoiding complete devascularization of the graft and limiting soft tissue and pectoralis minor release to no further than the tip of the coracoid process	Crossing the tunnels of the coracoid bone-block fixation screws and the glenoid anchors for the capsulorrhaphy Misplacement of the fixation screws to prevent bone block fracture Misevaluation of the screws' length (impingement with the infraspinatus muscle) A divergent axis of the screw fixation compared with the axis of the glenoid (lesion of the suprascapular nerve) Risk of entanglement and misrecognition of the threads

Table 14.3 Postoperative protocol and return to sport

Day 0–5	Day 5–45	Day >45	Week 8–12
Icing Active mobilization of elbow and wrist joints Passive shoulder abduction and scapular elevation Immediate self-rehabilitation	Icing Passive movement of the arm in abduction and anterior elevation No forced external rotation	Active without resistance Beginning of rotational movement	Active with resistance Stretching

14.8 Outcomes

- Until now, no statistical superiority of the open or the arthroscopic approach for the realization of the Latarjet procedure could have been demonstrated, both on recurrence or osteoarthritis incidence [3]. Both techniques have shown good functional and radiographic outcomes for the treatment of chronic osseous anterior shoulder instability.
- Ali et al., in a retrospective cohort of 48 patients, found a small statistically significant difference in favor of the open procedure concerning internal rotational loss, while the WOSI was superior in the arthroscopic techniques [16].
- Marion et al. made a prospective comparative study on 58 patients who underwent a Latarjet-Bristow procedure to compare the mini-open with the arthroscopic procedure. If the patients were significantly less painful during the first operative week, the results were comparable after at least 2 years of follow-up [17].
- With comparable clinical results compared to the open procedure, the direct costs of the arthroscopic Latarjet stay much higher, without a clear benefit for patients [18].
- The association of a capsular shift with the open Latarjet procedure aims to increase the postoperative mid-range and global stability of the shoulder. It also aims to prevent synovial fluid from altering the bone block between the bone-block and the glenoid rim and seems to prevent postoperative risk of glenohumeral arthritis.
- Favard and colleagues have evaluated the long-term results of the association of capsule reinsertion to enhance stability with the association of a Bankart effect to the open Latarjet procedure associated with strictly extra-articular positioning of the bone block. In a retrospective study of 76 patients with a minimum 10-year follow-up, they have demonstrated a low rate of recurrence with no revision surgeries and a significantly lower incidence of osteoarthritis (8.6%) compared to the previously published series with an equivalent follow-up [19].
- When anterior instability is associated with anterior capsular redundancy, the Latarjet procedure with a Neer capsulorrhaphy has shown good results in decreasing apprehension compared with Latarjet procedures without capsular repair.
- Ropars and colleagues proceeded to an additional Neer capsulorrhaphy for patients with anterior capsular redundancy associated with anterior shoulder instability and found excellent or good results, with a stability rate of 95% at a median follow-up of 55 months, without differences in the main clinical scores.
- These results confirm good efficiency of the discussed surgical procedure for patients who often present with a high Beighton score, an external rotation over 85°, and/or with a sulcus sign [20].
- Concerning the loss of external rotation, Itoi and colleagues compared capsular repair to the coracoid process versus the native glenoid in a cadaveric study regarding joint stability and range of motion. They found significantly greater abduction at 0° and 60° of abduction in the coracoid group. Even though the authors conclude that to avoiding limitation of external rotation may be an argument for repair to the coracoid process, they also acknowledge that repairing to the native glenoid appears to provide better mid-range stability. Capsular repair to the coracoid procedure might be a

risk factor for glenohumeral arthritis due to the intra-articular position of the bone block [21]. This conclusion was based on the results of the study by Mizuno et al., who found a rate of arthritis of approximatively 23.5% in patients with capsular repair to the coracoid 20 years after a Latarjet procedure.

- We also do not recommend practicing the capsular repair to the transferred coracoid bone-block to prevent the risk of coracoid fracture that may follow the tunnel realization that creates a bone loss [22].

14.9 Potential Complication

- The potential complications of the procedure are:
  - Recurrence (1–3%).
  - Neurological complication (axillary nerve).
  - Hematoma.
  - Infection.
  - Stiffness and loss of external rotation.
  - Bone block non-union/fracture/resorption.
  - Osteoarthritis.
  - Irritation due to implants and hardware removal.
- The most frequent complication of the procedure is the postoperative hematoma, which doesn't need any specific treatment in most of the cases.

Take Home Message

- With appropriate patient selection, the open capsular shift-Latarjet procedure is a reliable and safe technique for the treatment of patients with anterior instability to prevent the recurrence.
- The additional capsular repair seems to be an appropriate solution to better restore the anatomy and to prevent the long-term risk of arthritis of the glenohumeral joint.

References

1. Balg F, Boileau P. The instability severity index score. A simple pre-operative score to select patients for arthroscopic or open shoulder stabilisation. J Bone Joint Surg Br. 2007;89(11):1470–7. https://doi.org/10.1302/0301-620X.89B11.18962. PMID: 17998184.
2. Locher J, Wilken F, Beitzel K, Buchmann S, Longo UG, Denaro V, Imhoff AB. Hill-Sachs off-track lesions as risk factor for recurrence of instability after arthroscopic Bankart repair. Arthroscopy. 2016;32(10):1993–9. https://doi.org/10.1016/j.arthro.2016.03.005. Epub 2016 May 7. PMID: 27161511.
3. Metais P, Clavert P, Barth J, French Arthroscopic Society, et al. Preliminary clinical outcomes of Latarjet-Patte coracoid transfer by arthroscopy vs. open surgery: prospective multicentre study of 390 cases. Orthop Traumatol Surg Res. 2016;102:S271–6.
4. Longo UG, Loppini M, Rizzello G, Ciuffreda M, Maffulli N, Denaro V. Latarjet, Bristow, and Eden-Hybinette procedures for anterior shoulder dislocation: systematic review and quantitative synthesis of the literature. Arthroscopy. 2014;30:1184–211.
5. Hardy A, Sabatier V, Laboudie P, Schoch B, Nourissat G, Valenti P, Kany J, Deranlot J, Solignac N, Hardy P, Vigan M, Werthel JD. Outcomes after Latarjet procedure: patients with first-time versus recurrent dislocations. Am J Sports Med. 2020;48(1):21–6. https://doi.org/10.1177/0363546519879929. Epub 2019 Oct 24. PMID: 31647689; PMCID: PMC7052409.
6. Patte D, Debeyre J. Recurrent dislocation of the shoulder. Encycl Med Chir Paris Technique Chirurgical Orthopedie. 1980;44265:44–02.
7. Neer CS, Foster CR. Inferior capsular shift for involuntary and multidirectional instability of the shoulder. J Bone Joint Surg Am. 1980;62(6):897–908.
8. Altchek DW, Warren RF, Skyhar MJ, Ortiz G. T-plasty modification of the Bankart procedure for multidirectional instability of the anterior and inferior types. J Bone Joint Surg Am. 1991;73:105–12.
9. Hovelius L, Sandstrom B, Olofsson A, Svensson O, Rahme H. The effect of capsular repair, bone block healing, and position on the results of the Bristow-Latarjet procedure (study III): long-term follow-up in 319 shoulders. J Shoulder Elb Surg. 2012;21:647–60.
10. Kleiner MT, Payne WB, McGarry MH, Tibone JE, Lee TQ. Biomechanical comparison of the Latarjet procedure with and without capsular repair. Clin Orthop Surg. 2016;8(1):84–91. https://doi.org/10.4055/cios.2016.8.1.84. Epub 2016 Feb 13. PMID: 26929804; PMCID: PMC4761606.

11. Cohen BH, Thome AP, Tabaddor RR, Owens BD. Open surgical stabilization of glenohumeral dislocations. JBJS Essent Surg Tech. 2018;8:e17.
12. McHale KJ, Sanchez G, Lavery KP, et al. Latarjet technique for treatment of anterior shoulder instability with glenoid bone loss. Arthrosc Tech. 2017;6:e791–9.
13. Ranalletta M, Rossi LA, Bertona A, et al. Modified Latarjet procedure without capsulolabral repair for the treatment of failed previous operative stabilizations in athletes. Arthroscopy. 2018;34:1421–7.
14. Dekker TJ, Peebles LA, Grantham WJ, Akamefula RA, Hackett TR. Alternative Management of the capsule in the Bristow-Latarjet procedure. Arthrosc Tech. 2019;8(9):e1037–41. https://doi.org/10.1016/j.eats.2019.05.016. PMID: 31737481; PMCID: PMC6848964.
15. Milenin O, Sergienko R, Badtieva V. The combined arthroscopic revision technique after the Latarjet procedure. Arthrosc Tech. 2019;8(8):e917–21. https://doi.org/10.1016/j.eats.2019.04.007. PMID: 31700787; PMCID: PMC6823865.
16. Ali J, Altintas B, Pulatkan A, Boykin RE, Aksoy DO, Bilsel K. Open versus arthroscopic Latarjet procedure for the treatment of chronic anterior Glenohumeral instability with glenoid bone loss. Arthroscopy. 2020;36(4):940–9. https://doi.org/10.1016/j.arthro.2019.09.042. Epub 2019 Dec 20. PMID: 31870727.
17. Marion B, Klouche S, Deranlot J, Bauer T, Nourissat G, Hardy P. A prospective comparative study of arthroscopic versus mini-open Latarjet procedure with a minimum 2-year follow-up. Arthroscopy. 2017;33(2):269–77. https://doi.org/10.1016/j.arthro.2016.06.046. Epub 2016 Sep 8. PMID: 27617665.
18. Randelli P, Fossati C, Stoppani C, Evola FR, De Girolamo L. Open Latarjet versus arthroscopic Latarjet: clinical results and cost analysis. Knee Surg Sports Traumatol Arthrosc. 2016;24(2):526–32. https://doi.org/10.1007/s00167-015-3978-9. Epub 2016 Jan 8. PMID: 26745964.
19. Bouju Y, Gadéa F, Stanovici J, Moubarak H, Favard L. Shoulder stabilization by modified Latarjet-Patte procedure: results at a minimum 10 years' follow-up, and role in the prevention of osteoarthritis. Orthop Traumatol Surg Res. 2014;100(4 Suppl):S213–8. https://doi.org/10.1016/j.otsr.2014.03.010. Epub 2014 Apr 3. PMID: 24703796.
20. Ropars M, Cretual A, Kaila R, Bonan I, Hervé A, Thomazeau H. Diagnosis and treatment of anteroinferior capsular redundancy associated with anterior shoulder instability using an open Latarjet procedure and capsulorrhaphy. Knee Surg Sports Traumatol Arthrosc. 2016;24(12):3756–64. https://doi.org/10.1007/s00167-015-3621-9. Epub 2015 May 24. PMID: 26003480.
21. Itoigawa Y, Hooke AW, Sperling JW, Steinmann SP, Zhao KD, Yamamoto N, Itoi E, An KN. Repairing the capsule to the transferred coracoid preserves external rotation in the modified Latarjet procedure. J Bone Joint Surg Am. 2016;98(17):1484–9. https://doi.org/10.2106/JBJS.15.01069. PMID: 27605693.
22. Mizuno N, Denard PJ, Raiss P, Melis B, Walch G. Long-term results of the Latarjet procedure for anterior instability of the shoulder. J Shoulder Elb Surg. 2014;23(11):1691–9. https://doi.org/10.1016/j.jse.2014.02.015. Epub 2014 May 14. PMID: 24835298.

Surgical Techniques for Anterior Shoulder Instability: A Case and Video-Based Guide Arthroscopic Latarjet

15

Jean Kany

Key Point

- The "Latarjet bone" block can be used to treat almost every case of glenohumeral instability, especially significant glenoid bone loss, which is very common in post-traumatic injury.
- It can also be used with "off-track" lesions in the very frequent cases of combined bone loss on the humeral head (Hill-Sachs lesion) [6, 11].
- Finally, the hammock effect of the Latarjet can be equally effective in hyperlaxity.
- In comparison with the open technique, the arthroscopic-Latarjet has the double advantage of:
  - 1-positioning the bone block much more precisely, and
  - 2-treating associated lesions (cuff tear or SLAP).
- The literature does not reveal more neurological damage than the open technique, as long as the learning curve has been respected.

Supplementary Information The online version contains supplementary material available at https://doi.org/10.1007/978-3-662-73064-5_15.

J. Kany (✉)
Clinique de l'Union, Ramsay-GDS, Saint Jean, France
e-mail: jean.kany@clinique-union.fr

15.1 Introduction/Background

- Stabilization of glenohumeral joint instability using the Bankart technique (either open or arthroscopic) can lead up to 70% of failures in cases of significant bone defect [1].
- Sugaya showed that glenoid bone lesions could be observed in 90% of anterior instabilities [16].
- The French technique of "Latarjet" (open) was described in 1954 [10]. It consists of performing a coracoid process osteotomy at its base to re-fix it onto the area of glenoid bone loss through the muscular portion of the subscapularis using two screws.
- Patte showed that the "Latarjet" could stabilize the glenohumeral joint through a triple mechanism: the bone block effect as a stopper, the hammock effect with the conjoint tendon, and the ligament effect with the coracoacromial ligamentoplasty [14].
- In 2007, Lafosse proposed to perform this technique under a full arthroscopic procedure

L. Kovačič et al. (eds.), *Surgical Techniques for Anterior Shoulder Instability*, https://doi.org/10.1007/978-3-662-73064-5_15

taking the advantage for the associated lesions management (cuff ruptures, SLAP, filling, etc.) [9].
- In 2010, Boileau highlighted the difficulty of accurately positioning the bone block under arthroscopy and introduced the "suicide portal" [2].
- We have shown that it si possible to correctly position the bone block arthroscopically with proper orientation of the screws and without more complications than in the open procedure [8].

15.2 Indications

- The main indication is post-traumatic instability with bone loss.
- In a meta-analysis of the results of Bankart arthroscopic procedures, Hobby [7] showed that the risk of recurrence had greatly decreased since the Morgan transglenoid sutures (33% failures), staples (23%), the Caspari technique (22%), tags (17%), and anchors (11%). Over time, both improvements in equipment/implants and the learning curve for surgeons meant that the average failure rate was still around 10%, or even up to 12.5%, between 2004 and 2009, whereas the risk of recurrence with the Latarjet was only 3% over the same period.

15.3 Relevant Physical Findings

- The typical event is that of a young athlete (e.g., a rugby player) who comes up with an inaugural accident of anterior dislocated shoulder during a competition. This dislocation is demonstrated by a standard X-ray in a hospital emergency department, and the dislocation is reduced under general anesthesia. Despite proper rest and rehabilitation over a three-month period, dislocation can be repeatedly recurrent with increasingly simple movements that can justify a consultation with a shoulder surgeon. The clinical examination shows a positive apprehension test without any element of associated hyperlaxity but with a positive relocation test as well.
- In 2013, the French Shoulder Society conducted an 8-year follow-up of shoulder instabilities treated with an arthroscopic Bankart procedure and showed that the recurrence rate had worsened over time, up to 25%. The reason can be an underestimation of bony lesions, either on the glenoid side or on the humeral head side. We know from the ISIS score [1] that the failure rate of an isolated Bankart procedure is higher in case of an associated bone defect (37% with a glenoid defect, 31% with a Hill-Sachs lesion).

15.4 Relevant Imaging

- Sugaya [16] has shown that bone lesions on the glenoid side can be present in up to 90% of anterior recurrent instabilities, especially bony erosion onto the anterior margin of the glenoid that an arthroscopic Bankart procedure cannot repair.
- In addition, we now know that posterior bone lesions on the humeral head (Hill-Sachs lesion) can also exist in up to 90% of recurrent anterior instabilities [15, 19].
- A CT scan without injection, but with 3-dimensional reconstructions should be performed to analyze these bony lesions, as they may be underestimated with plain X-rays.
- Our experience has led us to calculate the Gerber index [3], as it is very simple and particularly reproducible: a Gerber index higher than 40% makes us decide to opt for a full-arthroscopic Latarjet procedure (Fig. 15.1).
- In case of hyperlaxity, bone loss is generally less significant, and it seems logicaly to propose a capsuloplasty instead of a bone block procedure. Nevertheless, capsuloplasty failures are numerous in this indication due to the pathologic elasticity of the soft tissues, which leads us to opt for a Latarjet procedure as well.
- The glenoid track concept described by Itoï [12] could be helpful, as it clearly explains the

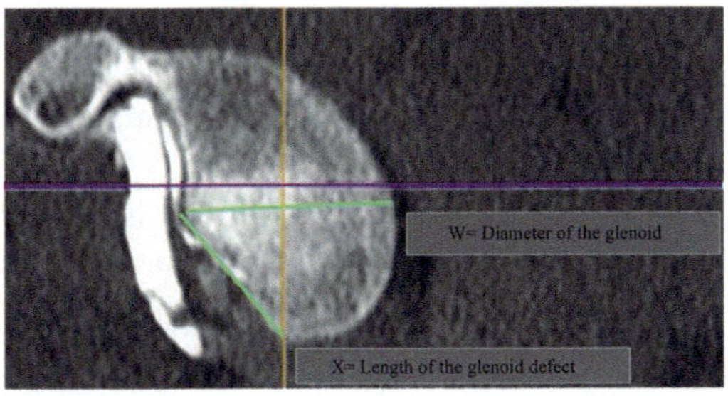

Fig. 15.1 Anterior glenoid bone loss. If the Gerber index is X/W>>40%, we opt for an arthroscopic Latarjet

biomechanical consequences of "bipolar" bone lesions ("kissing" lesions) on glenohumeral stability. Yet, in our hands, this index is not reproducible.

15.5 Goals of Surgical Procedure

- The advantages of the Latarjet procedure have been explained by Patte [14], especially the hammock effect that seems to be the most effective mechanism in stabilizing the joint. Moreover, this hammock effect could be of particular interest in the hyperlax patients, where capsuloplasty procedures have shown their limits due to tissue pathologic elasticity.
- The major advantage remains the effective treatment of post-traumatic instabilities with significant and combined humeral head/glenoid bone loss (Itoi's "off-track").
- We have shown that the positioning of the bone block was more precise arthroscopically than open [8], without any major risks of causing neurovascular complications [13].
- The "Latarjet" has the advantage over the "Bristow" published by Helfet in 1958 [5] due to a longer and more voluminous graft fixed with very effective bicortical screws, achieving compression and anti-rotation effect. Therefore, it is more efficient in reversed pear-shaped glenoids.
- Finally, the "Latarjet," thanks to its hammock effect with the conjoint tendon, is biomechanically much more efficient [4, 18, 20] than the artificial free graft or the "Eden-Hybbinette" procedure, which have the drawback of additional iliac crest harvesting with the risk of femoral cutaneous nerve lesion, aesthetic issues, and sometimes painful sequelae.
- On the other hand, the full arthroscopic Latarjet learning curve is very long (30–50 cases) and must be scrupulously observed, with an average operating time routinely reaching 45 min after 300 procedures [17].

15.6 Surgical Technique

- Lafosse [9] described the technique, and we added a few personal tips and tricks to it.
- In a beach-chair position, the arthroscope is inserted through the posterior portal and the probe through the anterior portal.
- The rotator interval is resected, and the debridement continues to allow exposure all around the coracoid process and conjoint tendon (CA ligament resection, pectoralis minor tenotomy, and conjoint tendon separation from deep deltoid aponeurosis).
- The debridement consists of exposure and subsequent resection of the anterior labrum where the bony lesion is, to position the bone block flush onto the precise location of the bone loss.
- The middle glenohumeral ligament is preserved and transversally incised only from its articular mid-portion surface (3:00 o'clock).
- The subscapularis split is now made from posterior to anterior.
- Then, the arthroscope is placed through the anterior portal (in front of the conjoint tendon).
- A switching stick is introduced through the posterior portal parallel to the glenoid and passes through the split in the subscapularis tendon to create room for the passage of the coracoid graft (by moving the upper part of the muscle superiorly as a lever arm).
- Instruments are introduced in the "suicide" (medial) portal [2], which is set in the same direction as the sagittal glenoid vault axis (switching stick direction).

- The axillary nerve is controlled at the switching stick tip but not closely dissected to avoid any thermal injury.
- With a needle, the coracoid portal is located and opened, midway between the base and the tip of the coracoid process.
- The inferior surface of the coracoid is debrided and prepared for osteotomy with a bur.
- With the use of a 2.9-mm drill and a specific guide, two drill holes are made 8 mm apart vertically into the coracoid, slightly medial to lateral, in order to position the two screws as parallel as possible with the glenoid vault axis after the bone block transfer. A top hat is implanted to prevent any bone fragmentation with a 3.5-mm drill.
- Coracoid osteotomy is performed 0.5 cm above the posterior tunnel at the union between the horizontal and vertical part of the coracoid, thanks to an osteotome and a mallet.
- Then, the arthroscope is positioned through the lateral portal.
- With the help of a special cannula (through the "suicide" portal), a specific cannulated guide is inserted and locks the coracoid process, thus allowing complete control during graft positioning.
- The graft is then mobilized through the split subscapularis tendon (helped by posterior and anterior switching sticks) and positioned onto the anterior rim of the glenoid onto the bone defect.
- For this final stage, the arthroscope is positioned through the anterior portal, as it is the best view to prevent any overhang of the bone block position (Fig. 15.2a).
- The posterior switching stick (that is parallel to the glenoid vault) is helpful to make the bone block perfectly flush with the cartilage glenoid vault surface (Fig. 15.2b). In case of an anterior step at the glenoid-graft interface, a bur can be used to obtain a flat graft, parallel to the glenoid surface.
- The patient is immobilized for 4 weeks with a Dujarrier, when he is allowed to make pendulum auto mobilization in addition to daily physiotherapy sessions with immediate work on passive external rotation without any limit except pain.
- Then active exercises will be authorized for the following 2 months, with gradual resumption of non-risky sports activities.
- Overhead activities and competitive sports with high kinetic energy will be resumed in the sixth month.
- Between 2010 and 2020, we treated 950 shoulder anterior instabilities, including 473 Bankart + Remplissage ("bipolar fixation") and 477 full arthroscopic Latarjet. The failure rate after bipolar fixation has progressively increased with follow-up (3% at 1 year, 6% at 2 years, 12% at 4 years, and almost 20% at 8 years). In the same period, we noted less than 2% of recurrence after arthroscopic

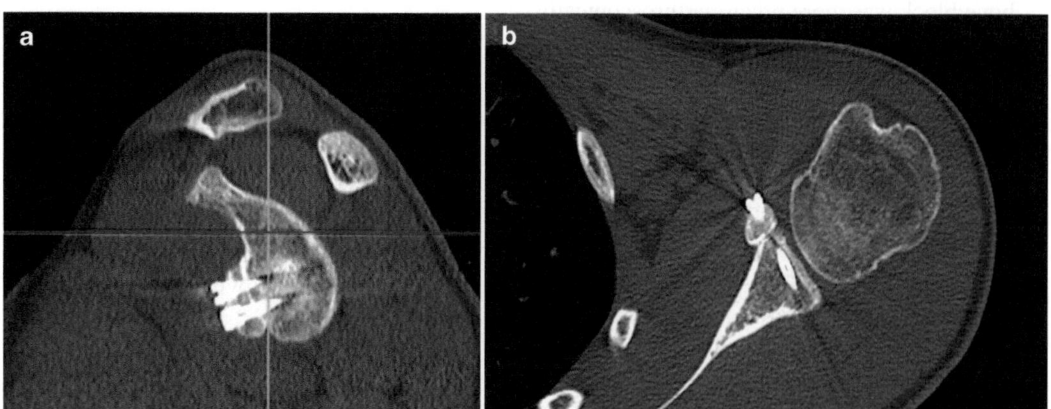

Fig. 15.2 CT scan after arthroscopic Latarjet (**a** - sagital plane, **b** - transverse plane). The bone block is flush onto the glenoid defect

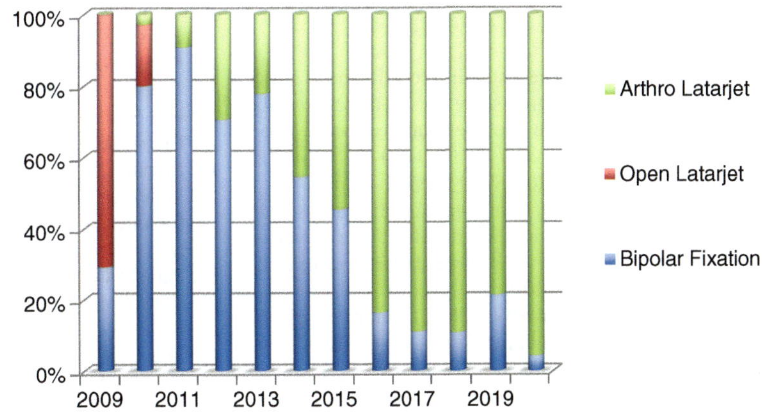

Fig. 15.3 Evolution of our indications for shoulder instability from 2009 to 2020. We abandoned open surgeries and arthroscopic soft tissue procedures to full-arthroscopic Latarjet

Latarjet. So far, over 90% of our indications are for arthroscopic Latarjet. We have abandoned the open Latarjet since 2010 (Fig. 15.3).

- We published our learning curve in 2015 [8]: we had no vascular injuries. We noticed only 1/104 patients with transitory axillary nerve palsy with full recovery after a 3-month follow-up. We did not report any musculocutaneous or suprascapular nerve lesions. No conversions to open surgery were needed, but 6/104 patients (5.7%) had to be revised: two patients to an open Latarjet procedure because of bone block dismantling or a mal-positioning, one patient to an immediate re-arthroscopic Latarjet because of mal-positioned screw, and three patients for screw removal after the bone block fusion because of posterior impingement (pain).

Pearls and Pitfalls

1. It is important to visualize both the musculocutaneous and the axillary nerve, which are the noble structures at risk.
2. The positioning of the bone block must be perfectly flush with the glenoid cartilage; it is therefore important to achieve two or even three different portal viewing controls before screwing.
3. Finally, the orientation of the two screws is important, as there is a risk of damage to the suprascapular nerve behind in the spinal notch (Laederman) if too oblique (angle greater than 30° relative to the axis of the glenoid). Our advice is to position the two coracoid tunnels slightly obliquely at an angle of 15° from inside to outside in relation to the direction of the joint tendon.

Take Home Message

- The full-arthroscopic Latarjet is a reliable, reproducible, and effective operation in most glenohumeral instability indications.
- So far, it has been our preference: we have used it on 90% of our patients.
- We have totally discarded the open Latarjet since it is outclassed by the full-arthroscopic technique on all criteria.

References

1. Balg F, Boileau P. The instability severity index score. A simple pre-operative score to select patients for arthroscopic or open shoulder stabilisation. J Bone Joint Surg Br Nov. 2007;89(11):1470–7. https://doi.org/10.1302/0301-620X.89B11.18962.
2. Boileau P, Mercier N, Roussanne Y, et al. Arthroscopic Bankart-Bristow- Latarjet procedure: the development and early results of a safe and reproducible technique. Arthroscopy. 2010;26:1434–50.
3. Gerber C, Nyffeler RW. Classification of glenohumeral joint instability. Clin Orthop Relat Res. 2002;2002(400):65–76.
4. Giles JW, Boons HW, Elkinson I, Faber KJ, Ferreira LM, Johnson JA, Athwal GS. Does the dynamic sling effect of the Latarjet procedure improve shoulder stability? A biomechanical evaluation. J Shoulder Elbow Surg. 2012;22(6):821–7. https://doi.org/10.1016/j.jse.2012.08.002.
5. Helfet AJ. Coracoid transplantation for recurring dislocation of the shoulder. J Bone Joint Surg Br. 1958;40-B(2):198–202.
6. Hill HA, Sachs. The grooved defect of the humeral head. A frequently unrecognized complication of dislocations of the shoulder joint. Radiology. 1940;35:690–700.
7. Hobby J, Griffin D, Dunbar M, Boileau P. Is arthroscopic surgery for stabilisation of chronic shoulder instability as effective as open surgery? A systematic review and meta-analysis of 62 studies including 3044 arthroscopic operations. J Bone Joint Surg Br. 2007;89(9):1188–96. https://doi.org/10.1302/0301-620X.89B9.18467.
8. Kany J, et al. Arthroscopic Latarjet procedure: is optimal positioning of the bone block and screws possible? A prospective computed tomography scan analysis. J Shoulder Elbow Surg. 2015, 2015:1–9. https://doi.org/10.1016/j.jse.2015.06.010.
9. Lafosse L, Lejeune E, Bouchard A, et al. The arthroscopic Latarjet procedure for the treatment of anterior shoulder instability. Arthroscopy. 2007;23:1242.e1–5.
10. Latarjet M. Treatment of recurrent dislocation of the shoulder. Lyon Chir. 1954;49:994–7.
11. Malgaigne JF. Traité des fractures et des luxations. Paris: JB Baillière ed; 1855.
12. Kurokawa D, Yamamoto N, Nagamoto H, Omori Y, Tanaka M, Sano H, Itoi E. The prevalence of a large Hill-Sachs lesion that needs to be treated. J Shoulder Elbow Surg. 2013;22:1285–9.
13. Mizuno N, Patrick J, Denard PJ, Raiss P, Melis B, Walch G. Longterm results of the Latarjet procedure for anterior instability of the shoulder. J Shoulder Elb Surg. 2014;2014(23):1691–9.
14. Patte D, Debeyre J. Luxations recidivantes de l'epaule. Encycl Med Chir Paris Tech Chir Orthop 1980;44265. 4.4–02.
15. Spatschil A, Landsiedl F, Anderl W, Imhoff A, Seiler H, Vassilev I, Klein W, Boszotta H, Hoffmann F, Rupp S. Posttraumatic anterior-inferior instability of the shoulder: arthroscopic findings and clinical correlations. Arch Orthop Trauma Surg. 2006. https://doi.org/10.1007/s00402-005-0006-4. Epub 2005 Oct 11.
16. Sugaya H, Moriishi J, Dohi M, Kon Y, Tsuchiya A. Glenoid rim morphology in recurrent anterior glenohumeral instability. J Bone Joint Surg Am. 2003;85(5):878–84. https://doi.org/10.2106/00004623-200305000-00016.
17. Valsamis M, Kany J, Bonnevialle N, Castricini R, Lädermann A, Cunningham G, Schwartz D, Athwal GS, Phadni J. The Arthoscopic Latarjet: a multi-surgeon learning curve analysis. J Shoulder Elbow Surg. 2020;29(4):681–8. https://doi.org/10.1016/j.jse.2019.10.022. Epub 2020 Jan 22.
18. Yamamoto N, Muraki T, An KN, Sperling JW, Cofield RH, Itoi E, et al. The stabilizing mechanism of the Latarjet procedure: a cadaveric study. J Bone Joint Surg Am. 2013;95:1390–7.
19. Yiannakopoulos CK, Mataragas E, Antonogiannakis E. A comparison of the spectrum of intra-articular lesions in acute and chronic anterior shoulder instability. Arthroscopy. 2007;23(9):985–90. https://doi.org/10.1016/j.arthro.2007.05.009.
20. Wellmann M, Petersen W, Zantop T, Herbort M, Kobbe P, Raschke MJ, et al. Open shoulder repair of osseous glenoid defects: biomechanical effectiveness of the Latarjet procedure versus a contoured structural bone graft. Am J Sports Med. 2008;37(1):87–94.

Arthroscopic Bone Block Procedure

16

Ettore Taverna, Vincenzo Guarrella, and Carlo Perfetti

Key Points

- Bone loss is an important risk factor for recurrency in anterior-inferior shoulder dislocation and after arthroscopic Bankart repair
- Bone stock reconstruction lower the risk of surgical failure
- Arthroscopic Bone Block procedure allows a guided anatomic bone and soft tissue repair without the need of screws

16.1 Introduction

- The aetiology of anterior-inferior glenohumeral instability is multifactorial. Successful treatment of this condition requires identification and repair of ll clinically significant lesions, which may be causing shoulder instability [1, 2].
- An erosion of the glenoid is quite a common phenomenon in chronic anterior shoulder instability [3–6]. Together with a Hill-Sachs lesion, a glenoid bone lesion often co-exists in anterior shoulder dislocation.
- Prevalence of fracture or erosion of the anterior-inferior part of the glenoid rim in shoulders with recurrent anterior dislocation has been reported up to 90% of cases [3, 4]. The lesions are caused by impaction of the posterior superior aspect of the humeral head on the anterior inferior glenoid rim during an episode of dislocation.
- Biomechanical studies have found an inverse relationship between the size of the glenoid defect and the stability of the shoulder: the stability of the shoulder progressively decreases as the size of the osseous defect increases [7–9]. Furthermore, clinical studies confirmed that a relationship does exist between the extent of the glenoid bone loss and the results of the treatment of recurrent anterior shoulder instability. Particularly, severe bony lesions (i.e. large Hill-Sachs lesions and/or glenoid bone loss) are associated with high risk of failure of arthroscopic shoulder stabilization and constituted in the recent past the real limit of the arthroscopic approach [7, 10].
- Treatments for patients with recurrent anterior shoulder instability have been grouped into two surgical categories: soft tissue repair and bone grafting. In cases involving bone loss from the humeral or the glenoid aspect of the shoulder, a bone graft procedure may be indicated [11–14].

Supplementary Information The online version contains supplementary material available at https://doi.org/10.1007/978-3-662-73064-5_16.

E. Taverna · V. Guarrella (✉) · C. Perfetti
IRCCS Istituto Ortopedico Galeazzi, Milano, Italy
e-mail: ettore.taverna@eoc.ch

L. Kovačič et al. (eds.), *Surgical Techniques for Anterior Shoulder Instability*,
https://doi.org/10.1007/978-3-662-73064-5_16

- Many authors recommend coracoid transfer if the glenoid rim deficiency involves 25% of the anterior-posterior diameter of the glenoid. Others suggest that measures to restore the arc of glenoid concavity may be beneficial, in terms of both stability and motion, for patients who have a glenoid defect greater than 20% of the area of the inferior glenoid [5, 7, 10]. The relationship between the size of the glenoid defect and the clinical outcome continues to be investigated. To date the exact size of the glenoid bone loss that contraindicates an arthroscopic soft tissue repair is still unknown [8].
- Optimally, the arthroscopic surgeon should be able to address all clinically relevant lesions, including bony defects, in all cases by incorporating techniques that allow restoration of both the anatomy and biomechanical function of damaged structures.
- If not properly addressed plastic deformation of the capsule and the ligaments and/or hyperlaxity could constitute another cause of failure of the arthroscopic treatment [8].
- Recently, some authors described techniques for arthroscopic positioning of a bone graft at the anterior-inferior aspect of the glenoid [15–17].

16.2 Indications

- Recurrence of instability represents the major complication of anterior shoulder stabilization.
- Currently, most surgeons use suture anchor techniques for arthroscopic soft tissue stabilization because of more reproducible results [1]. However, even with recent technical advances, a recurrence rate of between 5% and 20% still persists [8, 10].
- The best way would be to preoperatively identify patients whose risk factors preclude arthroscopic stabilization. Numerous prognostic factors have been reported in the literature. Younger patients are at risk, but no clear limit is proved. Athletes who practice contact or collision sports have higher recurrence rates after standard arthroscopic stabilization.
- Patients with significant glenoid bone loss, given the unacceptably high rate of recurrence after arthroscopic soft tissue repair, are good candidates for arthroscopic "bony procedures" [5, 8, 10, 15].

16.3 Decision-Making Algorithm

- Treatment algorithms depend on many factors, but size and type (fragment or erosion) of the bone defect of the glenoid are paramount.
- If a mobile bone fragment is associated with the labrum lesion, then the possibility for an arthroscopic reattachment does exist, despite the size of the fragment.
- In presence of bone erosion, no precise guidelines do exist. If the percent of bone loss is greater than 20% of the area of the intact contralateral glenoid, a bone grafting procedure, either open or arthroscopic, to fill the defect and restore the glenoid arc is recommended by most authors [5, 7, 8, 10–12, 15–17].
- Soft tissue quality is also important. In our practice, besides of imaging techniques, we don't rely on a soft tissue repair alone if more than 5 dislocations occurred or if the first dislocation occurred more than years before.
- If the missing area of the glenoid is less than 10% with good quality soft tissues, an arthroscopic soft tissue reconstruction is certainly an option for restoring the stability of the joint.
- If the bone loss is between 10% and 20% other factors should be considered. Certainly, a coexisting Hill Sachs lesion could constitute an indication for a bony procedure (Fig. 16.1).
- In case of bad quality soft tissues or hyperlaxity, arthroscopic subscapularis augmentation (ASA) should be considered [18]. Figure 16.1 outlines the treatment options based upon these factors.
- In addition to an accurate assessment of the possible presence of bone defect preoperatively, other risk factors that could preclude arthroscopic soft tissue stabilization must be verified [19].
- If the instability severity index score (ISIS) [20] is more than six points an isolated soft

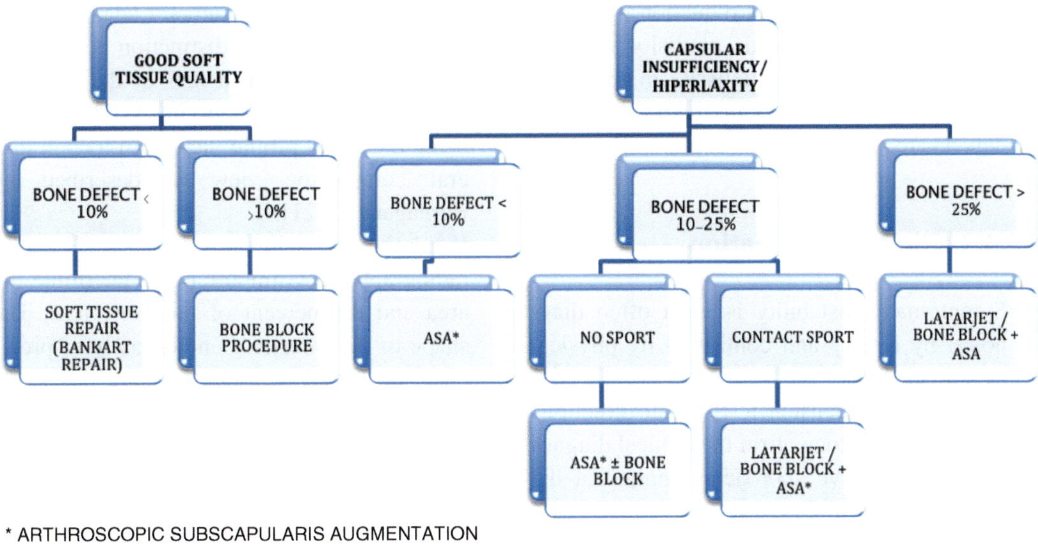

Fig. 16.1 Algorithm for selecting appropriate procedure for anterior glenohumeral instability

Table 16.1 The ISIS Score

	Prognostic Factors		Points
Questionnaire	Age at surgery	<= 20 yo > 20 yo	2 0
	Degree of sport practice (preop)	Competition Recreational or no sports	2 0
	Type of sports (preop)	Contact or forced ABD-ER Other	1 0
Exam	Shoulder hyperlaxity	Shoulder hyperlaxity Normal laxity	1 0
AP X-ray	Hill-Sachs on AP X-ray	In external rotation Not visible in ER	2 0
	Glenoid loss of contour on AP X-ray	Loss of contour No lesion	2 0
Total			10 pts

tissue reconstruction could be insufficient for stabilizing the shoulder (Table 16.1).

- In summary, the preoperative careful assessment of bony lesions, the ISIS scoring system, physical examination and history may help the surgeon to select patients who will benefit from an arthroscopic anterior soft tissue stabilization and those who will not.

16.4 Relevant Clinical Findings

16.4.1 History

- Patients presenting with glenohumeral anterior instability with bony lesions report various mechanisms of injury. These mechanisms often include individual whose arm is taken into forcible external rotation when abducted at 90°. A similar pattern can result from a fall on outstretched abducted arm. Direct distraction forces on the capsule and ligaments can be the mechanism of the injury.
- The amount of force required to create the instability is important. Atraumatic or minimally traumatic events lead generally to subluxation. In patients who sustain dislocation the force provoking the injury is generally greater and more likely show capsule and ligaments tear, and associated bony lesions.

- Individuals who required reduction by a physician at the first episode of dislocation are more likely to have soft tissue injuries, but with recurrent episodes of dislocation bony defects are more and more common [3, 5].

16.4.2 Clinical Examination

- Symptomatic instability is most often diagnosed by history and confirmed by physical examination.
- Shoulder apprehension tests in all directions should be done to confirm the clinical diagnosis. The operative approach is aimed at the direction of instability.
- Numerous instability tests have been described. In our practice, the drawer test is always performed. The examiner stabilizes the scapula with one hand and grasps the humeral head with the other hand. Anterior and posterior stresses are applied, the amount of translation and pain must be recorded. In case of significant glenoid bone loss, the anterior translation can determine a dislocation of the shoulder.
- The apprehension and relocation tests are also often positive in patients with glenoid bone deficits. With the patient supine the arm is taken into abduction and external rotation, and an anterior stress is applied until the patient's apprehension is reproduced. Posterior stress is then applied by pressing against the humeral head with reduction of the anterior subluxation and immediate decrease of the patient's apprehension.

16.4.3 Imaging

- Standard radiographs in the instability series include anterior-posterior (AP) views in three rotation positions (internal, neutral, and external). Presence of a Hill-Sachs lesion could be noted for each rotation (present or absent). If present on the external view, its location is more superior on the humeral head. Glenoid lesions are noted with distinction between an avulsion fracture and a loss of the anterior-inferior sclerotic contour in an AP view or using a glenoid profile view with a contralateral comparison view as described by Bernageau [3, 21].
- If a bone defect in the glenoid is shown on radiographs, it is important to determine the area and the percent of the bone loss. The shape of the inferior glenoid has been previously described as a circle; using this circle method with a 3D CT, spiral CT and MRI it is possible to measure the bone defect of the glenoid [4, 5, 21–25].

16.5 Surgical Technique

- The arthroscopic anterior bone block procedure described by Taverna [17, 26, 27] combines an arthroscopic Bankart repair with a bone grafting through the rotator interval and fixed on the glenoid rim under the equator.
- The efficacy of this procedure is related to the bone block effect provided by the bone graft that increases the size of the glenoid surface and the concavity re-creation provided by the labral repair and capsular and ligaments shift and repair.
- The goal of the procedure is to restore the normal anatomy of the unstable shoulder with bone defects.
- More recently the procedure has been performed with iliac crest allograft and with horse xenograft to avoid donor site pathology.

16.5.1 Equipment

- Standard artrhoscopic equipment, 30° optic, two cannulas (5 mm and 7.5 mm), shaver blade, radiofrequency, artroscopic guide, xenograft of autograft (if preferred over autograft), two double round endobuttons, tensioner device.

16.5.2 Bone Graft Harvesting (If Iliac Crest Autograft Is Preferred)

- With the patient in supine position a tricortical bone graft measuring 1 cm by 2 cm from the iliac crest is harvested. With a 1-mm Kirschner wire we create two holes at 0.5 cm from the ends.

16.5.3 Patient Positioning and Portals

- Surgical technique can be performed in the beach-chair or lateral decubitus position.
- Draping should allow access to the posterior and anterior aspects of the shoulder girdle.
- A high posterior lateral viewing portal is preferred for initial glenohumeral inspection so as to allow a subsequent posterior vector guide and double barrel guide sleeve to be inserted posteriorly into the joint. Standard anterior superior and anterior inferior portals are made utilizing 6 mm and 8 mm clear cannulas.

16.5.4 Step-by-Step Procedure

- Following joint inspection, the anterior labrum and capsule is detached from the anterior aspect of the glenoid utilizing the combination of an elevator, shaver and radiofrequency device. The capsule-labral complex is freed to view the subscapularis muscle fibers. Once detached a traction suture is placed into the capsule-labral tissue.
- The anterior glenoid bone defect is then smoothed with a motorized burr (Fig. 16.2).
- A spinal needle is then inserted posteriorly and rested against the face of the glenoid south of the equator. A second posterior portal is created, and the drill guide is inserted posteriorly, and its arm placed flush along the face of the glenoid with its hook passed over the edge of the glenoid (Fig. 16.3).
- Each drill sleeve of the guide is then advanced until it is flush to the posterior glenoid neck and two cannulated drill sleeves are inserted and advanced by power until exiting parallel

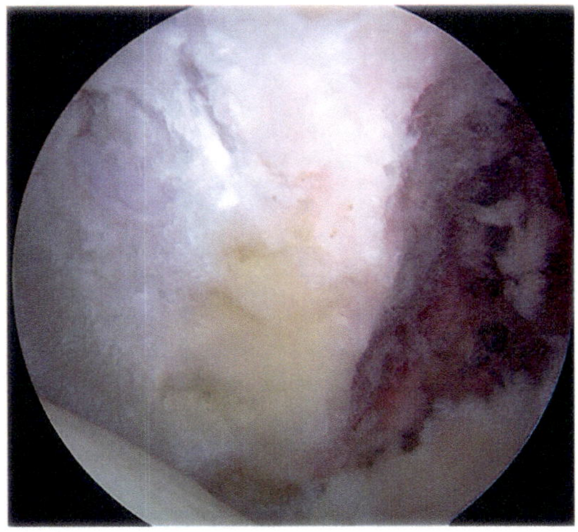

Fig. 16.2 The anterior glenoid bone defect is then smoothed with a motorized burr

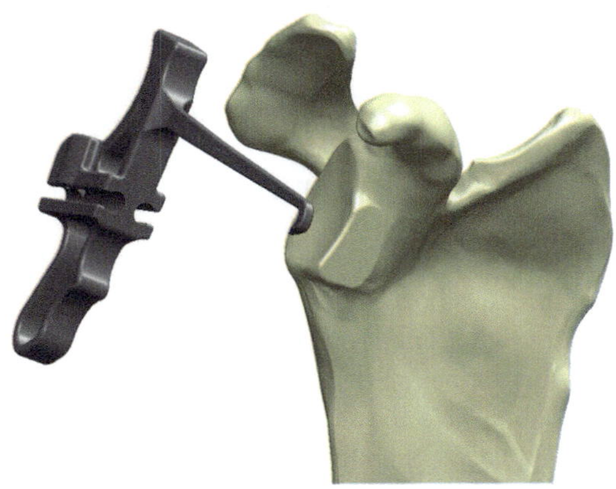

Fig. 16.3 Introduction of the glenoid guide from the posterior portal. (Courtesy of Smith & Nephew)

to one another 5 mm below the cortical edge of the anterior glenoid (Fig. 16.4). It is important to identify the cortex from the articular cartilage to ensure proper depth placement of the cannulated guide pins.
- At this point soft suture anchors can be placed on the anterior-inferior glenoid rim and the suture can be retrieved posteriorly.
- Using shuttle sutures two double round buttons (Smith & Nephew Inc., Andover, MA, USA) and the bone block (xenograft, iliac crest allograft or tricortical iliac crest bone autograft previously harvested and prepared) are inserted from the anterior portal through a metallic cannula.

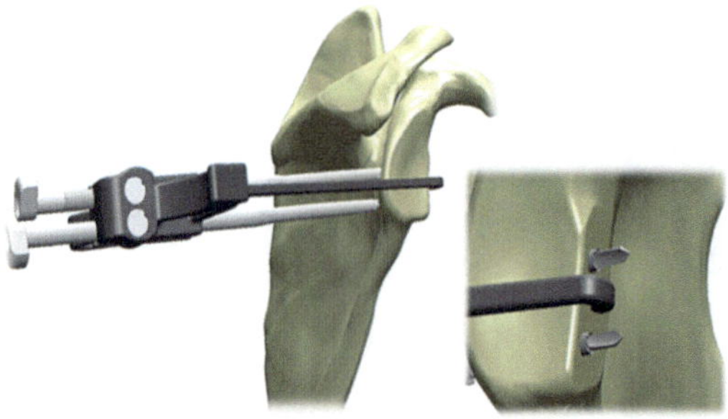

Fig. 16.4 Positioning of cannulated sleeves. (Courtesy of Smith & Nephew)

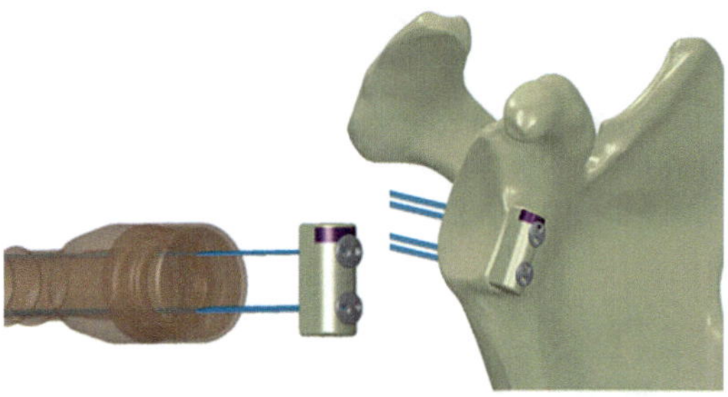

Fig. 16.5 Introduction and posizioning of the bone block. (Courtesy of Smith & Nephew)

- Once the bone graft is correctly positioned along the anterior glenoid neck (Fig. 16.5), posterior buttons are inserted and secured, and fixation is achieved with a tensioner device (Fig. 16.6). Stability of the graft is assessed with an arthroscopic probe.
- The anterior labrum and capsule can now be repaired in a standard fashion leaving the bone graft extraarticular.
- The advantages of this procedure are the associated repair of the glenoid labrum and tensioning and shift of capsule and ligaments. The bone block is placed in an extra-articular position avoiding the potential contact between the humeral head and the bone block which can cause pain and glenohumeral osteoarthritis. Screws have been substituted with buttons in order to avoid complication related to screw fixation [28].
- This is an anatomic procedure which restore normal glenohumeral anatomy, by increasing bony surface of the glenoid and recreating normal insertion of the labrum, ligaments and capsule.

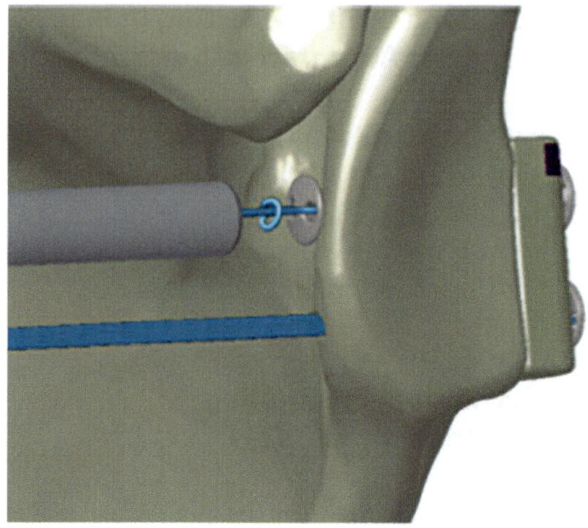

Fig. 16.6 Fixation of the bone block with the Double Round Endobutton system. (Courtesy of Smith & Nephew)

- The weakest point of this procedure is the impossibility to address instability due to glenoid bone defects combined with inconsistency of the labrum-capsule-ligaments complex. In this case the dynamic musculotendinous sling effect created by the conjoint tendon passing over the inferior part of the subscapularis of the Bristow-Latarjet procedure or ASA is preferable.

16.5.5 Top Technical Recommendations from the Expert

- Portal positioning and glenoid guide positioning are really important for good clinical and radiological results.
- The surgical procedure doesn't require exceptional surgical skills but an intermediate arthroscopical experience is recommended.
- To strictly follow the surgical steps is also highly recommended.

Pearls and Pitfalls

- Patient selection is critical for good clinical and radiological results
- It is the only arthroscopic procedure that allows guided bone and soft tissue restauration in an anatomic manner, avoiding screw fixation
- In case of chronic instability with multiple dislocation and major bone defect Latarjet procedure is a better solution.

16.6 Postoperative Protocol

- Postoperatively we recommend keeping the patients in a sling for a period of 3 weeks.
- After the immobilization there is no limitation in passive motion and the patients are allowed to a full recovering in elevation and external rotation.
- After complete wound healing is obtained, swimming pool active exercises are recommended and resumed working activities are allowed.
- Progressive strengthening exercises are started after 6–8 weeks.
- Return to overhead and contact sports are generally allowed after 4 to 6 months after surgery.

16.7 Outcomes

- Clinical and radiological results are very promising [26]. At a minimum 2-year follow-up, no recurrent anterior dislocations were described, excellent clinical results were observed [average Walch-Duplay score 93.2, (SD 7.8); average Rowe score, 96.4 (SD 6.5); average SSV, 87.4 (SD 12.1); satisfaction rate, 88.5%; average loss of external rotation, 4.4° (SD 8.7°)] and optimal graft positioning, and a healing rate of 92.3% on computed tomography scan were detected.

16.8 Potential Complications

- The main potential complication is recurrence of dislocation. With good patient selection and surgical technique, it can be easily limited.
- Other potential complications are graft resorption, graft non-union, nerve injury, vascular damage (very unlikely if the guide is properly positioned). Infection is another potential complication, rare after arthroscopic surgery.

Take Home Message

- When indicated, an arthroscopic bone block procedure is an effective and reproducible technique to manage shoulder instability with bone defect.
- It allows a guided anatomical extra articular bone grafting of the anterior glenoid with capsule-labral reconstruction.
- Double round Button fixation is used to achieve optimal compression and bone integration and avoid rotational graft instability and screw related complications.

References

1. Gartsman GM, Roddey TS, Hammerman SM. Arthroscopic treatment of anterior-inferior glenohumeral instability. J Bone Joint Surg. 2000;7A:991–1003.
2. Taverna E, Sansone V, Battistella F. Arthroscopic rotator interval repair: the three-step all-inside technique. Arthroscopy. 2004;20:105–9.
3. Edwards TB, Boulahia A, Walch G. Radiographic analysis of bone defects in chronic anterior shoulder instability. Arthroscopy. 2003;19:732–9.
4. Sugaya H, Morbshi S, Dodi M, Kon Y, Tsuchiya A. Glenoid rim morphology in recurrent anterior glenohumeral instability. J Bone Joint Surg. 2003;85A:878–84.
5. Piasecki DP, Verma NN, Romeo AA, Levine WN, Bach BR Jr, Provencher MT. Glenoid bone deficiency in recurrent anterior shoulder instability: diagnosis and management. J Am Acad Orthop Surg. 2009;17:482–93.

6. Ji JH, Kwak DS, Yang PS, Kwon MJ, Han SH, Jeong JJ. Comparisons of glenoid bony defects between normal cadaveric specimens and patients with recurrent shoulder dislocation: an anatomic study. J Shoulder Elb Surg. 2012;21:822–7.
7. Itoi E, Lee SS, Berglund LJ, Berge LL, An KN. The effect of a glenoid defect on anteroinferior stability of the shoulder after Bankart repair: a cadaveric study. J Bone Joint Surg. 2000;82A:35–46.
8. Beran MC, Donaldson CT, Bishop JY. Treatment of chronic glenoid defects in the setting of recurrent anterior shoulder instability: a systematic review. J Shoulder Elb Surg. 2010;19:769–80.
9. Ghodadra N, Gupta A, Romeo AA, Bach BR Jr, Verma N, Shewman E, et al. Normalization of glenohumeral articular contact pressures after Latarjet or iliac crest bone-grafting. J Bone Joint Surg. 2010;92A:1478–89.
10. Milano G, Grasso A, Russo A, Magarelli N, Santagada DA, Deriu L, et al. Analysis of risk factors for glenoid bone defect in anterior shoulder instability. Am J Sports Med. 2011;39:1870–6.
11. Moroder P, Hirzinger C, Lederer S, Matis N, Hitzl W, Tauber M, et al. Restoration of anterior glenoid bone defects in post-traumatic recurrent anterior shoulder instability using the J-bone graft shows anatomic graft remodeling. Am J Sports Med. 2012;40:1544–50.
12. Yamamoto N, Muraki T, Sperling JW, Steinmann SP, Cofield RH, Itoi E, et al. Stabilizing mechanism in bone-grafting of a large glenoid defect. J Bone Joint Surg. 2010;92A:2059–66.
13. Hybinette S. De la transposition d'un fragment osseux pour remedier aux luxations recidivantes de l'epaule constatations et resultats opératoires. Acta Chir Seand. 1932;71:411–45.
14. Latarjet M. A propos do traitement des luxations récidivantes de l'Ipaule. Lyon Chir. 1954;49:994–1003.
15. Boileau P, Bicknell RT, El Fegoun AB, Chuinard C. Arthroscopic Bristow procedure for anterior instability in shoulders with a stretched or deficient capsule: the "belt-and-suspenders" operative technique and preliminary results. Arthroscopy. 2007;23:593–601.
16. Lafosse L, Lejeune E, Bouchard A, Kakuda C, Gobezie R. The arthroscopic Latarjet procedure for the treatment of anterior shoulder instability. Arthroscopy. 2007;11:1242–5.
17. Taverna E, Golano P, Pascale V, Battistella F. An arthroscopic bone graft procedure for treating anterior-inferior glenohumeral instability. Knee Surg Sports Traumatol Arthrosc. 2008;16:872–5.
18. Maiotti M, Russo R, Zanini A, Schröter S, Massoni C, Bianchedi D. Arthroscopic Bankart repair and subscapularis augmentation: an alternative technique treating anterior shoulder instability with bone loss. J Shoulder Elb Surg. 2016;25(6):898–906.
19. Boileau P, Villalba M, Héry J, Balg F, Ahrens P, Neyton L. Risk factors for recurrence of shoulder instability after arthroscopic Bankart repair. J Bone Joint Surg. 2006;88A:1755–63.
20. Balg F, Boileau P. The instability severity index score. A simple pre-operative score to select patients for arthroscopic or open shoulder stabilisation. J Bone Joint Surg. 2007;89B:1470–7.
21. Charousset C, Beauthier V, Bellaïche L, Guillin R, Brassart N, Thomazeau H, et al. Can we improve radiological analysis of osseous lesions in chronic anterior shoulder instability? Orthop Traumatol Surg Res. 2010;96:S88–93.
22. Magarelli N, Milano G, Sergio P, Santagada DA, Fabbriciani C, Bonomo L. Intra-observer and interobserver reliability of the 'Pico' computed tomography method for quantification of glenoid bone defect in anterior shoulder instability. Skeletal Radiol. 2009;38:1071–5.
23. Huijsmans PE, de Witte PB, de Villiers RV, Wolterbeek DW, Warmerdam P, Kruger NR, et al. Recurrent anterior shoulder instability: accuracy of estimations of glenoid bone loss with computed tomography is insufficient for therapeutic decision-making. Skeletal Radiol. 2011;40:1329–34.
24. Magarelli N, Milano G, Baudi P, Santagada DA, Righi P, Spina V, et al. Comparison between 2D and 3D computed tomography evaluation of glenoid bone defect in unilateral anterior gleno-humeral instability. Radiol Med. 2012;117:102–11.
25. Bois AJ, Fening SD, Polster J, Jones MH, Miniaci A. Quantifying glenoid bone loss in anterior shoulder instability: reliability and accuracy of 2-dimensional and 3-dimensional computed tomography measurement techniques. Am J Sports Med. 2012;40:2569–77.
26. Taverna E, Garavaglia G, Perfetti C, Ufenast H, Sconfienza LM, Guarrella V. An arthroscopic bone block procedure is effective in restoring stability, allowing return to sports in cases of glenohumeral instability with glenoid bone deficiency. Knee Surg Sports Traumatol Arthrosc. 2018;26(12):3780–7.
27. Taverna E, D'Ambrosi R, Perfetti C, Garavaglia G. Arthroscopic bone graft procedure for anterior inferior glenohumeral instability. Arthrosc Tech. 2014;3(6):e653–60.
28. Zuckerman JD, Matsen FA. Complications about the glenohumeral joint related to the use of screws and staples. J Bone Joint Surg Am. 1984;66:175–80.

17 Open Trillat Procedure

Victor Housset and Geoffroy Nourissat

Key Points

- The Trillat procedure has shown to be a safe surgery to prevent recurrences of anterior shoulder instability, to restore range of motion, and allow a return to sport.
- It is composed of a partial superior osteotomy of the elbow of the coracoid process which is then positioned medially and downwards and fixed into the anterior scapular neck.
- As described in the "triple locking" concept for the Bristow-Latarjet procedure the transposition of the coracoid process leads to achieve a dynamic blocking function around and against the humeral head through a dynamic re-centering effect due to the anatomical modification of the conjoint tendon.
- No superiority of the arthroscopic techniques compared with the open procedure has been demonstrated until now.

17.1 Introduction

- Several treatments are available for patients with recurrent anterior shoulder instability [1, 2]. First described in 1954, the open Trillat procedure remains a very rarely performed procedure compared with the arthroscopic Bankart repair and the open or arthroscopic Latarjet procedure [3, 4].
- Incidence of anterior dislocation for middle-aged and elderly patients is increasing with the continuously increasing average population age and demand for participating in leisure sport [5, 6].
- Some studies demonstrate an incidence of almost 20% of shoulder dislocation for patients of 60 years of age and older [7, 8].
- Previous work concluded that hyperlaxity or pathological capsular ligamentous restraints due to a plastic deformation were not indication for a Bankart repair [9, 10].
- The rationale for this technique is based on the anatomical modification which reinforce the deficient capsule and to perform a "sling effect" to stabilize the humeral head and prevent the recurrence of the anterior shoulder instability [11].
- As for almost all the shoulder stabilization procedures, both open and arthroscopic techniques have been described and many fixation techniques have been used (screw, endobut-

Supplementary Information The online version contains supplementary material available at https://doi.org/10.1007/978-3-662-73064-5_17.

V. Housset · G. Nourissat (✉)
Clinique Maussins Nollet, Paris, France

L. Kovačič et al. (eds.), *Surgical Techniques for Anterior Shoulder Instability*,
https://doi.org/10.1007/978-3-662-73064-5_17

Table 17.1 Indication and contraindication for the open Trillat procedure

Indications	Contraindications
Elderly patient with recurrent dislocations, normal range of motion, a good subscapularis and irreparable rotator cuff tear	Intra articular lesion needing a surgical assessment
Patient with hyperlaxity (external rotation over 85° with the arm at side)	ISIS score < 3 with no plastic capsular deficiency
Capsular distension or deficiency without major bony defect of the glenohumeral joint	Important bone lesion on the glenoid or the humeral head
	Bipolar bone lesion with off track lesion following the glenoid track concept
	Pseudo-paralytic shoulder

ton) [12–15]. We present here the open Trillat procedure with a fixation using a screw.

17.2 Indications for Trillat Procedure (Table 17.1)

- This procedure is recommended for elderly patient presenting an irreparable rotator cuff tear with a history of recurrent shoulder instability.
- Patients with hyperlaxity (external rotation with arm at side >85°) or with a pathological capsular tissue can represent a good indication for the Trillat procedure [14, 16].
- Patients for which a Bankart repair or a Latarjet procedure remains indicated are considered as a relative contraindication for the Trillat procedure.

17.3 Relevant Physical Findings

- Clinical examination must be done bilaterally on an undressed patient with an inspection of the muscle trophicity, the research for scapular thoracic dyskinesia, the evaluation and register of the range of motion and the evaluation through specific tests of the rotator cuff muscles.
- The instability is confirmed with the finding of an anterior and/or posterior drawer test, a positive apprehension test in abduction and external rotation.
- A specific attention on the shoulder instability history (previous surgery; number of subsequent dislocation and/or subluxation, hand dominance, profession, type of sports and activities)
- The traumatic or atraumatic aspect of the shoulder instability must be established
- For younger patients, the research of a generalized hyperlaxity must be made, using if needed the Beighton Score.

17.4 Relevant Imaging

- Standard plain X-ray radiographs must be performed including a three rotations anterior and posterior view and a trans-scapular “Y” view. It is supposed to research bony lesions on both humeral (Hill-Sachs-lesion) and glenoid side (Bankart lesion). The presence of arthritis and its importance must be taken into account to discuss the feasibility of the Trillat procedure. Its benefit in that case, has to be compared with the benefit of proceeding to a reversed shoulder arthroplasty.
- For elderly patients, the statue of the rotator cuff muscle must be evaluated using an MRI or a CT-scan in order to determine the presence of a non-repairable degenerative rupture of the rotator cuff tendon, muscle retraction and atrophy.
- The 3D imaging can allow the visualization of intraarticular lesions that may modify the indication for the open Trillat procedure.
- In case of a generalized capsular and ligamentous hyperlaxity, many elements have been described on the 3D imagery as the presence of a patulous redundant inferior capsule, a capsular distention of a thickening of the capsular tissue.

17.5 Goals of Surgical Procedure

- The objective of the procedure is to tilt downward and medially the coracoid process to ensure a dynamic re-centering effect via the conjoint tendon on the humeral head.

- The transferred conjoint tendon aims to reinforce a deficient capsule by lowering the subscapularis tendon.
- The expected outcomes are to prevent the recurrence of anterior shoulder instability, to restore the full range of motion of the shoulder and to allow the patients to return to sport or work (for heavy workers).

17.6 Surgical Technique (Table 17.2)

- The patient is positioned in supine position under general anesthesia and with an interscalene block to minimize postoperative pain.
- The head of the patient is positioned in a regular head fixation device in a neutral position.
- The whole upper limb must be included in the surgical field to be able to apply rotational movement during the procedure and to allow the maximum range of motion of the shoulder.
- The arm is reposed on a separated moveable table which can be moved if posterior flexion of the shoulder is needed during the surgical procedure.
- The coracoid process is localized and marked to determine the skin incision which starts 1,5 centimeter above the apex and is generally of 4 cm length.

Table 17.2 Pearls and pitfalls of the open Trillat procedure

Pearls	Pitfalls
Make a good release of the both side of the coracoid process in order to get the best visualization during the osteotomy Apply the good rotation movement on the operated upper limb on each step to optimize visualization Precise control of the tilting of the coracoid process and soft control during the mobilization	Make bleed the coracohumeral ligament artery Apply compression while tightening the screw in the anterior scapular neck with a risk of breakage of the partial osteoclasia of the coracoid process Mispositioning of the screw at the level of the anterior scapular neck with a risk of conflict with the subscapularis

- A classical deltopectoral approach is performed with the arm positioned in neutral position.
- The conjoint tendon is exposed and dissected both medially and laterally with a specific caution in order to prevent any bleeding of the coracoacromial ligament artery during the section of the coracoacromial ligament.
- An anterior drilling of the coracoid process is the first performed right in the middle of the coracoid process in the medial to lateral and superior to inferior plans.
- A careful partial osteotomy of the anterior coracoid neck is performed using an osteotome. We recommend to perform a two third osteotomy to prevent any breakage of the inferior cortical.
- A careful two-finger maintenance of the bone block is recommended with a soft mobilization medially and downward of the coracoid process.
- The coracoid must be well maintained while drilling the anterior scapular neck above the superior border of the subscapularis muscle.
- We recommend the use of a guidewire not to lose the direction of the drilled holes and the coracoid process is fixed using a 4 millimeters cannulated screw with the arm positioned in internal rotation. The internal rotation aims to open the subcoracoid space and to prevent a subcoracoid impingement of the subscapularis muscle.
- The screw must be tightened carefully with no compression to avoid the breakage of the inferior cortical and not to over-tension the space between the deeper part of the coracoid process and the anterior scapular neck.
- After the fixation, the sling effect of the conjoint tendon against and around the humeral head must be controlled.
- We recommend to close the deltopectoral approach at the end of the procedure to prevent any risk of skin retraction secondary to a subcutaneous fibrosis.

17.7 Postoperative Protocol

- The postoperative cares include a shoulder immobilization with an abduction pillow position for 3 weeks.
- Pendulum exercises and passive range of motion rehabilitation is started at the third day to prevent shoulder stiffness.
- Clinical and radiological follow up (with AP view and trans-scapular "Y" view) are performed at the third and the sixth weeks postoperatively. The good positioning of the coracoid process and the screw are controlled.
- In the third week, Liotard protocol and active physiotherapy are started.
- At 6 months, the good healing of the coracoid process is evaluated using a computed tomography scan.
- Return to work for heavy workers and to sport (after a specific sport specific movements rehabilitation phase) is usually allowed at the third month.

17.8 Outcomes

- The open Trillat procedure presents the advantages of allowing an intraoperative assessment of the "sling effect" of the conjoint tendon on the humeral head as the control of the excursion of the subscapularis muscle to prevent conflict with the screw.
- The learning curve is fast and it remains a shorter and less expansive procedure compared with the arthroscopic techniques. It allows a precise control and a soft mobilization of the coracoid process during the surgical procedure.
- Compared with the arthroscopic techniques, the open procedure is less at risk for lesion of the brachial plexus. However, the open procedure does not allow the assessment and treatment of eventual intra-articular associated lesion unlike the arthroscopic techniques
- Its efficacy has been shown in 88–100% for the prevention of the recurrences [17–19]. Good functional results in terms of patient satisfaction, range of motion and return to sport are found with this procedure [18–20].
- Gerber et al., reported a high rate of postoperative arthritis of the shoulder after a Trillat procedure in elderly patients [19]. However, this result reflects the fact for these patients the glenohumeral joint is already damaged. That is one of the main reasons to not recommend performing this procedure arthroscopically.
- Jouve et al., studied a retrospective series of patients operated for recurrent anterior dislocation with a full thickness rotator cuff tear to determine the best timing and indication to treat the both pathologies [17]. They found at a mean follow-up of 73 and 5 months that 16% of the patients treated with an isolated open Trillat stabilization had recurrence (versus no recurrence in the group of patients treated with an open Latarjet procedure associated with a rotator cuff repair).
- The arthroscopic Trillat is technically challenging, especially concerning osteoclasia. If it remains less invasive it allows the assessment and treatment of the intra-articular lesions.
- Labattut et al., in an arthroscopy-assisted Trillat procedure found very satisfactory clinical outcomes with no recurrence and 94% of very satisfied and satisfied patients at 2 years mean follow-up [15].
- Until now, no study made a comparison between the classical open Trillat procedure and the arthroscopy technique which make it impossible to conclude to the superiority of one over the other.

17.9 Potential Complications

- One of the main per operative complications is the full osteotomy of the coracoid process. A specific caution must be made during the osteotomy and we recommend to perform a two third osteotomy and to be really careful while handling the coracoid during the procedure.
- Pain and weakness of the subscapularis muscle can be observed in case of mispositioning of the screw with a loss of external rotation.

An intraoperative control has to be performed after the fixation of the coracoid process.

- In case of mispositioning, bad healing of the coracoid process of mechanical failure of the fixation with a secondary breaking of the screw, the main complication remains the recurrence of shoulder instability.
- The release of the pectoralis minor tendon may have consequences on the scapula kinetic
- As for the open Latarjet procedure, this surgery exposes a risk of lesion of the musculocutaneous nerve.
- In case of a too long fixation screw, a conflict with the infraspinatus muscle may be responsible for postoperative pain and limitation of ROM.
- As for any open surgical procedure a risk of infection and wound complication exists.

17.10 Video

- Open Trillat procedure with tips and pearls is detailed in (Video 17.1).

Take Home Message

- The open Trillat procedure remains a safe and valid procedure in the treatment of shoulder instability when it is well indicated.
- The use of the open procedure presents the advantage of being a short time procedure which is less expansive compared with the arthroscopic techniques and presents a fast learning curve
- The crucial moment of the surgical procedure is the soft mobilization and the good positioning of the coracoid process to optimize the "sling effect on the humeral head while avoiding conflict with the subscapularis muscle
- Currently, there is no proof of the superiority of the open or the arthroscopic technique for the Trillat procedure for the treatment of recurrent shoulder instability.
- We strongly believe that no therapeutic strategy must be put aside in the complex entity that compose the shoulder instability

References

1. Arner JW, Peebles LA, Bradley JP, Provencher MT. Anterior shoulder instability management: indications, techniques, and outcomes. Arthroscopy. 2020;36:2791–3. https://doi.org/10.1016/j.arthro.2020.09.024.
2. Nazzal EM, Herman ZJ, Engler ID, Dalton JF, Freehill MT, Lin A. First-time traumatic anterior shoulder dislocation: current concepts. J ISAKOS Jt Disord Orthop Sports Med. 2023;8:101–7. https://doi.org/10.1016/j.jisako.2023.01.002.
3. Koh KH. Editorial commentary: the Trillat procedure may be (rarely) indicated instead of shoulder Latarjet for recurrent instability, irreparable cuff tear, no pain, preserved active motion, and no critical glenoid bone loss. Arthroscopy. 2023;39:946–7. https://doi.org/10.1016/j.arthro.2022.11.038.
4. Blomquist J, Solheim E, Liavaag S, Schroder CP, Espehaug B, Havelin LI. Shoulder instability surgery in Norway: the first report from a multicenter register, with 1-year follow-up. Acta Orthop. 2012;83:165–70. https://doi.org/10.3109/17453674.2011.641102.
5. Leroux T, Wasserstein D, Veillette C, Khoshbin A, Henry P, Chahal J, Austin P, Mahomed N, Ogilvie-Harris D. Epidemiology of primary anterior shoulder dislocation requiring closed reduction in Ontario, Canada. Am J Sports Med. 2014;42:442–50. https://doi.org/10.1177/0363546513510391.
6. Delgrande D, Lonjon G, Hardy P, Schoch B, Werthel J-D. Long-term results of arthroscopic Bankart repairs for anterior instability of the shoulder in patients aged thirty years or older. Int Orthop. 2021;45:1583–9. https://doi.org/10.1007/s00264-021-05014-4.
7. Murthi AM, Ramirez MA. Shoulder dislocation in the older patient. J Am Acad Orthop

Surg. 2012;20:615–22. https://doi.org/10.5435/JAAOS-20-10-615.
8. Gumina S, Postacchini F. Anterior dislocation of the shoulder in elderly patients. J Bone Joint Surg Br. 1997;79:540–3. https://doi.org/10.1302/0301-620x.79b4.7497.
9. Cole BJ, Millett PJ, Romeo AA, Burkhart SS, Andrews JR, Dugas JR, Warner JJ. Arthroscopic treatment of anterior glenohumeral instability: indications and techniques. Instr Course Lect. 2004;53:545–58.
10. Calvo E, Granizo JJ, Fernández-Yruegas D. Criteria for arthroscopic treatment of anterior instability of the shoulder: a prospective study. J Bone Joint Surg Br. 2005;87:677–83. https://doi.org/10.1302/0301-620X.87B5.15794.
11. Velasquez Garcia A, Chaney GK, Ingala Martini L, Valenti P. The Trillat procedure for anterior Glenohumeral instability. JBJS Rev. 2022;10 https://doi.org/10.2106/JBJS.RVW.22.00049.
12. Shekhbihi A, Bauer S, Walch A, Reichert W, Walch G, Boileau P. The Trillat procedure: the man and the technique revisited through the lens of arthroscopy. EFORT Open Rev. 2024;9:923–32. https://doi.org/10.1530/EOR-23-0208.
13. Housset V, Chevallier R, Nourissat G. Open Trillat procedure for recurrent anterior instability of the shoulder in elderly patients. Arthrosc Tech. 2021;10:e1211–6. https://doi.org/10.1016/j.eats.2021.01.021.
14. Boileau P, Clowez G, Bouacida S, Walch G, Trojani C, Schwartz DG. The arthroscopic Trillat procedure is a valuable treatment option for recurrent anterior instability in young athletes with shoulder hyperlaxity. Arthroscopy. 2023;39:948–58. https://doi.org/10.1016/j.arthro.2022.10.046.
15. Labattut L, Bertrand V, Reybet Degat PY, Arcens M, Trouilloud P, Baulot E, Martz P. Arthroscopy-assisted Trillat procedure for anterior shoulder instability: surgical technique and preliminary clinical results. Orthop Traumatol Surg Res OTSR. 2018;104:811–6. https://doi.org/10.1016/j.otsr.2017.12.022.
16. Kazum E, Martinez-Catalan N, Oussama R, Eichinger JK, Werthel JD, Valenti P. Arthroscopic Trillat procedure combined with capsuloplasty: an effective treatment modality for shoulder instability associated with hyperlaxity. Knee Surg Sports Traumatol Arthrosc Off J ESSKA. 2022;30:2067–73. https://doi.org/10.1007/s00167-021-06752-z.
17. Jouve F, Graveleau N, Nové-Josserand L, Walch G. Recurrent anterior instability of the shoulder associated with full thickness rotator cuff tear: results of surgical treatment. Rev Chir Orthop Reparatrice Appar Mot. 2008;94:659–69. https://doi.org/10.1016/j.rco.2008.03.032.
18. Walch G, Dejour H, Trillat AG. Recurrent anterior luxation of the shoulder occurring after the age of 40. Rev Chir Orthop Reparatrice Appar Mot. 1987;73:609–16.
19. Gerber C, Terrier F, Ganz R. The Trillat procedure for recurrent anterior instability of the shoulder. J Bone Joint Surg Br. 1988;70:130–4. https://doi.org/10.1302/0301-620X.70B1.3339045.
20. Trillat A. Treatment of recurrent dislocation of the shoulder; technical considerations. Lyon Chir. 1954;49:986–93.

Part III

Case Presentations

Combined Bankart and SLAP Lesion Repair/LHB Tenodesis

18

Oleg Milenin

Key Points

- Combined Bankart and SLAP lesion is a common problem of shoulder pathology.
- Labroplasty and simultaneous trans-subscapular transposition of the long head of the biceps can simultaneously treat biceps and anterior inferior labral lesion.
- This is our method of choice for treatment of SLAP and Bankart lesions with combination of poor quality gleno-humeral ligaments with or without sub-critical anterior-inferior bone loss.

18.1 Introduction

- Combined Bankart and SLAP lesions is a common finding in acute and chronic anterior shoulder instability. SLAP lesion in most cases spreads to the anterior-inferior direction (37% of all SLAP lesions [1].
- The frequency of combined Bankart and SLAP lesions is approximately 20 to 57% according to the publications of Moretti and Gartsman [2, 3].
- The refixation of glenoid labrum and SLAP repair is a golden standard of treatment for the young patients. The recurrence rate after combined SLAP/bankart repair was 6.47% [4].
- On the other side SLAP repair for middle-aged patients is still controversial and some authors recommend tenodesis of the long head of the biceps [5]. Thus, the combination of the Bankart repair and LHB tenodesis can be one of the possible options of the treatment of middle-aged patients.
- The treatment algorithm for the patients with combined Bankart and SLAP II tear associated with poor quality of gleno-humeral ligaments is still controversial. One of the possible options of the treatment for young patients with this type of lesion is combination of SLAP repair with Latarjet procedure. However, simultaneous LHB tenodesis and conjoint tendon transposition (Latarjet procedure) can disturb the proprioception and the function of the both biceps heads. A new alternative method of treatment of this combination is a dynamic anterior stabilization with the long head of the biceps (DAS-procedure) recently described by several authors [6–8].

Supplementary Information The online version contains supplementary material available at https://doi.org/10.1007/978-3-662-73064-5_18.

O. Milenin (✉)
National Medical Surgical Center, Moscow, Russia

L. Kovačič et al. (eds.), *Surgical Techniques for Anterior Shoulder Instability*,
https://doi.org/10.1007/978-3-662-73064-5_18

- In recent years, more and more results of dynamic anterior stabilization have been published, showing good results: low recurrence rate, return to full range of motion and athletic activity [9–12].
- For these patients, we described the repair augmentation by labroplasty and simultaneous trans-subscapular transposition of the long head of the biceps [13].
- This technique is our method of choice for treatment of SLAP and Bankart lesions with combination of poor quality gleno-humeral ligaments with or without subcritical anterior-inferior bone loss.

18.2 Clinical Case

- A 40 years-old female with chronic anterior-inferior instability of the right-shoulder with full range of motion. ROWE-score: 55.
- Complaints include moderate limitation of swimming and over-head work, anterior shoulder pain in over-head activities.
- Objective findings include pain in the bicipital groove, moderate pain during apprehension test, positive HERI test, O'Brien test—positive, sulcus-sign was negative, no hyperlaxity was observed, and the range of motion was full.
- SLAP II and Bankart lesions are presented on MRI. There is no Hill-Sachs lesion; subcritical anterior inferior glenoid bone loss is observed.(Fig. 18.1).

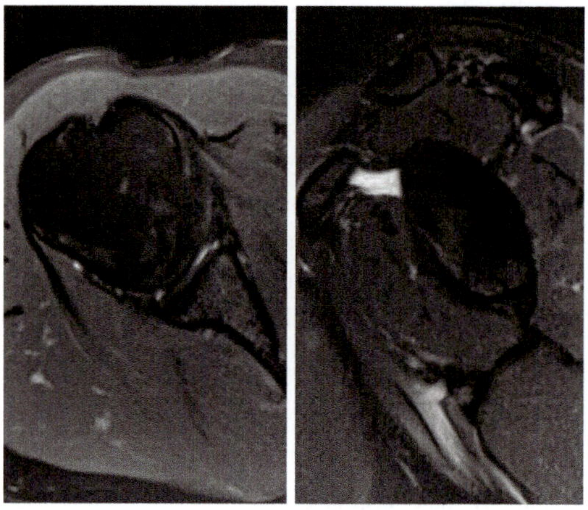

Fig. 18.1 Pre-operative MRI of the right shoulder

18.3 Surgical Technique

- The procedure is performed with the patient in the beach chair position and the injured arm (right arm herein) in a traction of 1.5 kg.
- Three standard portals are used. The posterior portal, anterosuperior, and anteromedial portal, and an additional suprapectoral portal, which is located 3–4 cm inferior from the standard anterosuperior portal in the projection of the cross-section of the biceps groove at the insertion site of the superior edge of the pectoralis major tendon.
- After diagnostic arthroscopy, the arthroscope is transferred to the anterior-superior portal (Fig. 18.2). After tenotomy of the long head of the biceps, the arthroscope is transferred into the subdeltoid space. The tendon of the long head is mobilized, captured, and passed through an additional lateral portal. The end of the tendon of the long head of the biceps is stitched 15 mm long with the nonabsorbable suture tape (Fig. 18.3).
- After mobilization of the capsule on front edge of the glenoid the drill-guide is placed on 4 o'clock position. 2.4 mm guide pin with eyelet is drilled through the glenoid from anterior to posterior direction.
- After that 4.5 mm tunnel through the scapula is drilled. The 4.5 mm button with self-locking clinch (ProClinch TM) is passed through the

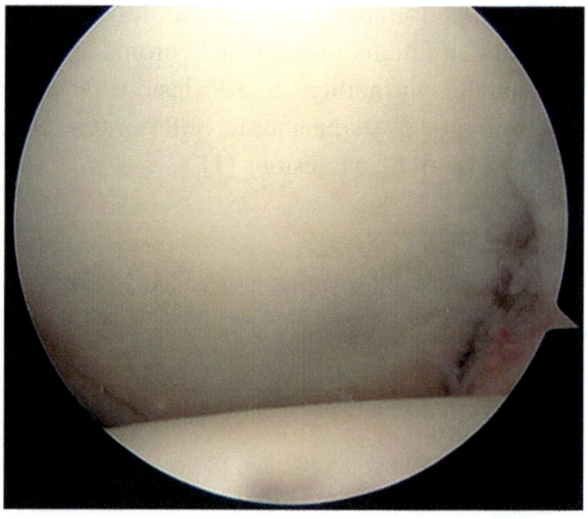

Fig. 18.2 Intra-articular view of Bankart lesion through the anterior superior portal

tunnel. Previously, to ease manipulation non-absorbable suture is passed through the ProClinch loop.

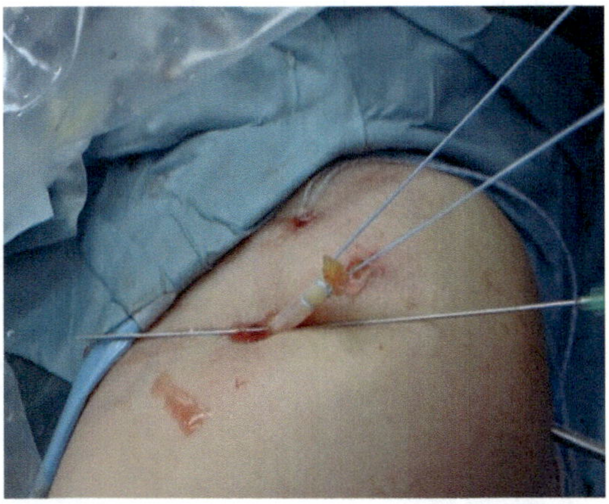

Fig. 18.3 Extra-articular view of the right shoulder. The end of the tendon of the long head of the biceps is stitched with non-absorbable sutures

- The suture manipulator is placed through posterior portal and passed through the threads of the ProClinch device. After that ProClinch is a little bit tightened for better visualization, then the tip of the suture manipulator gently perforates the subscapularis muscle.
- After that arthroscope is transferred to the subdeltoid space. After the dissection of the space between conjoint tendon and the subscapular muscle, we inspect the axillary nerve. With second suture manipulator that is placed through the additional suprapectoral portal threads which are fixed to the tips of the biceps are passed to the first suture manipulator and further passed through the joint (Fig. 18.4).
- After dissection of adhesions and mobilization of the biceps under the pectoralis muscle, we observe the sling-effect of the biceps.
- The ProClinch device is completely tightened, and the tip of the biceps is additionally fixed

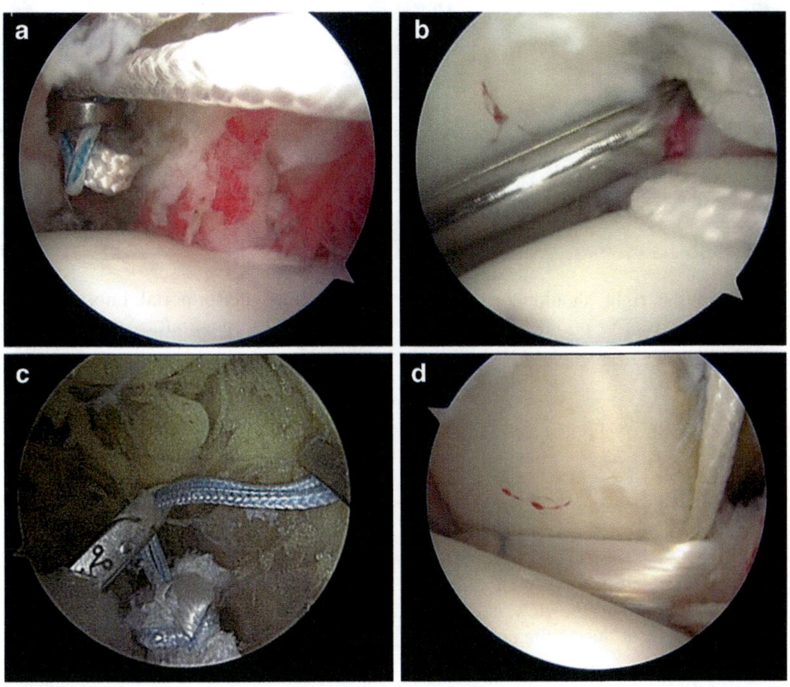

Fig. 18.4 Intra-articular view of the right shoulder from anterior superior portal. (**a**) The button with self-locking clinch is passed through the pre-drilled tunnel. (**b**) The suture manipulator is placed through posterior portal and passed through the threads of the ProClich device. (**c**) The suture manipulator is inserted from the posterior portal, the tip of the suture manipulator gently perforates the subscapular muscle in the 5 o'clock position of the glenoid, and captures the sutures attached to the tip of LHB tendon. (**d**) Biceps is transported into the joint and through ProClinch loop

with the knotless 2.9 mm pushlock anchor on the 1 o'clock position.
- The sutures previously placed in the 1 and 4 o'clock position for biceps fixation are used for labrum fixation (Fig. 18.5).
- Additionally, capsule is fixed at 5 o'clock position with the knotless anchor. At the end of the procedure the position and tightness of the button is visualized through the posterior portal. Additional knots can be made if necessary (Fig. 18.6).
- All the steps are demonstrated in Video 18.1.
- Pearls and pitfalls are shown in the Table 18.1.

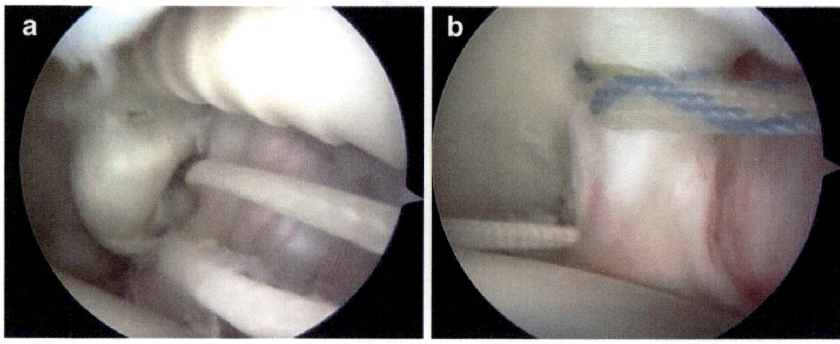

Fig. 18.5 Intra-articular view of the right shoulder. (**a**) The tip of the tendon is fixed with a knotless anchor at 1 o'clock position. (**b**) The capsule is additionally fixed to same sutures

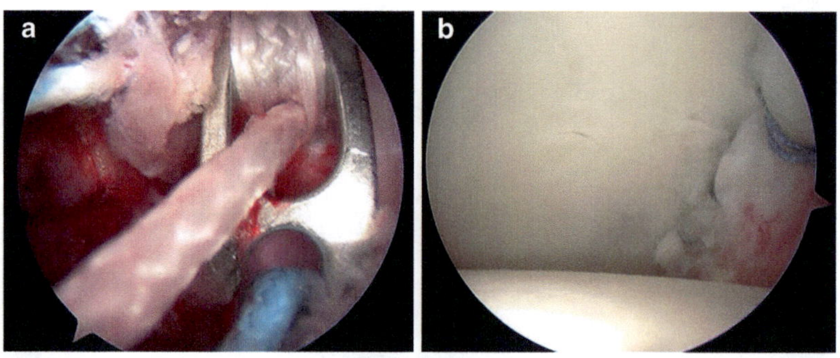

Fig. 18.6 The view of the right shoulder. (**a**) Extra-articular view through the posterior portal. The button is placed on the subscapular neck. (**b**) Final view through the anterior superior portal. Labrum and capsule are fixed above the biceps graft. Acceptable bumper effect is achieved

Table 18.1 Pearls and pitfalls of surgical technique

Pearls	Pitfalls
Preparation of glenoid bed is critical for strong graft healing to the glenoid	Perforation of the subscapularis should always be performed under visualization because of a very high risk of vascular injuries
Use of a switching stick as an elevator from an additional portal creates more space, improves the view, and protects neurovascular structures during the perforation of the subscapularis muscle	Mobilization of the biceps tendon should be far from the under pectoralis major muscle because it is critical for prophylaxis of postoperative biceps pain
Accurate placement of the button on the posterior surface of the glenoid neck is critical and should be expected extra-articullary through the posterior portal	

18.4 Post-Op Protocol and Clinical Results

- Four to six weeks of immobilization in 15 degrees abduction sling with neutral rotation is recommended. Time of immobilization depends on the quality of the tissue.
- Standard Bankart procedure rehabilitation protocol is recommended.
- Six weeks after procedure good bumper and sling effect can be observed on MRI (Fig. 18.7).
- Twelve weeks after the procedure acceptable range of motion is achieved (Fig. 18.8), ROWE-score: 95.
- Participation in active and competitive sports and overhead activities are not recommended 4–6 months after the procedure.

Disadvantages and possible complications:

- There is a risk of axillary nerve injury during the perforation of subscapularis muscle from the inside-out direction.
- Theoretically, there is a possibility of biceps pain after the procedure.
- Procedure is not recommended in cases of poor quality of the biceps tendon or previous procedures with biceps tenodesis or tenotomy.
- In cases of glenoid bone loss >20% or significant Hill-Sachs lesions, it is not recommended to perform described technique as a single procedure without any additional techniques including bone graft.
- Procedure is not recommended in case of total absence of the capsule structure.

Expert recommendation

- In case of SLAP lesion, described procedure simultaneously treats this pathology.
- Procedure can significantly reinforce the Bankart procedure in cases of poor-quality glenohumeral ligaments by the synergy of the anterior labroplasty and sling effect of dynamic tenodesis.

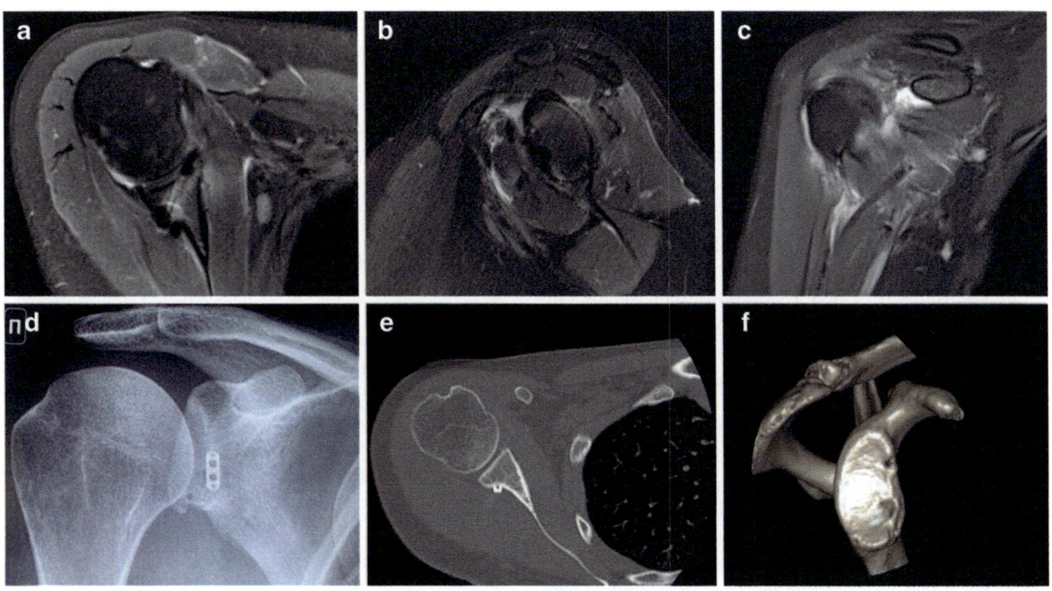

Fig. 18.7 (**a**) MRI 6 weeks after the surgery. Axial view. Good bumper effect and capsular healing is achieved. (**b**) MRI 6 weeks after the surgery. Saggital view. Labroplasty and good anterior interior bone defect filling with biceps are achieved. (**c**) MRI 6 weeks after the surgery. Frontal view. The sling effect of the procedure is achieved. (**d**) Post-operative X-ray. Anterior posterior view. Good position of the button is observed. (**e**) Post-operative CT scan. Axial view. Good position of the button is observed. (**f**) Post-operative 3D CT scan. Positions of the 1 o'clock anchor and 4 o'clock tunnel are observed

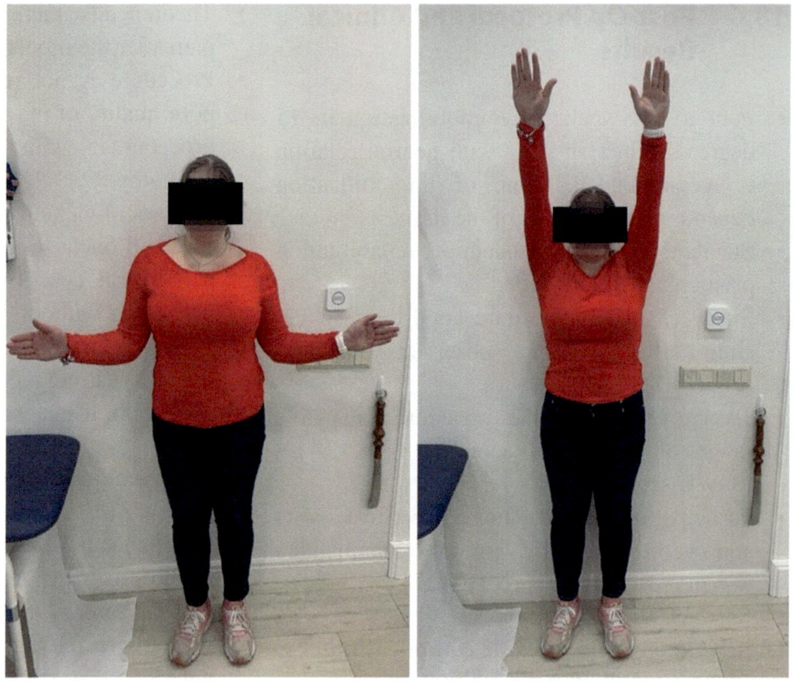

Fig. 18.8 The patient 12 weeks after the procedure. Full range of motion is achieved

- Procedure can be performed in cases of subcritical glenoid bone loss if there are any doubts in choosing soft-tissue or bone reconstruction procedure.
- Procedure can be performed together with bone block or remplissage techniques.

References

1. Morgan CD, Burkhart SS, Palmeri M, Gillespie M. Type II SLAP lesions: three subtypes and their relationships to superior instability and rotator cuff tears. Arthroscopy. 1998;14(6):553–65.
2. Garofalo R, Mocci A, Moretti B, Callari E, Di Giacomo G, Theumann N, et al. Arthroscopic treatment of anterior shoulder instability using knotless suture anchors. Arthroscopy. 2005;21(11):1283–9.
3. Gartsman GM, Roddey TS, Hammerman SM. Arthroscopic treatment of anterior-inferior glenohumeral instability: two to five-year follow-up. JBJS. 2000;82(7):991.
4. Feng S, Song Y, Li H, Chen J, Chen J, Chen S. Outcomes for arthroscopic repair of combined bankart/SLAP lesions in the treatment of anterior shoulder instability: a systematic review and meta-analysis. Orthop J Sports Med. 2019;7(10):2325967119877804.
5. Boileau P, Parratte S, Chuinard C, Roussanne Y, Shia D, Bicknell R. Arthroscopic treatment of isolated type II SLAP lesions: biceps tenodesis as an alternative to reinsertion. Am J Sports Med. 2009;37(5):929–36.
6. Tang J, Zhao J. Arthroscopic transfer of the long head of the biceps brachii for anterior shoulder instability. Arthrosc Tech. 2017;6(5):e1911–7.
7. Collin P, Lädermann A. Dynamic anterior stabilization using the long head of the biceps for anteroinferior glenohumeral instability. Arthrosc Tech. 2018;7(1):e39–44.
8. de Campos Azevedo CI, Ângelo AC. Dynamic anterior stabilization of the shoulder: Onlay biceps transfer to the anterior glenoid using the double double-pulley technique. Arthrosc Tech. 2023;12(7):e1097–106.
9. Collin P, Nabergoj M, Denard PJ, Wang S, Bothorel H, Lädermann A. Arthroscopic biceps transfer to the glenoid with Bankart repair grants satisfactory 2-year results for recurrent anteroinferior glenohumeral instability in subcritical bone loss. Arthroscopy. 2022;38(6):1766–71.
10. de Campos Azevedo C, Ângelo AC. Onlay dynamic anterior stabilization with biceps transfer for the treatment of anterior glenohumeral instability produces good clinical outcomes and successful healing at a minimum 1 year of follow-up. Arthrosc Sports Med Rehabil. 2023;5(2):e445–57.
11. Jain N, McKeeman J, Higgins M, Johnson A, Smith T, Waterman B. Dynamic anterior shoulder stabilization using a long head of the biceps transfer and Bankart repair improves clinical outcomes in patients with subcritical bone loss: a systematic review. Arthrosc Sports Med Rehabil. 2025;7(3):101141.

12. Avram G, Neculau DC, Tomescu H, et al. Dynamic anterior stabilization for recurrent anterior shoulder instability improves postoperative patient-reported outcomes without restricting shoulder range of motion: a meta-analysis. Int Orthopaed (SICOT). 2025;49(9):1931–41.
13. Milenin O, Toussaint B. Labral repair augmentation by labroplasty and simultaneous trans-subscapular transposition of the long head of the biceps. Arthrosc Tech. 2019;8(5):e507–12.

19 HAGL Lesions

Naman Wahal, Abdullah Alabbasi, and Frank Martetschläger

Key Points

HAGL lesions are relatively uncommon lesions that can lead to shoulder instability

High index of clinical suspicion in cases of traumatic instability can prevent missing these injuries

Classic J shaped appearance of the axillary pouch on MRI

Should be looked for in cases with recurrence of instability after failed surgical management

Open and Arthroscopic repair of HAGL lesions have excellent outcomes

19.1 Introduction/Background

- The term HAGL or the Humeral Avulsion of Glenohumeral Ligaments was coined by Wolf et al. in 1995 [1] describing an injury of the capsuloligamentous attachments to the Humerus leading to shoulder instability.
- In comparison to the tear of the labrum complex, HAGL is a relatively rare cause of shoulder instability, resulting from the tear or avulsion of the most important static stabilizer i.e. the Inferior Glenohumeral Ligament (IGHL) at its humeral attachment [2, 3].

19.2 Epidemiology

- HAGL is a relatively uncommon diagnosis with a reported incidence of 2.1 to 9.3% in cases of anterior instability [1, 4]. Mostly occurring in combination with other lesions such as Labrum tear, Subscapularis tear and Hill Sachs lesions, it can also occur in isolation [2, 5]. The incidence can be higher (up to 40%) when looking at specific subgroups of anterior instability with no labrum lesions [6].
- Overwhelming majority of cases are associated with a history of trauma causing dislocation or subluxation of shoulder. However, some reports claim repetitive microtrauma as another possible mechanism [7].

Supplementary Information The online version contains supplementary material available at https://doi.org/10.1007/978-3-662-73064-5_19.

N. Wahal
Fortis Escorts Hospital, New Delhi, India

A. Alabbasi
King Fahad Armed Forces Hosh, Jeddah, Saudi Arabia

F. Martetschläger (✉)
German Center of Shoulder Surgery, Atos Clinic Munich, Munich, Bayern, Germany
e-mail: f.martetschlaeger@d-s-z.de

L. Kovačič et al. (eds.), *Surgical Techniques for Anterior Shoulder Instability*, https://doi.org/10.1007/978-3-662-73064-5_19

- Male predominance [8].
- Average age of 25–35 years but has been reported in 12–79 years of age [2, 4].

19.3 Pathophysiology

- IGHL is the primary static stabilizer of the shoulder joint. It functions as a 'hammock' with its anterior and posterior bands inserting on Humerus in a 'collar' like or a 'V-shaped' manner with an interposed axillary pouch [9, 10].
- Anterior band is the primary stabilizer in abduction and external rotation while the posterior band is the primary stabilizer in flexion and internal rotation.
- Hyperabduction of the arm along with external rotation is considered the possible mechanism of injury. In contrast, Bankart lesion is associated with hyperabduction only or with less degrees of external rotation [11, 12].
- Bui et al. [8] gave the West Point nomenclature for classification of HAGL lesions depending on the band of IGHL involved (posterior or anterior), presence or absence of bony fragment and the associated labrum disruption.
- Disruption of axillary pouch of IGHL as a cause of instability was reported in a short case series of 4 female volleyball players by Taljanovic et al. [7].

19.4 History

- Complaints of instability along with nonspecific shoulder complaints in a male patient of 25–35 years of age is the usual presentation.
- Mechanism of trauma especially the position of arm in hyperabduction and external rotation at the time of injury.
- A note should be made of the direction of instability, history and number of dislocations or subjective feeling of instability.
- Previous surgeries especially a failed shoulder stabilization surgery (Bankart repair or capsular shift) can indicate a previously missed HAGL lesion [13].
- Presence or absence of neurological symptoms such as paraesthesia should also be mentioned in the report.

19.5 Physical Findings

- Indicative of instability. Not specific or sensitive for HAGL lesions.
- Inspection for muscle atrophy; diffuse in cases of disuse or focal in cases of associated neurological injury.
- Positive provocative manoeuvres such as:
  - Apprehension test and relocation test.
  - The load and shift test.
  - the Jerk test.
- Neurological examination to rule out brachial plexus or axillary nerve injury [14].

19.6 Relevant Imaging

- Radiographs
  - Bony avulsion can be seen occasionally [12].
  - True Antero-Posterior (AP) view in neutral and internal rotation.
  - Scapular Y films.
  - Axillary view to evaluate Hill-Sachs and glenoid fractures.
  - Garth view (optional) taken as 15 degree oblique view to visualize the bony HAGL (BHAGL) [15].
- MRI with or without contrast is the gold standard
  - Sensitivity of 70% and a specificity of 100% [4].
  - J sign—pathognomonic sign for HAGL on coronal T-2 fat suppressed images.
  - The axillary pouch appears J shaped instead of the usual U shape in HAGL lesion due to the escape of dye or the joint fluid.
  - In chronic cases due to scarring the J sign may not be visible.

19.7 Treatment Options and Indications

- Non-operative:
  - Sling treatment with physiotherapy.
  - Recurrence rate reported to be as high as 90% [5, 16].
- Surgical management:
  - Young, active and high demand individuals.
- Open repair and arthroscopic repair:
  - Satisfactory outcomes with low recurrence rates in both techniques [2, 16].
  - Presence of concomitant lesions such as rotator cuff tear may prevent the return to previous sport levels [17].
- Mini open technique has also been described sparing the superior 50% of the Subscapularis tendon by making a L shaped incision [18].

19.8 Decision-Making Algorithm (Fig. 19.1)

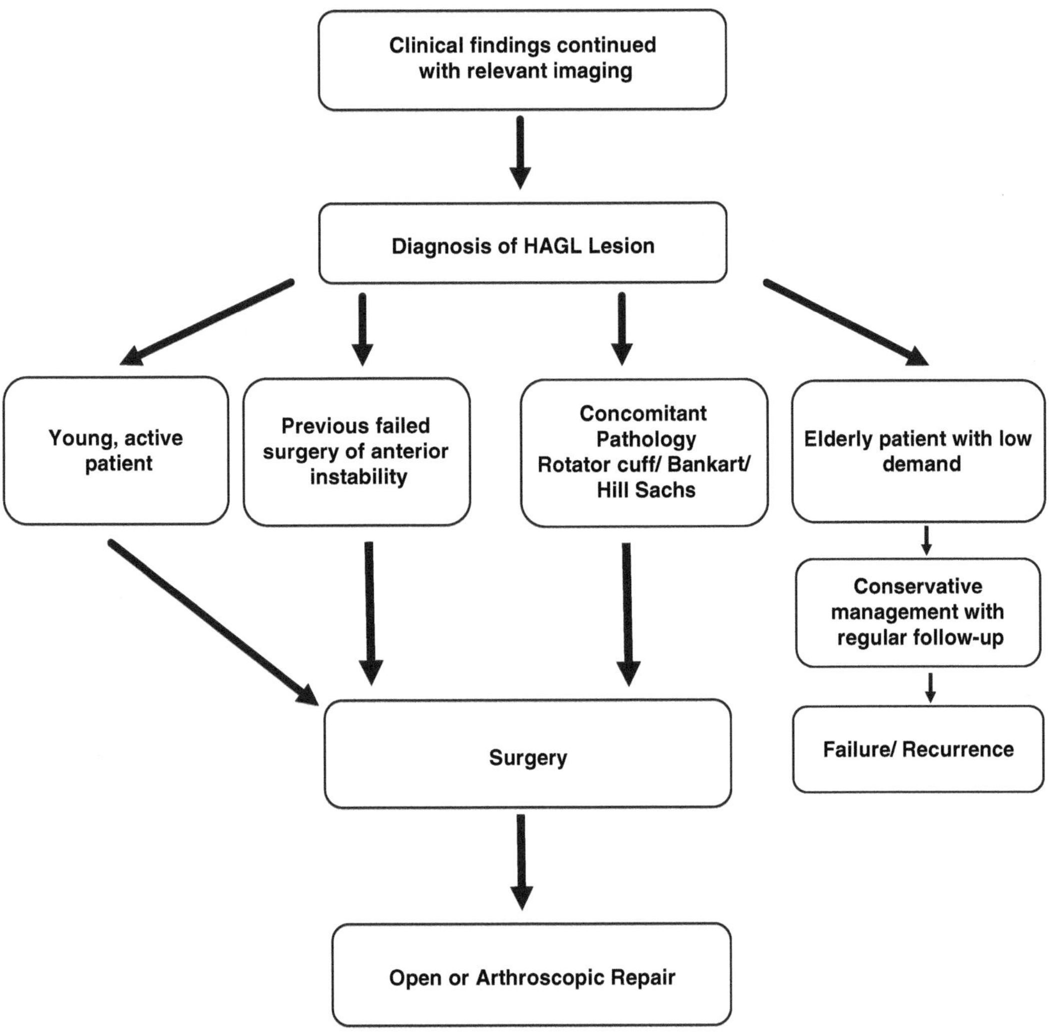

Fig. 19.1 Decision making algorithm for HAGL lesion. HAGL Humeral Avulsion of Glenohumeral Ligament

19.9 Clinical Case

A 52-year-old male presented to our Shoulder Center with complaints of

- Recurrent Right shoulder dislocation—the first episode of dislocation 6 years ago, following a mountain bike accident. The dislocation was reduced at the emergency department of the nearby hospital under sedation. No operative intervention was performed and patient was managed conservatively with a sling and physiotherapy.
- The patient suffered multiple spontaneous dislocations of the shoulder which he was able to reduce spontaneously.
- There was reduced function of shoulder with limitation of external rotation.
- No complaints of pain. No complaints of any paraesthesia suggestive of neurological involvement.
- Physical examination revealed—a positive apprehension test and relocation test. No neurological deficit was observed.

19.10 Xray Findings (Fig. 19.2)

- Anteroposterior (AP), Y-Scapular, and axillary views were obtained. No significant bone loss; no fractures were observed.

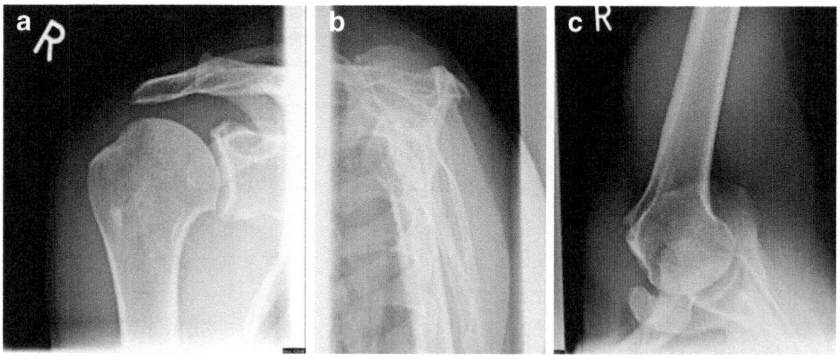

Fig. 19.2 Showing the standard Radiographs with no abnormal findings. (**a**) Antero-posterior View, (**b**) Scapular View and (**c**) Axillary view

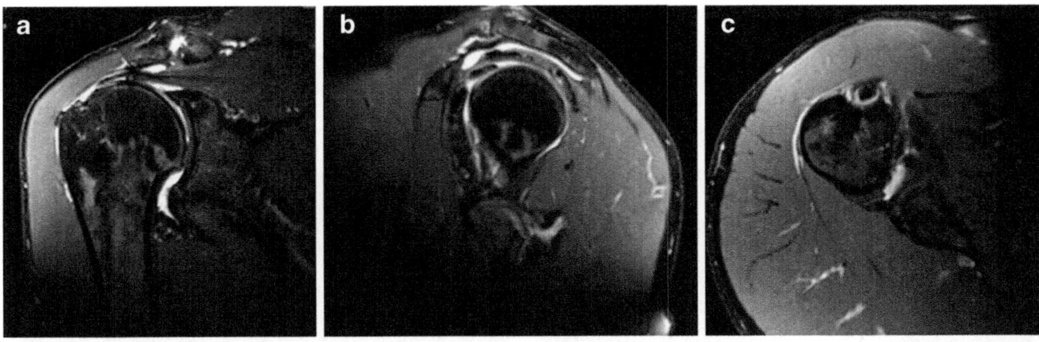

Fig. 19.3 Showing the MRI images. (**a**) Coronal T2 image showing the J-shaped axillary pouch. (**b** and **c**) showing the avulsion of Glenohumeral Ligament from the humeral attachment side

19.11 MRI Findings (Fig. 19.3)

- J-Shaped inferior pouch known as J-sign seen on coronal T2 weighted fat suppressed MRI.
- Avulsion of the gleno-humeral ligament seen on the humeral site in other sagittal and axial slides.
- Presence of Biceps Pulley lesion, SLAP lesion, Supraspinatus and subscapularis tear were also seen on the MRI.

19.12 Operative Technique (Video 19.1)

- Patient was placed in the standard Beach chair position under general anaesthesia and additional suprascapular nerve block for the right shoulder.
- Range of motion under anaesthesia was full and free in all planes. Anterior translation of humeral head relative to glenoid was observed.
- After cleaning and draping by the sterile technique, a standard posterior portal was established for performing a diagnostic arthroscopy.
- A note of the Biceps Pulley lesion, SLAP lesion, Supraspinatus tear and Subscapularis tear was made along with the presence of HAGL lesion (Fig. 19.4). The muscle striations of the Subscapularis were visible in the anterior inferior corner.
- An anterosuperior portal was created under direct visualization through rotator interval for management of the pulley lesion and the SLAP lesion.
- An anteroinferior portal (5 o'clock position, trans-subscapularis portal) was then established using 'outside-in' technique and biceps tenotomy followed by tenodesis was performed.
- Next the HAGL lesion was addressed. First the humeral bone bed for the attachment of anterior band of IGHL was prepared through the antero-inferior portal.
- Adhesiolysis was performed meticulously to aid visualization and mobilization of the IGHL and the capsule.
- Fiberwire (Arthrex, Naples, FL) sutures were then passed through the IGHL from antero-superior portal using the right sided Suture lasso (Arthrex, Naples, FL) and shuttled through the Antero-inferior portal. Using a drill-sleeve, a drill hole was created at the prepared site (distal to the lesser tuberosity anteriorly) for the insertion of 2.9 mm Push-Lock Anchor (Arthrex, Naples, FL) (Fig. 19.5). The fixation of anteroinferior capsule and the IGHL was achieved through knotless sutures (Figs. 19.6 and 19.7). Arthroscopic probe was used to test the tension and integrity of the repair.
- Subscapularis repair followed by Supraspinatus repair was then performed by the standard double row repair technique using Suture Anchors (Arthrex, Naples, FL) and Swivel Lock (Arthrex, Naples, FL).

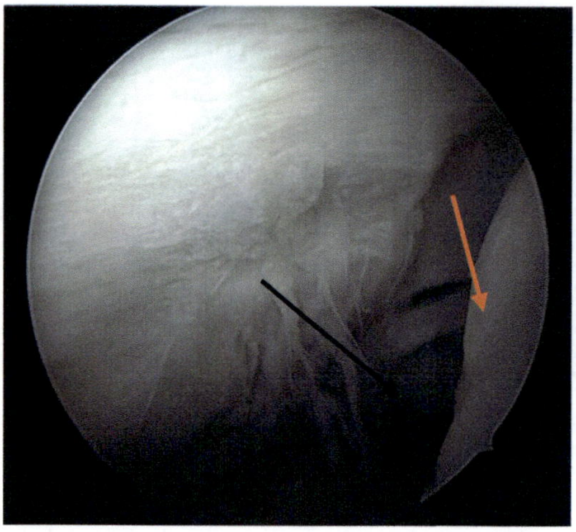

Fig. 19.4 Showing the arthroscopic image. Diagnostic arthroscopic image through the standard posterior portal showing the detached Anterior Band (black arrow) of Inferior Glenohumeral Ligament (IGHL) from the Humeral (orange arrow) side

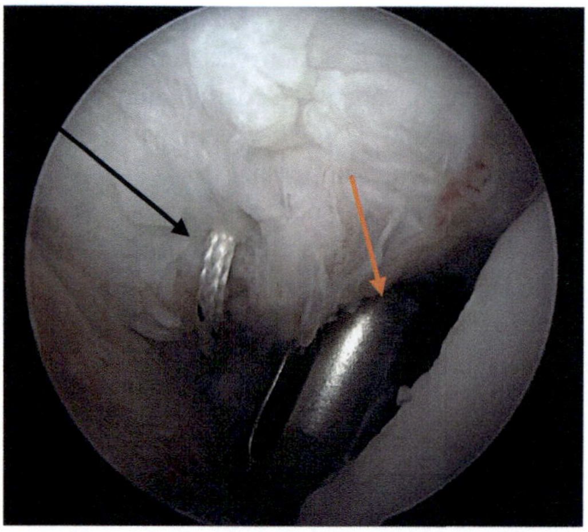

Fig. 19.5 Showing the suture through the Inferior Gleno humeral ligament (black arrow) and the drill sleeve (orange arrow) after removing the drill used for drilling hole for insertion of 2.9 mm Push-Lock Anchor (Arthrex, Naples, FL)

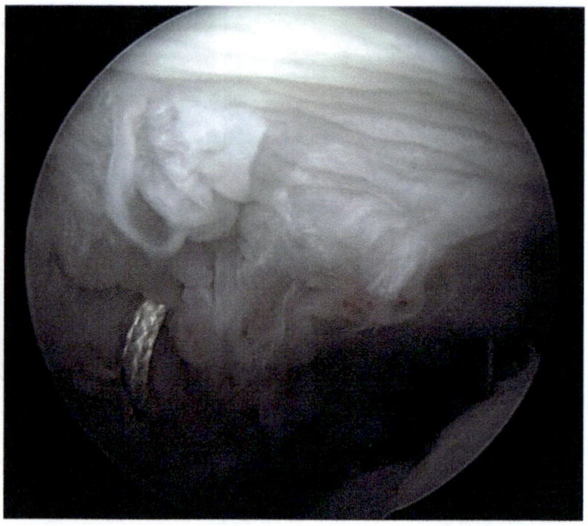

Fig. 19.6 Showing the insertion of the insertion of 2.9 mm Push-Lock Anchor (Arthrex, Naples, FL) with the suture

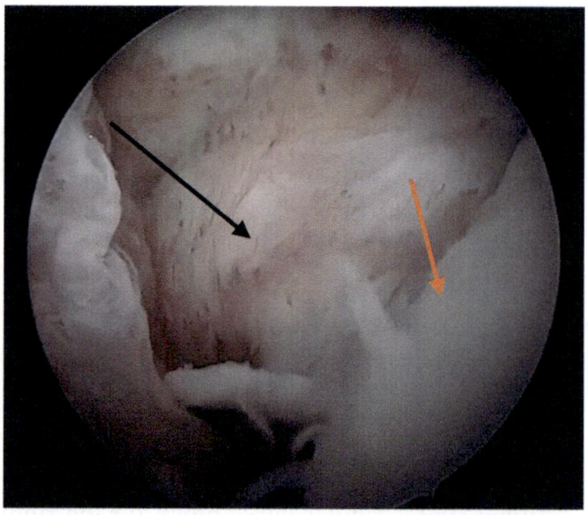

Fig. 19.7 Showing the attached Inferior Glenohumeral Ligament (black arrow) to the Humerus (orange arrow)

19.13 Post-operative Rehabilitation Protocol [19]

- A shoulder immobilizer with abduction pillow is used for 6 weeks. Elbow and wrist mobilization exercises should be started immediately with adequate pain management.
- Gradually progressive passive range of motion is initiated at 3 weeks with avoidance of anterior loading of IGHL complex.
- Active range of motion is usually started at 6 weeks with gradual weaning of the orthosis.
- Strengthening exercises for the rotator cuff, deltoid trapezius and biceps can be started from 8th–10th week.

19.14 Tips and Tricks

1.	Patient Positioning	Lateral preferred by some surgeons for better visualization Adaptable water pump to maintain a bloodless working field Arm abducted by 50 degree and flexed by 20 degree facilitates accurate reduction of IGHL Posterior force on the head by assistant aids the proper placement of anchors
2.	Accessory portals	If necessary use of postero-inferior (7 o'clock) described by Davidson and Rivenburgh [20] as visualizing portal
3.	Avoid nerve injury	Using spinal needle with outside-in technique to establish portals [19]
4.	Knotless sutures	To prevent glenohumeral cartilage abrasion
5.	Reducing the surgical time	Familiarity with the instruments and implants
6.	Concomitant pathologies	Thorough diagnostic arthroscopy to visualize all the possible pathologies and then treat them in stepwise manner

19.15 Outcomes

- Owing to the relative rarity of the lesion, there is a paucity of literature on outcomes.
- Mostly restricted to short case series and reports, the studies report excellent outcomes with 0% recurrent rates and return to sports after both open and arthroscopic procedures [15, 21–24]. On the other hand the recurrence rates after non-surgical management has been reported as high as 90–100% [1, 16, 21]. The systemic review of 11 studies by Longo et al. [16] established the odds ratio of 0.05 for recurrence after surgical repair as compared to conservative management. They also reported some loss of external rotation following the surgical repair. These results were confirmed by a systemic review of 18 studies by Bozzo et al. [2].
- Provencher et al. [25] compared the outcomes after open and arthroscopic repair of HAGL and reported excellent outcomes and full return to sporting activity with both procedures at a mean follow-up of 32 months. Schmiddem et al. [17] reported some loss of external rotation and decrease in the level of sporting activity after arthroscopic repair of IGHL in 4 female volleyball athletes at a long term follow-up of 5 years.

19.16 Potential Complications/ Difficulties

- Stiffness and decreased external rotation:
  - Adherence to a strict physiotherapy and rehabilitation program can prevent stiffness.
- Axillary nerve injury
- Chondrolysis

   - Avoid overtightening of the capsule. Use knotless sutures.
- Recurrence of instability
   - Very rare with both open and arthroscopic procedures.

19.17 Expert Recommendation

- High suspicion of HAGL lesion in patients with recurrent instability and failed initial stabilization procedure.
- Thorough history and clinical examination.
- Surgical complications can be avoided by preoperative planning. Planning the sequence of repair for HAGL and the concomitant lesions along with the use of accessory portals makes the surgery less challenging.

References

1. Wolf EM, Cheng JC, Dickson K. Humeral avulsion of glenohumeral ligaments as a cause of anterior shoulder instability. Arthrosc J Arthrosc Relat Surg. 1995;11(5):600–7.
2. Bozzo A, Oitment C, Thornley P, Yan J, Habib A, Hoppe DJ, et al. Humeral avulsion of the Glenohumeral ligament: indications for surgical treatment and outcomes—a systematic review. Orthop J Sports Med. 2017;5(8):232596711772332.
3. Bigliani LU, Pollock RG, Soslowsky LJ, Flatow EL, Pawluk RJ, Mow VC. Tensile properties of the inferior glenohumeral ligament. J Orthop Res. 1992;10(2):187–97.
4. Magee T. Prevalence of HAGL lesions and associated abnormalities on shoulder MR examination. Skeletal Radiol. 2014;43(3):307–13.
5. Ferguson M. Humeral avulsion of the Glenohumeral ligaments (HAGL) in shoulder instability. In: Imhoff A, Savoie IIIF, editors. Shoulder instability across the life span. Berlin/Heidelberg: Springer; 2017. https://doi.org/10.1007/978-3-662-54077-0_14.
6. Bokor DJ, Conboy VB, Olson C. Anterior instability of the glenohumeral joint with humeral avulsion of the glenohumeral ligament. J Bone Joint Surg Br. 1999;81-B(1):93–6.
7. Taljanovic MS, Nisbet JK, Hunter TB, Cohen RP, Rogers LF. Humeral avulsion of the inferior Glenohumeral ligament in college female volleyball players caused by repetitive microtrauma. Am J Sports Med. 2011;39(5):1067–76.
8. Bui-Mansfield LT, Banks KP, Taylor DC. Humeral avulsion of the Glenohumeral ligaments: the HAGL lesion. Am J Sports Med. 2007;35(11):1960–6.
9. Burkart AC, Debski RE. Anatomy and function of the Glenohumeral ligaments in anterior shoulder instability. Clin Orthop Relat Res. 2002;400:32–9.
10. O'Brien SJ, Neves MC, Arnoczky SP, Rozbruck SR, Dicarlo EF, Warren RF, et al. The anatomy and histology of the inferior glenohumeral ligament complex of the shoulder. Am J Sports Med. 1990;18(5):449–56.
11. Nicola T. Acute anterior dislocation of the shoulder [Internet]. J Bone Joint Surg Am. 1949. https://pubmed.ncbi.nlm.nih.gov/18106758/
12. Bui-Mansfield LT, Taylor DC, Uhorchak JM, Tenuta JJ. Humeral avulsions of the glenohumeral ligament: imaging features and a review of the literature. AJR Am J Roentgenol. 2002;179(3):649–55. https://doi.org/10.2214/ajr.179.3.1790649.
13. George MS, Khazzam M, Kuhn JE. Humeral avulsion of glenohumeral ligaments. J Am Acad Orthop Surg. 2011;19(3):127–33. https://doi.org/10.5435/00124635-201103000-00001.
14. Gutkowska O, Martynkiewicz J, Urban M, Gosk J. Brachial plexus injury after shoulder dislocation: a literature review. Neurosurg Rev. 2020;43(2):407–23.
15. Oberlander MA, Morgan BE, Visotsky JL. The BHAGL lesion: a new variant of anterior shoulder instability. Arthrosc J Arthrosc Relat Surg. 1996;12(5):627–33.
16. Longo UG, Rizzello G, Ciuffreda M, Locher J, Berton A, Salvatore G, et al. Humeral avulsion of the Glenohumeral ligaments: a systematic review. Arthrosc J Arthrosc Relat Surg. 2016;32(9):1868–76.
17. Schmiddem U, Watson A, Perriman D, Liodakis E, Page R. Arthroscopic repair of HAGL lesions yields good clinical results, but may not allow return to former level of sport. Knee Surg Sports Traumatol Arthrosc. 2019;27(10):3246–53.
18. Grimm NL, Jimenez AE, Levy BJ, Bell R, Arciero RA. The original mini-open technique for repair of humeral avulsion of the Glenohumeral ligament. Arthrosc Tech. 2020;9(12):e1865–70.
19. Martetschläger F, Ames JB, Millett PJ. HAGL and reverse HAGL lesions. In: Milano G, Grasso A, editors. Shoulder arthroscopy. London: Springer London; 2014. p. 411–8. [cited 2021 Apr 10]; http://link.springer.com/10.1007/978-1-4471-5427-3_33.
20. Davidson PA, Rivenburgh DW. The 7-o'clock Posteroinferior portal for shoulder arthroscopy. Am J Sports Med. 2002;30(5):693–6.
21. Rothberg DL, Burks RT. Capsular tear in line with the inferior Glenohumeral ligament: a cause of anterior Glenohumeral instability in 2 patients. Arthrosc J Arthrosc Relat Surg. 2009;25(8):934–6.
22. Bhatia DN, DasGupta B. Surgical treatment of significant glenoid bone defects and associated humeral avulsions of glenohumeral ligament (HAGL) lesions in anterior shoulder instability. Knee Surg Sports Traumatol Arthrosc. 2013;21(7):1603–9.
23. Rhee YG, Cho NS. Anterior shoulder instability with humeral avulsion of the glenohumeral ligament lesion. J Shoulder Elb Surg. 2007;16(2):188–92.

24. Kon Y, Shiozaki H, Sugaya H. Arthroscopic repair of a humeral avulsion of the Glenohumeral ligament lesion. Arthrosc J Arthrosc Relat Surg. 2005;21(5):632.e1–6.
25. Provencher M, McCormick F, LeClere LE, Dewing CB, Solomon DJ. A prospective outcome evaluation of humeral avulsions of the Glenohumeral ligament (HAGL) tears repairs in an active population. Orthop J Sports Med. 2014;2(3_suppl):2325967114S0001.

Locked Chronic Anterior Dislocation

20

Ladislav Kovačič

Key Points

- Chronic shoulder dislocation should be suspected in a patient with shoulder pain and limited range of motion in the circumstances of low compliance associated with dementia, alcohol or drug abuse, seizure disorders and multiple trauma and in cases of low accessibility to the health system.
- A quality x-ray imaging and careful evaluation is necessary to rule out dislocation.
- Closed reduction of a chronic shoulder dislocation after 3 weeks can be very difficult. Additional injuries can be caused by vigorous attempt of joint reduction like proximal humerus fracture.
- If the dislocation is unreducible or more than 3 weeks old, open reduction should be considered in sufficiently compliant patient.
- CT scan is mandatory to evaluate bone injury such as anteroinferior glenoid bone loss and posterolateral humeral impaction. Significant bone defect and bone loss are usually present.
- If reconstructive surgical treatment is selected, bone loss has to be addressed to achieve postoperative stability. Additional soft tissue release is necessary due to adhesions and muscle contraction.
- Arthroplasty may be considered in patients with significant glenoid bone loss, greater than 50% humeral head destruction, osteopenia and arthritis.

20.1 Introduction/Background

- There is no clear consensus on the period when the dislocation is considered chronic. Inexact terms such as old, neglected, ancient, locked are used to describe the same condition [4, 7, 10, 25].
- Some authors suggested that any dislocation which is not initially recognized and receives delayed treatment should be considered chronic [17].
- The incidence of anterior chronic dislocation is not lower to the posterior one [16, 17].
- Chronic glenohumeral dislocation arises in patients with multiple distracting injuries (polytrauma patients), patients that may not

L. Kovačič (✉)
Arbormea - Artro Center, Ljubljana, Slovenia

L. Kovačič et al. (eds.), *Surgical Techniques for Anterior Shoulder Instability*,
https://doi.org/10.1007/978-3-662-73064-5_20

explain a thorough history (sedation, brain injury, postictal, dementia) and patients that do not seek immediate medical attention (alcohol or drug abuse).
- Patients are often complex with medical comorbidities and questionable compliance so their functional demands, outcomes expectations, rehabilitation potential and comorbidities must be taken in consideration when developing treatment plan.
- Coexisting shoulder pathology and concomitant injuries must be recognized (rotator cuff tears—often massive, subscapularis tear, dislocation of long head of biceps, glenoid bone loss, humeral head defects, nerve injuries).
- Significant soft tissue contractures and adhesions with glenoid bone loss and humeral head defect and osteoporosis with damage to the joint cartilage make achieving postoperative stability challenging.
- Some patients with low functional demands can tolerate pain and loss of shoulder function and careful neglection should be considered as a treatment option.

20.2 Clinical Evaluation

20.2.1 History

- Patients complain of pain and restricted range of motion (ROM).
- Loss of shoulder motion and subsequent dysfunction often prompts patients to see medical attention.
- Patients has to be questioned about history of trauma, seizure or electrical shock.
- Specific timing of injury is important as it has implication to treatment, however initial event and period of disability is sometimes difficult to determine.
- To make appropriate decision about treatment we have to consider patient's age, hand dominance, activity level, occupation, level of dysfunction, expectations and medical comorbidities.

20.2.2 Relevant Physical Findings

- Visual inspection reveals asymmetric contour. It is of outmost importance to examine the patient undressed.
- Chronic dislocations are often accompanied with muscular atrophy which provide easier physical examination.
- The humeral head can be palpated in the subcoracoid region.
- Despite loss of ROM patients may present with functional mobility due to impression fracture, progressive bony erosion and scapulothoracic compensation.
- Careful attention must be paid to assess motor and sensory function of brachial plexus, especially the function of axillary nerve.
- Specific testing of the rotator cuff is difficult and full thickness tears or even massive tears of rotator cuff are not uncommon.

20.2.3 Relevant Imaging

- Complete trauma series x-ray (AP view in scapular plane, scapular Y view and axillary view) is mandatory to assess direction of the dislocation and status of the bony defects.
- CT is necessary and valuable tool to assess status of the bone—glenoid erosion, humeral head defect, reactive bone formation and ossification of the soft tissues. Those information are crucial for preoperative planning.
- Chronic dislocations can be distinguished from acute by the presence of reactive bone formation around the glenoid neck or ossification of the rotator cuff and capsule.
- Soft tissue status can be evaluated by MRI. While the bone incongruency is so marked, the value of MRI is limited.
- In the event of neurovascular injury electrodiagnostic studies should be considered. They are helpful to distinct preoperative vs postoperative nerve disfunction. Serial studies can compare potential nerve recovery.

- The incidence of vascular injuries is low; however, it is necessary to exclude it in every patient. If necessary, angiogram may be performed. One should keep in mind that vascular injury can occur during reduction manoeuvrers as well.

20.3 Treatment Options and Indications

- A wide variety of treatment options exist for the management of chronic glenohumeral dislocations. Treatment plan is individualized. Factors considered are: patient comorbidities, patient dysfunction, patient compliance, patient expectations, chronicity of dislocation, status of articular cartilage, bony defects on glenoid and humeral head and soft-tissue status.
- Careful neglection can be considered in patients with serious medical comorbidities and low compliance especially when they have low functional demands and if they tolerate pain and loss of shoulder function. This is important to consider in patients with history more than 1 year of shoulder dislocation [5, 14].
- Closed reduction is seldom possible. It might be attempted in the first 4 weeks after injury [17]. Humeral head is usually locked in front of the glenoid. Reduction attempt, if indicated, has to be carried out very carefully to avoid possible additional injuries to proximal humerus and humeral head.
- Arthroscopic reduction has been described [22, 24], however further scientific reports are required. Potential benefit is lower morbidity and treatment of soft-tissue intraarticular pathology at the same time.
- Dislocations with bony defects larger than 20–25% of articular surface are more likely to remain unstable following closed reduction [6, 11, 17].
- Open reduction is favourable if dislocation cannot be reduced by closed means. Supplemental surgical procedures will likely be required.
- Surgical treatment includes glenohumeral joint preserving treatment options with various techniques for joint stabilization and possible additional procedures. In some cases, arthroplasty is indicating including humeral head replacement, anatomic arthroplasty or reverse shoulder arthroplasty.
- Glenohumeral joint preserving techniques are used in young, active individuals. Surgical techniques used are: capsulolabral repair, infraspinatus remplissage, disimpaction and bone grafting, allograft reconstruction, greater tuberosity transfer, glenoid bone block procedures or coracoid transfer.
- In some patients who are dissatisfied with their function but cannot tolerate invasive surgical procedures or follow the postoperative instructions and rehabilitation, resection arthroplasty or glenohumeral arthrodesis may be considered.
- Prosthetic replacement is suitable for older patients with humeral head impaction fractures larger then 40% of articular surface [8, 26]. Additional indications are significant cartilage damage and osteopenic bone that cannot adequately support hardware. Reverse shoulder arthroplasty is an option in patients with coexisting irreparable rotator cuff tear, significant bone loss or elderly with poor bone quality.

20.4 Decision-Making Algorithm

- It is important to consider patient related factors together with bony status before decision (Fig. 20.1).

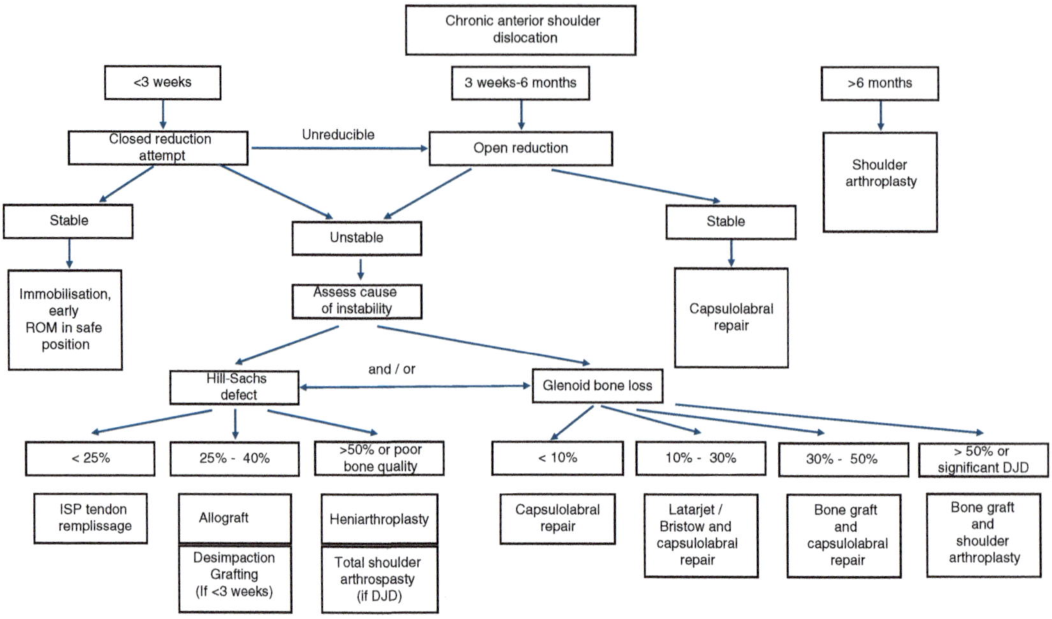

Fig. 20.1 Decision-making algorithm for the treatment of chronic locked anterior shoulder dislocation

20.5 Clinical Case/Example/ Preferred Treatment Option

- Sixty-seven years old women presented at Emergency department 2 months after injury. He complained because of pain in the right shoulder. He was not seeking the medical help because of Covid epidemy.
- Diagnostic studies (x-ray and CT scan) revealed anterior shoulder dislocation with glenoid rim avulsion, Hill-Sachs lesion and periscapular calcification (Fig. 20.2).
- Closed reduction was not attempted based on the duration of history and changes seen on CT scan. It was considered that it will not be successful.
- Patient was scheduled for open reduction in OR, however he could not be operated on because of respiratory insufficiency due to COPD. She was transferred to Department of pulmology for the respiratory treatment.
- After additional 6 weeks, her respiratory function was better and she was scheduled again for consultation. Shoulder was still painful, and ROM was significantly reduced (Fig. 20.3).
- The choice of treatment was Reverse Shoulder Prosthesis based on the bone loss, soft tissue contracture and her comorbidities (Fig. 20.4).

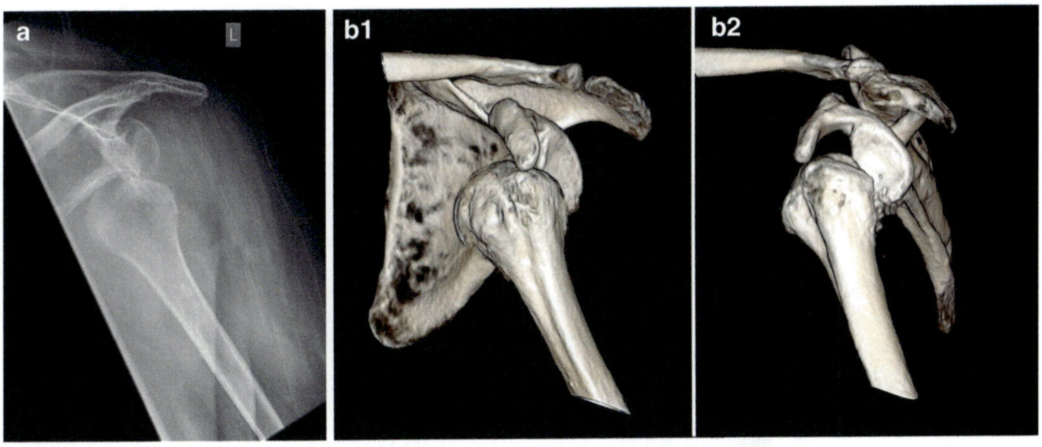

Fig. 20.2 (A) X-ray of the patient with chronic anterior shoulder dislocation. (B1–2). CT 3D reconstruction in the same patient showing locking of the humeral head against glenoid and medially to the coracoid process from lateral (B!) and anterolateral view (B2)

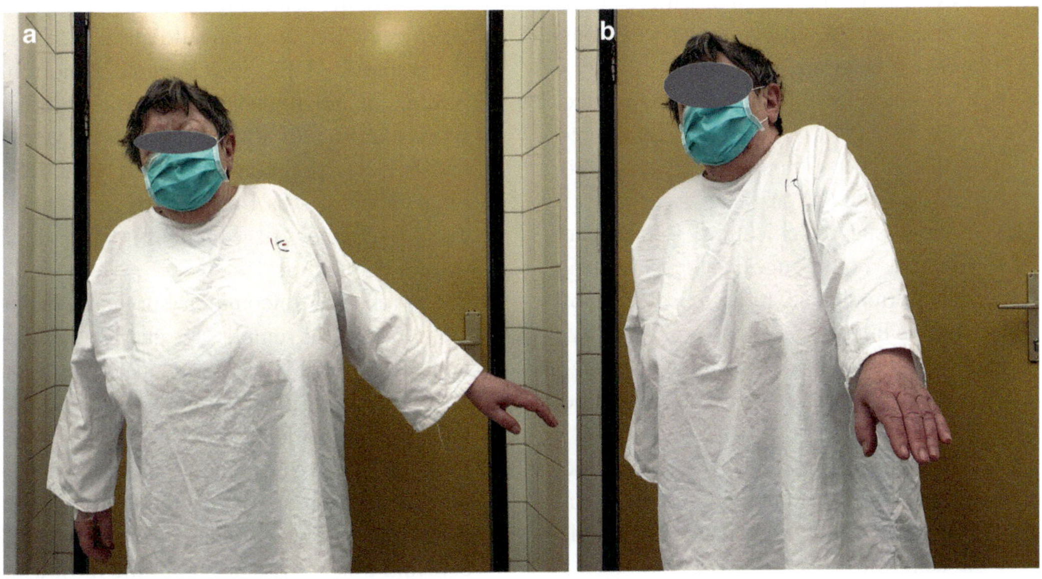

Fig. 20.3 Significantly reduced ROM in patient with chronic shoulder dislocation of 4 months duration. (**a**) Limited abduction. (**b**) Limited forward flexion

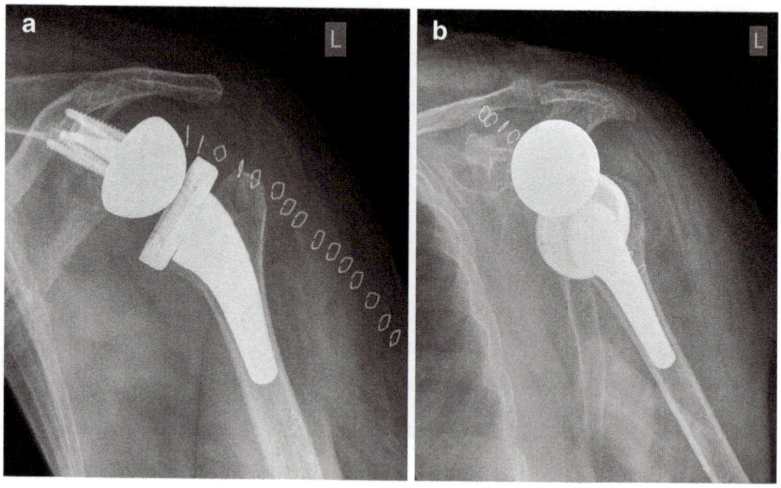

Fig. 20.4 Treatment of chronic anterior shoulder dislocation with reverse shoulder arthroplasty using large glenosphere positioned with inferior inclination to improve stability. X-ray in ap (**a**) and lateral (**b**) view

Pearls and Pitfalls

- Low compliant patients with alcohol abuse or other psychiatric conditions may not be aware of injury.
- Low compliant patients may be treated with nonoperative management, especially if the symptoms are small (no pain, limited ROM).
- Soft tissue calcification, blunt and rounded bony edges, and periosteal bone formation are radiological signs of chronic injury.
- Determining time from injury to diagnosis is important for decision about the management.
- The longer the delay in treatment, the greater the soft tissue deformities. In this cases, soft tissue balance is difficult to achieve.
- Chronic cases with glenoid bone loss and soft tissue deformities are probably best treated with reverse shoulder arthroplasty.

20.6 Outcomes

- Although nonoperative treatment may be an option in low compliance patients with limited pain and attempted ROM, results of surgical treatment are superior to those of the nonoperative group [3, 8, 10].
- Closed reduction may be attempted, but successful reduction in chronic cases with more than 3 weeks of dislocation are unlikely [10, 23].
- Open reduction and capsulolabral repair is rarely reported [3, 15]. Specific cohort of patients in one of the studies has mean rather short duration of dislocation of 10 weeks and Hill-Sach's defect less than 40% [15]. Final elevation was 140°. Out of eight shoulders, five achieved excellent result, three good and one fair.
- Some reported uncommon surgical options are infraspinatus remplissage and K wire fixation [1, 2]. ROM was reported as elevation 135° after infraspinatus remplissage and 91° after K wire fixation.
- In cases of anterior glenoid bone loss, a glenoid reconstruction may be required to repair the glenoid surface. Glenoid bone block and coracoid transfer (Latarjet) are the most used reconstructive surgical procedures. However, there is a wide variation in outcomes.
- Smaller defects of the glenoid surface may be reconstructed with a capsulolabral repair reinforced with a Bristow procedure [10].
- Latarjet can be successful if the shoulder reduction can be performed without requiring a subscapularis tenotomy. If this is not possible, then other surgical reconstruction options should be considered. Re-dislocation rate after subscapularis tenotomy is up to 56% [13].
- If the glenoid bone loss is greater than 20% than reconstruction with a tricortical iliac crest

bone graft may be required. Graft must be placed flush with the articular surface. The reconstruction should create a smooth transition between graft and glenoid cartilage and stable surface for the humeral head to articulate.

- In the reconstructive surgical options, attention must be given to humeral head defects as well [9]. Defects larger than 25% of the humeral head should be addressed. The choices for treatment of glenoid defects up to 45% are following: disimpaction and bone grafting if the injury is less than 3 weeks old or allograft reconstruction of the injury is more than 3 weeks old. If the bone stock is not adequate, if there is marked osteopenia or articular cartilage wear, then arthroplasty is recommended. Any defect involving more than 50% of the humeral head should be treated with arthroplasty.
- In patients important glenoid bone loss or/and with marked involvement of articular surface of the humeral head, shoulder arthroplasty is the treatment of choice. Arthroplasty is also treatment of choice in patients with marked osteopenia or loss of articular surface integrity.
- Analysis of shoulder arthroplasty for locked anterior shoulder dislocation shows better results and lower complication rate with reverse shoulder arthroplasty [18, 20, 21]. It provides greater pain relief, and improvement in range of motion (ROM) compared to total shoulder arthroplasty or hemiarthroplasty. Anatomic arthroplasty is associated with a higher rate of instability and subsequent revision surgery than with reverse arthroplasty. Therefore, anatomic prosthesis is likely not indicated in these difficult circumstances.

20.7 Potential Complications/Difficulties

- Collapse of the articular surface of the humeral head after reduction of a long-standing dislocation has been reported [8].

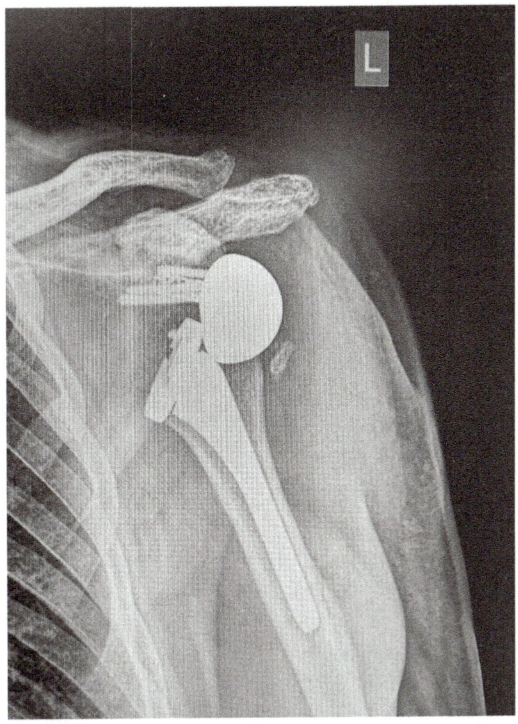

Fig. 20.5 Dislocation of reverse shoulder prothesis implanted after chronic dislocation is one of the main complications of this treatment option

- Expected range of motion following surgical reconstruction is elevation 130–140 deg. and ER 30–35°. Reported final Constant score varied from 58 +/− 24 to 82 +/− 9 [19].
- Described complications following joint preserving reconstructive surgical options are subluxation or redislocation, superior head migration and osteoarthritis [19]. Redislocation rate is reported up to 56% and arthritis is reported from 20% to 93% [13].
- Compared to total shoulder arthroplasty or hemiarthroplasty, reverse shoulder arthroplasty provides greater pain relief and better functional outcomes. Also, re-operation rate and re-dislocation rate is notably lower (Fig. 20.5) [20]. However, patients treated with reverse shoulder arthroplasty after chronic anterior dislocation have lower outcome scores and less improvement in elevation and rotation compared to classic reverse shoulder indications [12].

20.8 Expert Recommendations

- Consideration of non-surgical treatment options is important, especially in low compliance patients.
- Closed reduction in patients with shoulder dislocation longer than 1 months is rarely successful.
- The choice of treatment for patients with subcritical glenoid bone loss and less than 25% of humeral head involvement is rather straightforward. Repair or reconstruction procedures should include anterior capsuloligamentous repair when possible.
- Reconstruction procedures in patients with significant glenoid bone loss and 25–50% of humeral head involvement are associated with important complication rate. Reconstruction procedures in these cases are warranted in young population.
- Reverse shoulder arthroplasty is preferred treatment option in patients with significant glenoid bone loss, Injuries involving 50% of the humeral head, older patients and long duration of dislocation.

Take Home Message

- Chronic locked dislocations of shoulder are rare injuries. Therefore, small number of serries are available.
- Chronic anterior shoulder dislocation is encountered when diagnosis of acute dislocation is initially missed, normally there is a reason related to patients which compliance is low.
- Time from injury to diagnosis and bone injury of the glenoid and humeral head in addition to other patient's related factors are most important for decision about the management.
- In some patients nonoperative intervention may be the best option.
- Injuries with significant bone loss on glenoid side and/or humeral head require that the surgeon understand the benefits and limitations of each of the treatment options discussed.

References

1. Abdelhady AM, AbouElsoud MM. Neglected anterior shoulder dislocation: open remplissage of the Hill-Sachs lesion with the infraspinatus tendon. Acta Ortop Belg. 2015;76:162–5.
2. Akinci O, Kayali C, Akalin Y. Open reduction of old unreduced anterior shoulder dislocations: a case series including 10 patients. Eur J Orthop Surg Traumatol. 2010;20:123–9.
3. Babalola OR, Vrgoč G, Idowu O, Sinidik J, Čoklo M, Marinović M, et al. Chronic unreduced shoulder dislocations: experience in a developing country trauma centre. Injury. 2015;46:S100–102.
4. Bennett GE. Old dislocations of the shoulder. J Bone Joint Surg. 1936;18:594–606.
5. Chung H, Yoon YS, Shin JS, Shin JJ, Kim D. Chronic irreducible anterior dislocation of the shoulder without significant functional deficit. Clin Orthop Surg. 2016;8:333–8.
6. Cicak N. Posterior dislocation of the shoulder. J Bone Joint Surg Br. 2004;86:324–32.
7. Cubbins WR, Callahan JJ, Scuderi CS. The reduction of old or irreducible dislocations of the shoulder joint. Surg Gynecol Obstet. 1934;58:129–35.
8. Flatow EL, Miller SR, Neer CS. Chronic anterior dislocation of the shoulder. J Shoulder Elb Surg. 1993;2:2–9.
9. Gerber C. Chronic, locked anterior and posterior dislocations. In: Warner JJ, Iannotti JP, Gerber C, editors. Complex and revision problems in shoulder surgery. Philadelphia: Lippincott-Raven; 1997. p. 99–113.
10. Goga IE. Chronic shoulder dislocations. J Shoulder Elb Surg. 2003;12:446–50.
11. Hawkins RJ, Neer CS, Pianta RM, Mendoza FX. Locked posterior dislocation of the shoulder. J Bone Joint Surg Am. 1987;60:9–18.
12. Kurowicki J, Triplet JJ, Momoh E, Moor MA, Levy JC. Reverse shoulder prosthesis in the treatment of locked anterior shoulders: a comparison with classic reverse shoulder indications. J Shoulder Elb Surg. 2016;25:1954–60.
13. Li Y, Jiang C. The effectiveness of the Latarjet procedure in patients with chronic locked anterior shoulder dislocation: a retrospective study. J Bone Joint Surg Am. 2016;98:813–23.
14. Novi M, Tarallo L, Colozza A, Paladini P, Micheloni G, Catani F, Porcellini G. Locked anterior glenohumeral dislocation: is it always recommendable a conservative treatment? Musculoskelet Surg. 2022;106:239–45.
15. Rouhani A, Navali A. Treatment of chronic anterior shoulder dislocation by open reduction and simultaneous Bankart lesion repair. Sports Med Arthrosc Rehabil Ther Technol. 2010;16(2):15.
16. Rowe CR, Zarins B. Chronic unreduced dislocations of the shoulder. J Bone Joint Surg Am. 1982;64:494–505.

17. Sahajpal DT, Zuckerman JD. Chronic glenohumeral dislocation. J Am Acad Orthop Surg. 2008;16:385–98.
18. Sahu D, Rathod V, Phadnis A. Instability, complications, and functional outcomes after reverse shoulder arthroplasty and anatomic shoulder arthroplasty for chronic neglected shoulder dislocation: a systematic review. JSES Rev Rep Tech. 2020;13:17–25.
19. Sahu D, Rathod V, Phadnis A, Shyam A. Results and complications of head-preserving techniques in chronic neglected shoulder dislocation: a systematic review. J Shoulder Elb Surg. 2021;30:685–94.
20. Statz JM, Schoch BS, Sanchez-Sotelo J, Sperling JW, Cofield RH. Shoulder arthroplasty for locked anterior shoulder dislocation: a role for the reversed design. Int Orthop. 2017;41:1227–34.
21. Van Tongel A, Claessens T, Verhofste B, De Wilde L. Reversed shoulder arthroplasty as treatment for late or ancient chronic glenohumeral dislocation. Acta Orthop Belg. 2016;82:637–42.
22. Verma NN, Sellards RA, Romeo AA. Arthroscopic reduction and repair of a locked posterior shoulder dislocation. Arthroscopy. 2006;22(1252):e1–5.
23. Yang YL, Li QH, Zhang Q, Jia HL, Wang BM, Dong JL, Zhou DS, Wang XM, Li LX. Treatment of chronic anterior shoulder dislocation by coracoid osteotomy with or without Bristow-Latarjet procedure. Orthop Surg. 2020;12:1478–88.
24. Yanmis I, Komurcu M, Oguz E, Basbozkurt M, Gur E. The role of arthroscopy in chronic anterior shoulder dislocation: technique and early results. Arthroscopy. 2003;19:1129–32.
25. Schultz T, Jacobs B, Patterson RL. Unrecognized dislocations of the shoulder. J Trauma 1969;9:1009–23.
26. Loebenberg MI, Cuomo F. The treatment of chronic anterior and posterior dislocations of the glenohumeral joint and associated articular surface defects. Orthop Clin North Am. 2000;31:23–34.

Bony Bankart Lesions

21

Claudio Rosso, Stefan Loske,
and Andreas Marc Müller

Key Points/Take Home Messages

- Recognition of glenoid bone injury is paramount.
- Instability does not only depend on the amount of bone loss but also on the location of the defect and the centering of the humeral head.
- Recommendation: repairable bony Bankart injuries not associated with other intraarticular pathologies and less than 3 weeks since trauma might be appropriate for arthroscopic reduction and internal fixation (ARIF).
- Arthroscopic techniques allow for minimally invasive reconstruction of glenoid bone defects and osteosynthesis of glenoid fractures.

Supplementary Information The online version contains supplementary material available at https://doi.org/10.1007/978-3-662-73064-5_21.

C. Rosso (✉)
ARTHRO Medics, Shoulder and Elbow Center, Basel, Switzerland

University of Basel, Basel, Switzerland
e-mail: c.rosso@arthro.ch

S. Loske
ARTHRO Medics, Shoulder and Elbow Center, Basel, Switzerland

A. M. Müller
Department of Orthopaedic Surgery, University Hospital Basel, Basel, Switzerland

21.1 Introduction

- Gleno-humeral joint is intrinsically susceptible to instability by its bony architecture (golf ball on a "t").
- Proper early identification of glenoid bone injury will guide safe and successful conservative or operative treatment, specifically in the athlete [1].
- The lesion significantly predisposes the patient to recurrent instability [14].
- Presence of a defect is significantly associated with recurrence [15].
- Difficulty to precisely define the size of the fracture fragment as a percentage of the glenoid.
- Arthroscopy allows for minimally-invasive reconstruction of glenoid bony reconstruction including osteosynthesis of glenoid fractures.

L. Kovačič et al. (eds.), *Surgical Techniques for Anterior Shoulder Instability*,
https://doi.org/10.1007/978-3-662-73064-5_21

21.2 Pathoanatomy

- Reattachment of small bony fragments fixed in the anatomical position together with labrum can be successful [18] while the size of the reconstructed glenoid is crucial to the success of the surgery [9].
- When reviewing imaging, a CT may be useful for assessing the bony lesion and labrum but not so helpful when it comes to looking at the ligamentous tissue, for which an MRI is more appropriate.
- The importance of soft tissue lesions around the glenoid should not be overlooked.
- The size of the defect is significantly associated with recurrent dislocation, increasing number of dislocations, timing from first dislocation, manual work, male gender, age at first dislocation and type of sport [6, 15].
- Threshold of 21% of glenoid length to result in instability even after Bankart repair [8].
- In delayed cases
  - The fragment can be considerably smaller than it was initially and therefore too small to succeed in recuperating glenohumeral stability [17].
  - Severe absorption of the fragment within 1 year after the primary shoulder dislocation is common.
  - Before arthroscopic Bankart repair, bony glenoid defects and bone fragment resorption should be assessed [17].

21.3 Clinical Presentation and Essential Examination

21.3.1 Essential Radiology

- Plain radiographs
  - antero-posterior (AP)
  - Bernageau or axillary view
  - Y-Neer
- Computed tomography (CT) and/or magnetic resonance imaging (MRI).
  - similar accuracy of MRI when compared to CT and 3D CT, using the circle method [7]
- Glenoid track: in the presence of a Hill-Sachs lesion, the glenoid track should be estimated [26]

21.4 Disease Specific Clinical and Arthroscopic Pathology

- Comprehensive and specific history of the patient.
- Record Demographic parameters such as age, gender, job, type of sport (contact vs. non-contact) and level of sport (competitive vs. recreational).
- Details of the dislocations should be taken including:
  - Number of shoulder dislocations
  - Direction
  - Who reduced the shoulder joint (patient, physician, physician in operating room) and time to reduction?
  - Previous shoulder operations
- Clinical evaluation:
  - Range of motion
  - Internal and external rotation at 90° of humeral abduction (ABIR and ABER).
  - apprehension at ABER at 90 and 140° position?
  - Gagey test gives an estimate of inferior glenohumeral ligament laxity [5]
  - Rotator cuff integrity is tested with the Jobe (supraspinatus), resisted external rotation (infraspinatus) and the belly-press test (subscapularis).
- Arthroscopic evaluation:
  - Arthroscopy is performed in a beach chair or lateral decubitus position; a 70° scope can be used to better peek around the glenoid from a posterior view

- Two portals:
  - Posterior portal for the camera
  - Rotator interval portal for instrumentation
- Diagnostic arthroscopy for the presence of concomitant lesions:
  - Amount of labral detachment, posterior labrum intact?
  - SLAP tears
  - Course of the biceps
  - Rotator cuff
  - Hill-Sachs lesion
  - HAGL (Humeral Avulsion of the Glenohumeral Ligament)
  - ALPSA (Anterior Labral Periosteal Sleeve Avulsion) lesion
  - Presence of an "inverted pear" suggesting a glenoid width loss of at least 25–27% [13]
  - Percentage of glenoid osseous is measured at the height of the bare spot [2]
  - For better estimation of the lesion, the camera is inserted into the rotator interval portal using a switching stick

21.5 Treatment Options

Treatment Algorithm (see PPT)

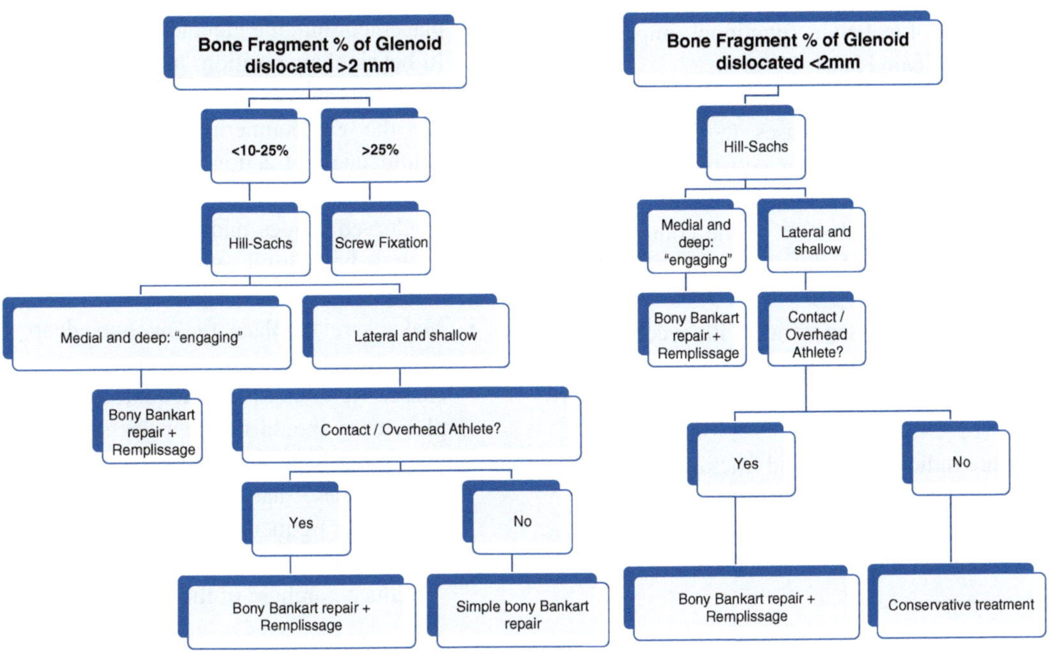

21.5.1 Non-operative Treatment

- Small bony fragment in an anatomical position.
- Meta-analysis has shown no benefit if the arm is immobilized in external rotation [25].

21.5.2 Operative Treatment

- Open and arthroscopic surgical approaches have been published, with equivalent results [3].
- Arthroscopic soft-tissue repair for small glenoid bony fragments in an acute setting is associated with successful treatment [3, 19, 20, 21].
- In <u>small</u> bony Bankart lesions (<12.5%), restoration of capsulolabral soft tissue tension alone is enough [11].
- In <u>medium</u> lesions (12.5–25%), the osseous architecture of the glenoid should be reconstructed for better functional improvement and less pain [11].
- For bigger fragments and small Bankart fragments in chronic cases (> 3 weeks post-trauma), outcomes for soft-tissue repairs are less favorable and associated with failure [3, 4, 17, 19] as 38–49% of the contribution to stability is due to bony reconstruction of the glenoid area [27].
  - thus an osseous glenoid reconstruction using the Latarjet, Bristow or free bone graft techniques is preferred [12, 14, 16, 22–24, 26, 28],
- Rare indication: glenoid fracture with a single fragment after shoulder dislocation.
  - an acute reduction of the fragment using cannulated screws can be achieved [10, 19].

Pearls and Pitfalls

- In arthroscopic surgery, make sure to fully mobilize the labral or osteolabral Bankart defect.
  - Additional portals and portal switches can be helpful (e.g. anterolateral portal) to fully visualize the defect, especially if no 70° scope is available.
  - A landmark for a good mobilisation can be the visualization of the subscapularis muscle belly between the anterior glenoid and the Bankart defect.
- In acute trauma, be prepared for a highly traumatized glenohumeral joint. A good arthroscopic overview may be much harder to obtain compared to chronic instabilities.
- Smaller cartilage injuries adjacent to labral Bankart lesions may be covered with a slightly more posterior anchor placement into the glenoid surface.
- In beach chair position, inferior anchor placement may be facilitated by widening the glenohumeral joint space by gentle lateral traction at the proximal upper arm by an assistant.
  - Curved guides and flexible anchors may be helpful as well to avoid a trans-subscapularis portal.
- Make sure to place the anchors deep enough into the bone for proper purchase. Reference for adequate anchor placement should be the bony surface, not the cartilage surface.
  - Be aware that the strong cortical bone is frequently injured in osteolabral Bankart defects, which may reduce purchase of the anchors.

References

1. Bhatia S, Ghodadra NS, Romeo AA, Bach BR, Verma NN, Vo ST, Provencher MT. The importance of the recognition and treatment of glenoid bone loss in an athletic population. Sports Health. 2011;3(5):435–40. https://doi.org/10.1177/1941738111414126.
2. Burkhart SS, Debeer JF, Tehrany AM, Parten PM. Quantifying glenoid bone loss arthroscopically in shoulder instability. Arthroscopy. 2002;18(5):488–91. https://doi.org/10.1053/jars.2002.32212.
3. Bushnell BD, Creighton RA, Herring MM. Bony instability of the shoulder. Arthroscopy. 2008;24(9):1061–73. https://doi.org/10.1016/j.arthro.2008.05.015.
4. Dumont GD, Russell RD, Robertson WJ. Anterior shoulder instability: a review of pathoanatomy, diagnosis and treatment. Curr Rev Musculoskelet Med. 2011;4(4):200–7. https://doi.org/10.1007/s12178-011-9092-9.
5. Gagey OJ, Gagey N. The hyperabduction test. J Bone Joint Surg Br. 2001;83(1):69–74.
6. Gerometta A, Rosso C, Clouche S, Hardy P. Arthroscopic bankart shoulder stabilization in athletes: return to sports and functional outcomes at 2 years mean follow-up. Knee Surg Sports Traumatol Arthrosc. 2014. Accepted January 2014.
7. Gyftopoulos S, Hasan S, Bencardino J, Mayo J, Nayyar S, Babb J, Jazrawi L. Diagnostic accuracy of MRI in the measurement of glenoid bone loss. AJR Am J Roentgenol. 2012;199(4):873–8. https://doi.org/10.2214/AJR.11.7639.
8. Itoi E, Lee SB, Berglund LJ, Berge LL, An KN. The effect of a glenoid defect on anteroinferior stability of the shoulder after Bankart repair: a cadaveric study. J Bone Joint Surg Am. 2000;82(1):35–46.
9. Jiang CY, Zhu YM, Liu X, Li FL, Lu Y, Wu G. Do reduction and healing of the bony fragment really matter in arthroscopic bony bankart reconstruction?: a prospective study with clinical and computed tomography evaluations. Am J Sports Med. 2013;41(11):2617–23. https://doi.org/10.1177/0363546513499304.
10. Kim KC, Rhee KJ, Shin HD. Arthroscopic three-point double-row repair for acute bony Bankart lesions. Knee Surg Sports Traumatol Arthrosc. 2009;17(1):102–6. https://doi.org/10.1007/s00167-008-0659-y.
11. Kim YK, Cho SH, Son WS, Moon SH. Arthroscopic repair of small and medium-sized bony bankart lesions. Am J Sports Med. 2014;42(1):86–94. https://doi.org/10.1177/0363546513509062.
12. Lafosse L, Lejeune E, Bouchard A, Kakuda C, Gobezie R, Kochhar T. The arthroscopic Latarjet procedure for the treatment of anterior shoulder instability. Arthroscopy. 2007;23(11):1242 e1241–1245. https://doi.org/10.1016/j.arthro.2007.06.008.
13. Lo IK, Parten PM, Burkhart SS. The inverted pear glenoid: an indicator of significant glenoid bone loss. Arthroscopy. 2004;20(2):169–74. https://doi.org/10.1016/j.arthro.2003.11.036.
14. Martetschlager F, Kraus TM, Hardy P, Millett PJ. Arthroscopic management of anterior shoulder instability with glenoid bone defects. Knee Surg Sports Traumatol Arthrosc. 2013;21(12):2867–76. https://doi.org/10.1007/s00167-012-2198-9.
15. Milano G, Grasso A, Russo A, Magarelli N, Santagada DA, Deriu L, Baudi P, Bonomo L, Fabbriciani C. Analysis of risk factors for glenoid bone defect in anterior shoulder instability. Am J Sports Med. 2011;39(9):1870–6. https://doi.org/10.1177/0363546511411699.
16. Mochizuki Y, Hachisuka H, Kashiwagi K, Oomae H, Yokoya S, Ochi M. Arthroscopic autologous bone graft with arthroscopic Bankart repair for a large bony defect lesion caused by recurrent shoulder dislocation. Arthroscopy. 2007;23(6):677 e671–674. https://doi.org/10.1016/j.arthro.2006.01.024.
17. Nakagawa S, Mizuno N, Hiramatsu K, Tachibana Y, Mae T. Absorption of the bone fragment in shoulders with bony Bankart lesions caused by recurrent anterior dislocations or subluxations: when does it occur? Am J Sports Med. 2013;41(6):1380–6. https://doi.org/10.1177/0363546513483087.
18. Park JY, Lee SJ, Lhee SH, Lee SH. Follow-up computed tomography arthrographic evaluation of bony Bankart lesions after arthroscopic repair. Arthroscopy. 2012;28(4):465–73. https://doi.org/10.1016/j.arthro.2011.09.008.
19. Porcellini G, Campi F, Paladini P. Arthroscopic approach to acute bony Bankart lesion. Arthroscopy. 2002;18(7):764–9.
20. Porcellini G, Paladini P, Campi F, Paganelli M. Long-term outcome of acute versus chronic bony Bankart lesions managed arthroscopically. Am J Sports Med. 2007;35(12):2067–72. https://doi.org/10.1177/0363546507305011.
21. Rhee YG, Cho NS, Cho SH. Traumatic anterior dislocation of the shoulder: factors affecting the progress of the traumatic anterior dislocation. Clin Orthop Surg. 2009;1(4):188–93. https://doi.org/10.4055/cios.2009.1.4.188.
22. Scheibel M, Kraus N, Diederichs G, Haas NP. Arthroscopic reconstruction of chronic anteroinferior glenoid defect using an autologous tricortical iliac crest bone grafting technique. Arch Orthop Trauma Surg. 2008;128(11):1295–300. https://doi.org/10.1007/s00402-007-0509-2.
23. Taverna E, Golano P, Pascale V, Battistella F. An arthroscopic bone graft procedure for treating anterior-inferior glenohumeral instability. Knee Surg Sports Traumatol Arthrosc. 2008;16(9):872–5. https://doi.org/10.1007/s00167-008-0541-y.
24. Thomazeau H, Courage O, Barth J, Pelegri C, Charousset C, Lespagnol F, Nourissat G, et al. Can we improve the indication for Bankart arthroscopic repair? A preliminary clinical study using the ISIS score. Orthop Traumatol Surg Res. 2010;96(8 Suppl):S77–83. https://doi.org/10.1016/j.otsr.2010.09.007.

25. Vavken P, Sadoghi P, Quidde J, Lucas R, Delaney R, Mueller AM, Rosso C, Valderrabano V. Immobilization in internal or external rotation does not change recurrence rates after traumatic anterior shoulder dislocation. J Shoulder Elb Surg. 2014;23(1):13–9. https://doi.org/10.1016/j.jse.2013.07.037.
26. Yamamoto N, Itoi E, Abe H, Minagawa H, Seki N, Shimada Y, Okada K. Contact between the glenoid and the humeral head in abduction, external rotation, and horizontal extension: a new concept of glenoid track. J Shoulder Elb Surg. 2007;16(5):649–56. https://doi.org/10.1016/j.jse.2006.12.012.
27. Yamamoto N, Muraki T, An KN, Sperling JW, Cofield RH, Itoi E, Walch G, Steinmann SP. The stabilizing mechanism of the Latarjet procedure: a cadaveric study. J Bone Joint Surg Am. 2013;95(15):1390–7. https://doi.org/10.2106/JBJS.L.00777.
28. Young AA, Maia R, Berhouet J, Walch G. Open Latarjet procedure for management of bone loss in anterior instability of the glenohumeral joint. J Shoulder Elb Surg. 2011;20(2 Suppl):S61–9. https://doi.org/10.1016/j.jse.2010.07.022.

22 Return to Sports: Specialized Rehabilitation and Isokinetic Evaluation

Hélder Fonte, Gaetano Rossi, Flórido Pereira, Marília Ventura, and Nuno Gomes

Key Points

- Isokinetic testing is a valuable tool for objectively assessing muscle strength and function in patients with shoulder instability, especially post-surgery.
- Isokinetic evaluation can identify specific muscle imbalances (e.g., internal vs. external rotation) and weaknesses, guiding targeted rehabilitation programs.
- Using Biodex, rehabilitation protocols can be tailored to strengthen specific muscle groups (internal and external rotators) at different speeds to maximize recovery.
- Recent evidence establishes specific strength thresholds (ER ≥0.32 Nm/kg concentric at 240°/s; ≥0.51 Nm/kg eccentric at 30°/s) that correlate with successful return to sport.
- Isokinetic testing helps track patient progress during rehabilitation, ensuring optimal recovery and a safe return to sports.
- Integration of isokinetic testing and rehabilitation can lead to improved recovery times and reduced absence from sports.

Supplementary Information The online version contains supplementary material available at https://doi.org/10.1007/978-3-662-73064-5_22.

H. Fonte · N. Gomes (✉)
Hospital Forças Armadas – Pólo do Porto, Porto, Portugal

Hospital Luz Arrábida, Porto, Portugal

G. Rossi
Facoltà Medicina e Chirurgia San Luigi Gonzaga, Orbassano, TO, Italy
e-mail: gaetano.rossi@edu.unito.it

F. Pereira · M. Ventura
Hospital Forças Armadas – Pólo do Porto, Porto, Portugal

22.1 Introduction

- Isokinetic or isospeed exercise is a dynamic muscle exercise performed at constant speed with the help of appropriate equipment that, by means of a robotic or hydraulic mechanism, adapt the resistance to the variation of the tension developed by the muscle. In this way, when the set speed is reached, the isokinetic device absorbs excess applied force and transforms it into resistance so that the power developed by the muscle cannot increase the speed of the lever to produce acceleration. It is therefore possible to work at maximum load throughout the movement.

L. Kovačič et al. (eds.), *Surgical Techniques for Anterior Shoulder Instability*, https://doi.org/10.1007/978-3-662-73064-5_22

- Biodex→ is the system used for this paper, following the guidelines suggested by the official operation manual of the machinery [1]. It is a type of workout that involves specialized machines, and it is mostly used to train athletes to improve their running or throwing by improving the speed at which they can move their limb/body or a weight. With isokinetic equipment it is possible to evaluate the strength of a muscle and then build a rehabilitation protocol that points out the reinforcement of the correct muscle from the early post-operative phases, associated with traditional physiotherapy isokinetic muscle exercise.
- Isokinetic testing and evaluation are a valuable tool for assessing muscle strength and function following shoulder instability surgery and it is useful in the identification of muscle imbalances and weaknesses that may be contributing to shoulder instability and for tracking progress during rehabilitation.
- The literature is scarce about Isokinetic testing and evaluation regarding shoulder pathology. For this chapter, scientific articles (originals and reviews) were searched in electronic databases (Pubmed, Cochrane and Epistemonikos) and by non-electronic search, based on the references of the selected articles, without restriction of the year of publication. The sources of the highest scientific evidence between 2000 and 2025 were used and integrated with the data collected at our institution. Most literature refers to studies conducted by Todd S. Ellenbecker and George J. Davies [2]. where a total of 111 patients were tested in the 90/90° position for shoulder internal and external rotation with Isokinetics to specifically evaluate torque acceleration energy, emphasizing the primordial importance of muscle strengthening in the post-operative period.
- This chapter offers an overview of the usage of Isokinetic in the shoulder, particularly in the post-operative rehabilitation of the unstable shoulder. Correlation with data collected at our institution demonstrates and supports the usage of Isokinetic to substantially improve recovery time and reduce absence from sports.

22.2 Shoulder Instability and Isokinetic Testing

- Shoulder instability is a common condition that occurs when the shoulder joint becomes too loose or unstable, leading to a feeling of looseness or "giving way" during certain movements. It can be caused by a variety of factors, including trauma, overuse injuries, and congenital conditions. Surgery is often necessary to stabilize the shoulder joint and restore normal function. After shoulder instability surgery, it is important to undergo a thorough rehabilitation program to help restore strength, range of motion, and function to the shoulder. Isokinetic testing can be a valuable part of this process, as it allows for precise measurement of muscle strength and function at different speeds and ranges of motion.
- One of the key benefits of isokinetic testing is that it allows for objective measurement of muscle strength. Traditional methods of muscle testing, such as manual muscle testing or resistance testing, rely on the subjective judgment of the therapist or clinician. Isokinetic testing, on the other hand, uses a machine to measure muscle strength and output, providing more accurate and reliable results. Another benefit of isokinetic testing is that it allows for evaluation of muscle imbalances and weaknesses. After shoulder instability surgery, it is common for certain muscles to become weaker or more imbalanced compared to others. Isokinetic testing can identify these imbalances and help guide the rehabilitation process by targeting specific muscle groups for strengthening.
- Isokinetic testing is also useful for tracking progress during rehabilitation. By regularly performing isokinetic testing, therapists and clinicians can monitor changes in muscle strength and function over time and adjust the rehabilitation program as needed to ensure optimal progress. In addition to improving the strength and function of the shoulder, isokinetic testing can also be used to assess the muscle imbalances and asymmetries that may

be present in an athlete's shoulder. These imbalances can lead to increased risk of injury and reduced performance. By identifying and addressing these imbalances, isokinetic testing can help to improve the overall function and performance of the shoulder.

- Recent developments in shoulder instability research have emphasized the need for standardization of outcome measures. A modified Delphi consensus study (2023) involving 44 healthcare providers and 30 patients identified 11 critical domains for evaluation in shoulder instability studies—including range of motion, return to sport status, and objective strength parameters [3]. Importantly, all these domains can be measured through comprehensive isokinetic testing protocols, which reinforces the clinical relevance of this assessment tool. However, the study also highlighted considerable variation in how these measurements are performed across institutions; this underscores the importance of adopting validated, reproducible protocols like those described in this chapter.
- The evidence base for isokinetic testing in return-to-sport decision-making has been expanded considerably. Moussa et al. [4] published a prospective cross-sectional study of 96 patients who underwent the Latarjet procedure; they performed isokinetic testing (Biodex System 4) at 6-month follow-up and correlated strength measurements with actual return-to-sport outcomes [4]. Their analysis revealed specific strength thresholds with high predictive value: patients who achieved concentric external rotation strength ≥0.32 Nm/kg at 240°/s demonstrated 100% sensitivity for successful sport resumption (though specificity was moderate at 47.1%). For eccentric external rotation, a threshold of ≥0.51 Nm/kg at 30°/s provided 94.1% sensitivity with 41.2% specificity. While these findings require validation across different surgical procedures and patient populations, they represent an important step toward establishing objective, evidence-based return-to-sport criteria.
- Isokinetic testing can also be used to track progress and ensure that an athlete's shoulder is healing properly after an injury or surgery. By measuring the strength and range of motion of the shoulder at regular intervals, it is possible to determine if the shoulder is healing at an appropriate rate and to make any necessary adjustments to the rehabilitation program. Overall, isokinetic testing and evaluation can be a useful tool for improving sports performance by identifying and addressing areas of weakness, muscle imbalances, and asymmetries in the shoulder, as well as tracking progress during rehabilitation.

22.2.1 Recent Advances and Emerging Technologies

- The past years have witnessed refinements in isokinetic assessment methodology. Multi-joint isokinetic systems now demonstrate excellent test-retest reliability (ICC >0.90 for both concentric and eccentric contractions) [5], which provides confidence for their use in longitudinal monitoring during rehabilitation. These newer systems also offer enhanced data visualization capabilities and improved patient feedback mechanisms, factors that may contribute to better patient engagement during testing sessions.
- Beyond traditional ER:IR ratio measurements, the concept of "dynamic control ratios" has gained attention. These ratios incorporate both concentric and eccentric components of muscle action; proponents argue they provide better insight into neuromuscular control patterns essential for overhead athletic activities [6]. Whether these refined measurements offer clinically meaningful advantages over conventional ratios remains an open question, but they illustrate the ongoing evolution in how we conceptualize shoulder muscle balance.
- Looking further ahead, machine learning applications are beginning to appear in shoulder assessment research. Recent work has explored AI-enhanced evaluation of scapular dyskinesis [7], which could potentially be combined with isokinetic data to provide more comprehensive shoulder function profiles.

While these applications remain largely experimental at present, they point toward interesting possibilities for future rehabilitation monitoring systems.

22.3 Isokinetic Evaluation

- Isokinetics testing can be a relevant tool in the patient's objective dynamic muscular power evaluation. That includes observation of posture, referral and related joints, neurologic examination, sensation and reflexes, kinesthetic and proprioceptive testing, palpation, scapular assessment, active range of motion (ROM), physiologic passive ROM flexibility tests, resisted ROM and Manual muscle testing (MMT), special tests, computerized isokinetic testing and reliability, functional testing, and imaging studies.
- In the data collected by Todd and George, a total of 111 patients were tested in the 90°/90° position for shoulder internal and external rotation with Isokinetics to specifically evaluate torque acceleration energy, that is the total work performed in the first 125 milliseconds of a muscular contraction and indicates the patient's ability to generate force quickly [2]. Knops et al. conducted a test-retest reliability study of the modified neutral position for internal and external rotation of the glenohumeral joint. This position places the arm in a 30°/30°/30° position. Velocity-spectrum testing at 600, 1800, and 3000°s-1 was performed with intraclass correlation coefficients applied to determine the degree of test-retest reliability. This position of testing produced a high test-retest reliability, with intraclass correlation coefficients ranging between 0.91 and 0.96 [8]. During rehabilitation primary emphasis is placed on the assessment of internal and external rotation strength. The rationale for this apparently narrow focus is provided by an isokinetic training study by Quincy et al. [9] Six weeks of isokinetic training of the internal and external rotators produced statistically significant improvements, not only in internal and external rotation strength, but also in flexion and extension and abduction and adduction strength as well.
- A maximum limb dominance of the internal and external rotators of 5–10% is assumed in nonathletic and recreational-level upper extremity sport athletes. In the article of Malavolta et al. the isokinetic test was performed at around 36 months after the *Latarjet procedure*, with a minimum of 17 months. The patients were submitted to the assessments using a Biodex System 3 isokinetic dynamometer and the *Rowe Scale*. In the isokinetic evaluation of the shoulder, they found a 13.5% decrease in external rotation strength at 60°/s and 4.5% at 180°/s ($p = 0.009$ and $p = 0.040$, respectively). The internal rotation strength was not decreased, either at 60°/s or at 180°/s ($p = 0.575$ and $p = 0.794$, respectively). The patients showed a significant improvement with the procedure, from 30.5 ± 11.9 to 93.8 ± 9.3 on the *Rowe Scale* ($p < 0.001$). None of them presented recurrence of instability. The comparison between surgeries performed on the dominant side versus the non-dominant side showed no statistically significant difference for any of the studied outcomes [10].
- In support of an article published on the website "The shoulder channel TV" written by Giovanni Di Giacomo [11] claims that at the time when the patient is able to tolerate isotonic exercises with 0.90–1,40 kg and can perform rotational reinforcement exercises without experiencing pain, using an average resistance level, isokinetic exercises can be performed for rotations in the modified base position with the glenohumeral articulation at 30° of flexion and 30° of abduction, and uses an inclination of 30° of the dynamometer with respect to the horizontal plane which allows the patient to proceed from sub-maximum resistance levels to maximum levels. In particular, the progression of the patient to the 90°/90° position in the iso-inertial exercise as well as the exercise with the isokinetic dynamometry with shoulder elevated

to 90° on the scapular plane, provides an additional stimulus for optimal training for increasing the strength of the rotator cuff in sport and activity-specific positions.

- In accordance with the various selected works and with the literature, our study was based on the test of IR/ER in the scapula plane, the safest and recommended to safeguard the joint integrity avoiding, for example, the impingement and the apprehension, situations that can occur in the IR/ER at 90° of abduction, flexion and abduction. We have used what is suggested by the Biodex brand and the available literature with angular speeds of 60°, 180° and 300°/s, using 5–10 repetitions at 180°, 300°, and 450°/sec and the optimal period of rest between each isokinetic test speed is 90 s. In general terms the applying isokinetic test data are [2, 10, 12]:
  - Bilateral comparison—the evaluation of the involved to the uninvolved extremity is probably the most common comparison.
  - Bilateral differences of 10–15% are considered sensitive for significant asymmetry. However, this single parameter, if used by itself, has limitations.
  - Unilateral strength ratios—comparison of agonist-antagonist muscle groups are typically obtained by dividing the value of the weaker of the 2 muscle groups into the value of the stronger muscle group to obtain a ratio.
  - Torque—and work-to-body-weight ratios.
  - Relative fatigue ratios.

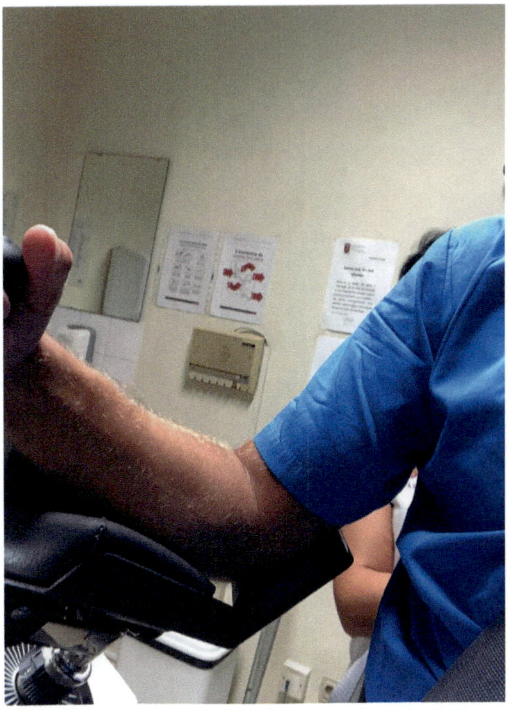

Fig. 22.1 Tested position: external e internal rotation of the shoulders in *neutral position*. Several studies show this to be the most reliable movement for the assessment

22.4 Clinical Case

22.4.1 Testing

- The main parameters that can be evaluated using Biodex→ are:
  - *Peak Torque*: Gives us information about Maximum Strength. These values are read at low speeds (e.g., 60°/s) and few repetitions. A normal test should show a difference between the right and left sides below 10%.
  - *Average Power*: Gives information on Power. These values are read in the test at intermedium speeds (e.g., 180°/s) and few repetitions. A normal test should show a difference between the right and left sides below 10%.
  - *Total Work*: Gives information about the Resistance. These values are read at high speeds (e.g., 300°/s) and many repetitions. A normal test should show a difference between the right and left sides below 10%.
  - *Agon/Antag Ratio*: These values should be approximated to the number G.
- In our study we tested external e internal rotation of the shoulders in *neutral position* (Figs. 22.1 and 22.2) because several studies show this to be the most reliable position. The test starts with the counter-lateral limb and

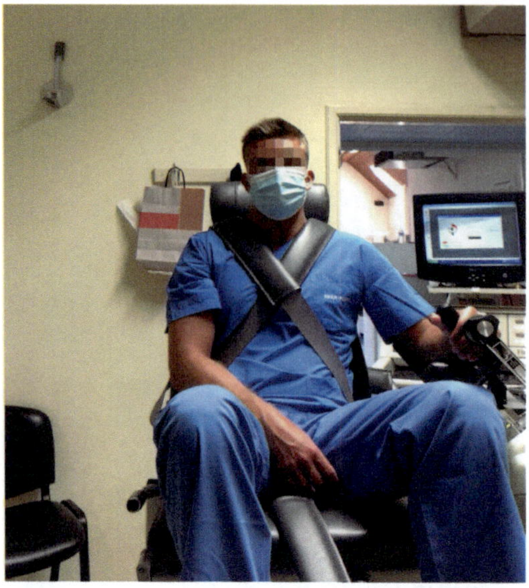

Fig. 22.2 Starting position. The preoperative test always begins by weighing the two limbs to check that there are no weight differences

then the injured shoulder. The test is performed the same way for both limbs and was carried out in the following manner:

- Ten minutes of warm-up on pulleys.
- Before each test speed, three repetitions to familiarize with the speed to be tested are performed.
- Then, at each speed, the patient is instructed to perform the movement with the greatest speed and force possible. He is motivated throughout the test with verbal and visual stimuli (biofeedback graphics on the computer monitor where the isokinetic device is connected).

60°/s: 5 repetitions Rest: 60 s
180°/s: 10 repetitions Rest: 60 s
300°/s: 15 repetitions

Results

- The results of the test show that the patient in question has a strength deficit (peak torque) of the right shoulder compared to the left at low, medium, and high speeds. Focusing on the injured shoulder (left) it is also evident that there is a greater deficit of force in internal rotation (IR) at low and medium speeds, while at high speeds the deficit is greater in external rotation (ER). (Figs. 22.3, 22.4 and 22.5).
- There is a gap of forces between the healthy limb (Right) and the affected one (Left). This deficit is greater in IR than in ER. The peak torque in relation to body weight is not reached both in ER and IR (Fig. 22.6).
- The gap of forces is more pronounced compared to the test at 60°/s, both in ER and IR. The deficit of the left limb is greater in IR and the goal, the peak torque in relation to body weight, is not reached in IR or ER (Fig. 22.7).
- At high speeds the graph shows that the force gap is more significant in ER than in IR (Fig. 22.8).

22.4.2 Post-operative

22.4.2.1 Immediate Post-operative

- Many types of exercise programs are currently in widespread use for the rehabilitation of the injured athlete. We give an example of a rehabilitation protocol to implement after a shoulder stabilization surgery, with a resisted rehabilitation program that can be implemented using Biodex. This resisted rehabilitation programs include isometric, concentric and eccentric isotonics, concentric and eccentric isokinetics, and isoacceleration and isodeceleration types of programs. More training would be implemented in the terminal phases of rehabilitation, using exercises such as plyometrics and neuromuscular control exercises. The resisted rehabilitation program encompasses personalized setting according with patient deficits.

		EXT ROTATION 60 DEG/SEC			INT ROTATION 60 DEG/SEC		
# OF REPS: Right 5		UNINVOLVED	INVOLVED	DEFICIT	UNINVOLVED	INVOLVED	DEFICIT
# OF REPS: Left 5		RIGHT	LEFT		RIGHT	LEFT	
PEAK TORQUE	N-M	34.8	29.6	15.1	49.6	41.1	17.2
PEAK TQ/BW	%	43.6	37.0		62.0	51.4	
TIME TO PK TQ	MSEC	420.0	400.0		960.0	930.0	
ANGLE OF PK TQ	DEG	-17.0	2.0		-23.0	-14.0	
TORQ @ 30.0 DEG	N-M	0.0	0.0	0.0	0.0	0.0	0.0
TORQ @ 0.18 SEC	N-M	31.2	28.2	9.6	38.8	28.8	25.7
COEFF. OF VAR.	%	2.1	2.3		7.1	5.5	
MAX REP TOT WORK	J	42.1	39.9	5.3	58.9	56.0	4.9
MAX WORK REP #	#	5	1		5	3	
WRK/BODYWEIGHT	%	52.7	49.9		73.7	70.1	
TOTAL WORK	J	205.4	191.8	6.6	278.8	258.6	7.2
WORK FIRST THIRD	J	73.5	71.5		102.0	92.3	
WORK LAST THIRD	J	60.5	58.0		87.1	77.9	
WORK FATIGUE	%	17.7	18.9		14.6	15.6	
AVG. POWER	WATTS	25.9	22.3	14.0	36.6	29.7	19.1
ACCELERATION TIME	MSEC	40.0	60.0		60.0	60.0	
DECELERATION TIME	MSEC	100.0	200.0		70.0	230.0	
ROM	DEG	89.9	92.2		89.9	92.2	
AVG PEAK TQ	N-M	34.1	28.8		46.2	38.4	
AGON/ANTAG RATIO	%	70.3	72.0	G: 64.5			

Fig. 22.3 The test shows a deficit of Peak Torque in external and internal rotation of 15.1/17.2 N-M respectively

		EXT ROTATION 180 DEG/SEC			INT ROTATION 180 DEG/SEC		
# OF REPS: Right 10		UNINVOLVED	INVOLVED	DEFICIT	UNINVOLVED	INVOLVED	DEFICIT
# OF REPS: Left 10		RIGHT	LEFT		RIGHT	LEFT	
PEAK TORQUE	N-M	28.4	23.5	17.2	43.7	35.2	19.4
PEAK TQ/BW	%	35.5	29.4		54.7	44.1	
TIME TO PK TQ	MSEC	170.0	210.0		390.0	220.0	
ANGLE OF PK TQ	DEG	-10.0	1.0		-25.0	-45.0	
TORQ @ 30.0 DEG	N-M	0.0	0.0	0.0	0.0	0.0	0.0
TORQ @ 0.18 SEC	N-M	28.1	22.9	18.3	38.4	33.3	13.3
COEFF. OF VAR.	%	7.6	8.5		14.4	6.3	
MAX REP TOT WORK	J	30.5	24.9	18.4	52.8	40.7	22.9
MAX WORK REP #	#	6	2		10	4	
WRK/BODYWEIGHT	%	38.2	31.2		66.1	51.0	
TOTAL WORK	J	285.3	235.4	17.5	458.5	356.8	22.2
WORK FIRST THIRD	J	92.0	78.4		121.8	111.2	
WORK LAST THIRD	J	82.3	70.7		152.8	110.5	
WORK FATIGUE	%	10.6	9.8		-25.5	0.7	
AVG. POWER	WATTS	43.6	33.9	22.2	66.3	48.0	27.6
ACCELERATION TIME	MSEC	100.0	130.0		120.0	130.0	
DECELERATION TIME	MSEC	120.0	130.0		130.0	150.0	
ROM	DEG	89.3	91.6		89.3	91.6	
AVG PEAK TQ	N-M	27.2	22.4		38.0	30.9	
AGON/ANTAG RATIO	%	64.8	66.6	G: 66.0			

Fig. 22.4 The test shows the patient has a deficit of power in left ER and IR of 22.2/27.6 watts respectively

		EXT ROTATION 300 DEG/SEC			INT ROTATION 300 DEG/SEC		
# OF REPS: Right 15		UNINVOLVED	INVOLVED	DEFICIT	UNINVOLVED	INVOLVED	DEFICIT
# OF REPS: Left 15		RIGHT	LEFT		RIGHT	LEFT	
PEAK TORQUE	N-M	21.9	17.7	19.1	39.8	34.8	12.5
PEAK TQ/BW	%	27.4	22.2		49.8	43.6	
TIME TO PK TQ	MSEC	200.0	220.0		230.0	230.0	
ANGLE OF PK TQ	DEG	-20.0	-10.0		-38.0	-32.0	
TORQ @ 30.0 DEG	N-M	0.0	0.0	0.0	0.0	0.0	0.0
TORQ @ 0.18 SEC	N-M	21.0	14.3	31.7	39.0	29.4	24.5
COEFF. OF VAR.	%	20.0	23.7		14.4	19.9	
MAX REP TOT WORK	J	17.7	13.6	23.2	39.0	33.0	15.3
MAX WORK REP #	#	6	4		13	15	
WRK/BODYWEIGHT	%	22.1	17.0		48.8	41.3	
TOTAL WORK	J	229.4	168.1	26.8	505.3	404.5	20.0
WORK FIRST THIRD	J	75.0	59.0		139.0	122.0	
WORK LAST THIRD	J	69.0	47.0		181.2	142.0	
WORK FATIGUE	%	8.0	20.4		-30.3	-16.5	
AVG. POWER	WATTS	31.5	20.2	35.8	67.2	47.6	29.1
ACCELERATION TIME	MSEC	160.0	190.0		130.0	160.0	
DECELERATION TIME	MSEC	110.0	140.0		130.0	160.0	
ROM	DEG	87.9	90.8		87.9	90.8	
AVG PEAK TQ	N-M	20.0	15.9		35.6	28.6	
AGON/ANTAG RATIO	%	55.0	50.9	G: N/A			

Fig. 22.5 The test shows the patient has a deficit of total work in left ER and IR of 26.8/20.0 J respectively

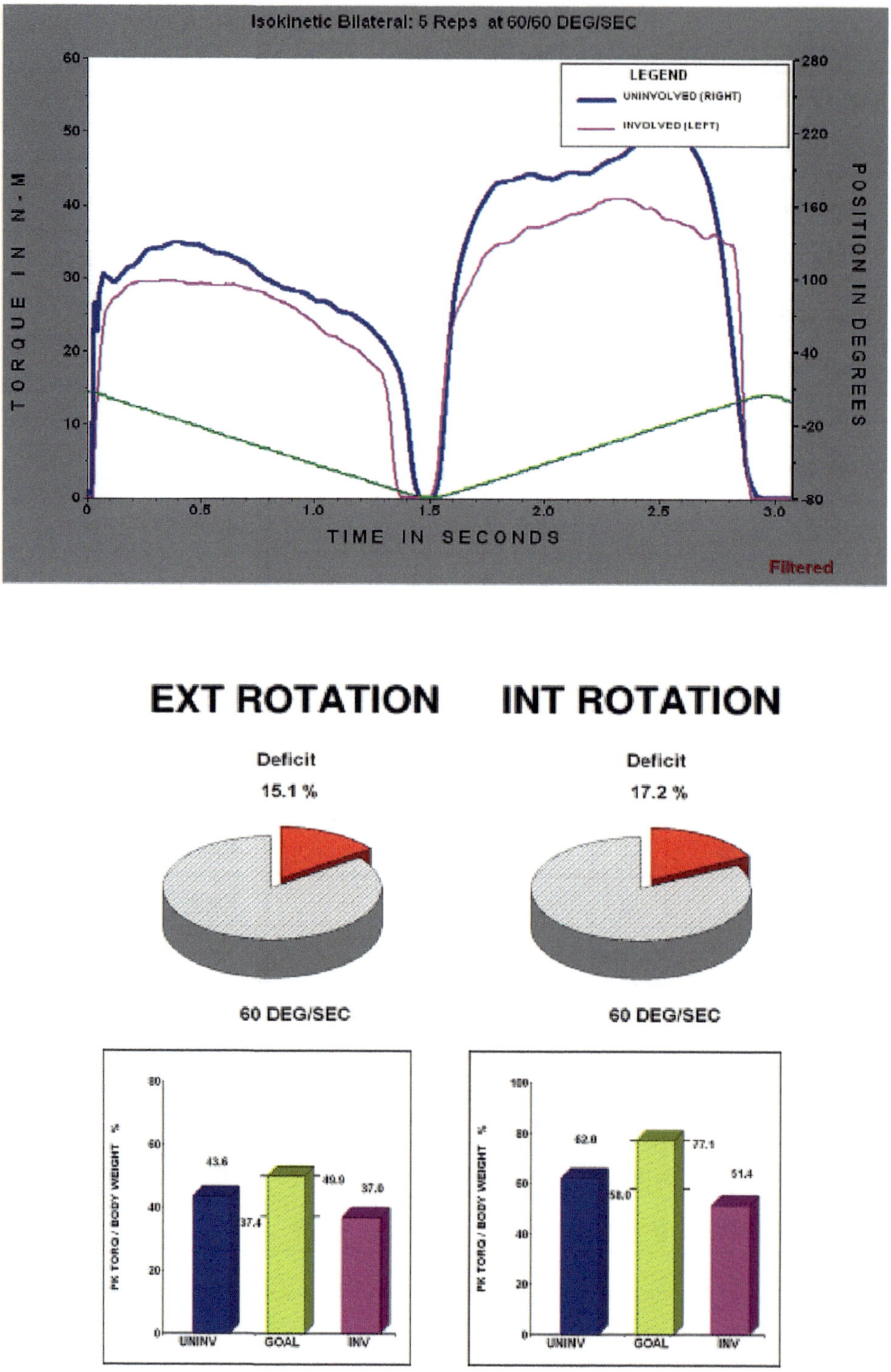

Fig. 22.6 The graph illustrates the gap of forces between the healthy limb (Right) and the affected one (Left). The pie chart shows that this deficit is greater in internal rotation than in ER. The Bar charts show that the goal, the peak torque of the left shoulder in relation to body weight (yellow bars) is not reached either in ER than in IR

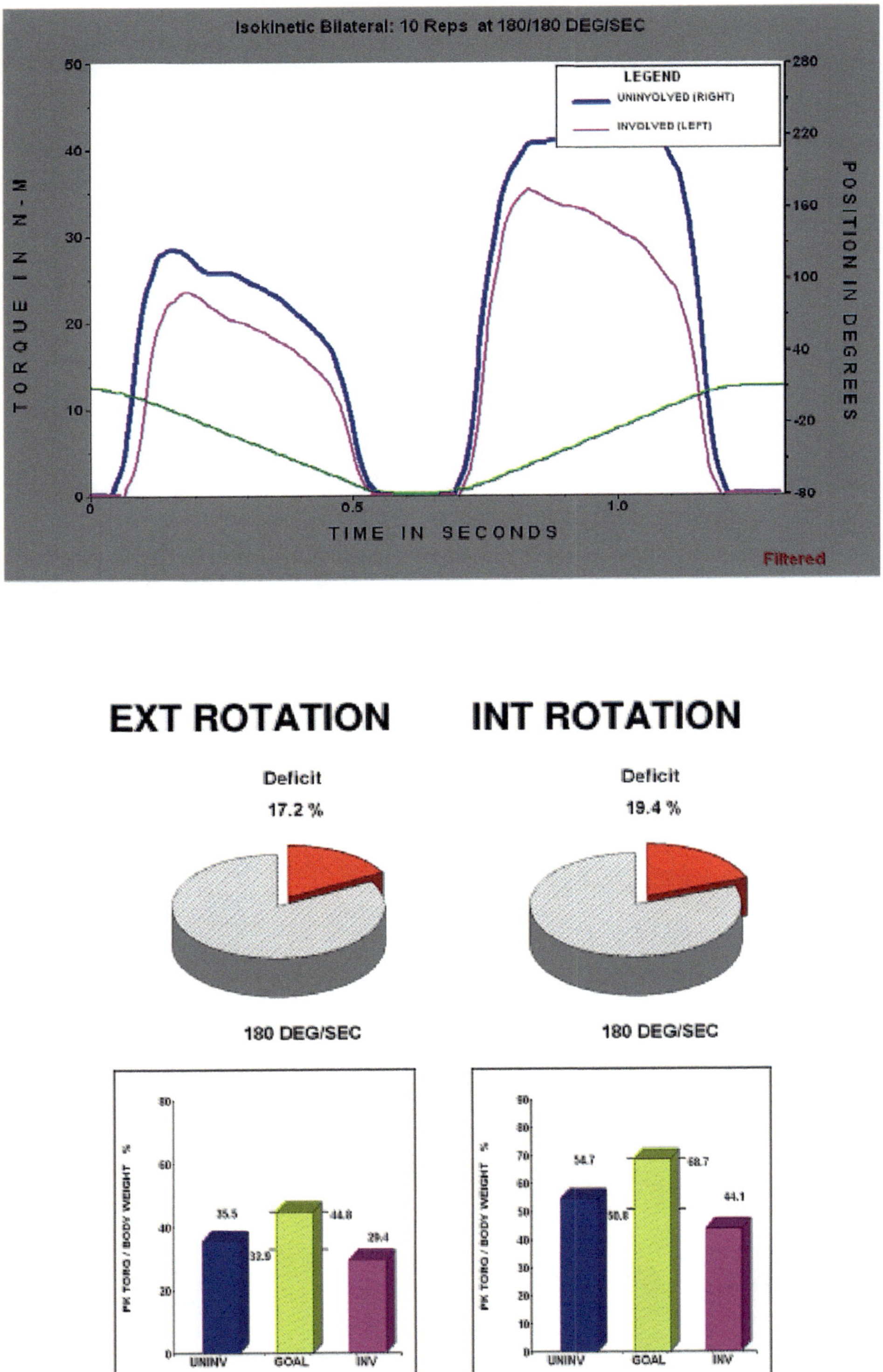

Fig. 22.7 The graph illustrates the gap of forces between the healthy limb (Right) and the affected one (Left), which is more pronounced at 180 Deg/Sec than at 60 deg./sec, both in ER and IR. Pie charts show again that the deficit of the left limb is greater in IR than in ER and the goal, the peak torque of the left shoulder in relation to body weight (yellow bars), is not reached both in ER and IR

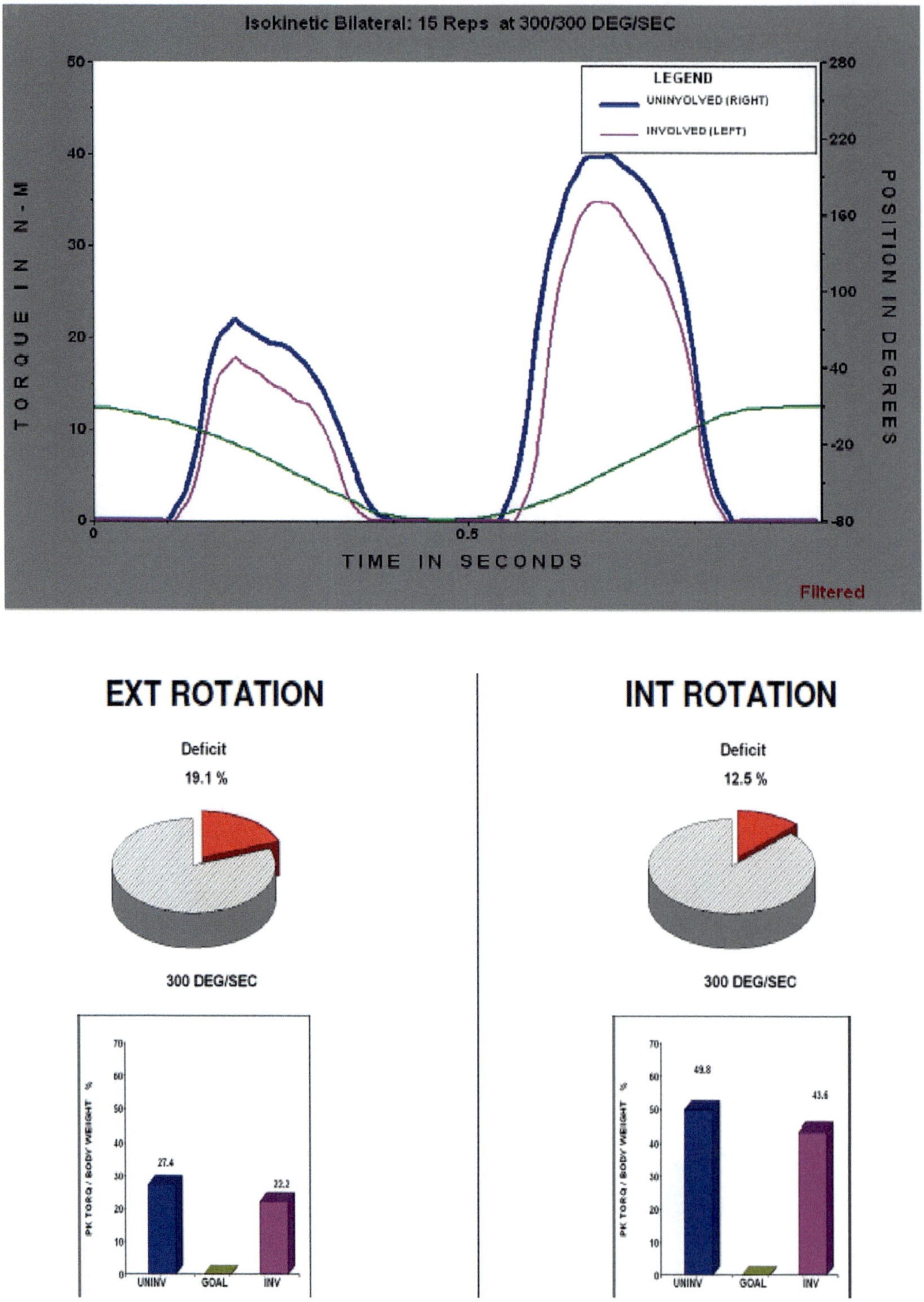

Fig. 22.8 The graph shows that the gap of force at high speeds is more significant in ER than in IR

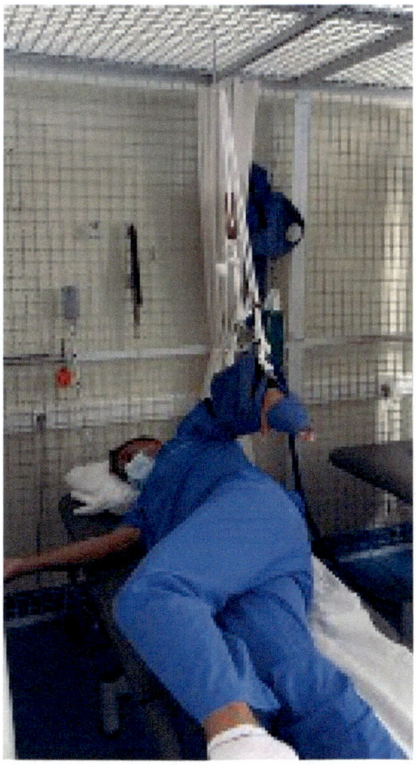

Fig. 22.9 Doing this exercise as part of a warmup before performing upper body exercise can improve mobility and flexibility in shoulders and upper back

- The goal in the immediate post-operative is to gain mobility. This, in addition to use of Biodex, is achieved through several methods:
  - Active movements with complete weight discharge (Fig. 22.9)
  - Shoulder pass-through (Fig. 22.10)
  - Electrostimulation (Fig. 22.11)
  - Biodex→ (Fig. 22.12, 22.13 and 22.14, Video 22.1)
- The duration of each exercise is between 5 and 15 min. Each exercise is performed passively, and the range of movement varies in relation to the patient's clinic. In the present case, the patient has complete ROM.

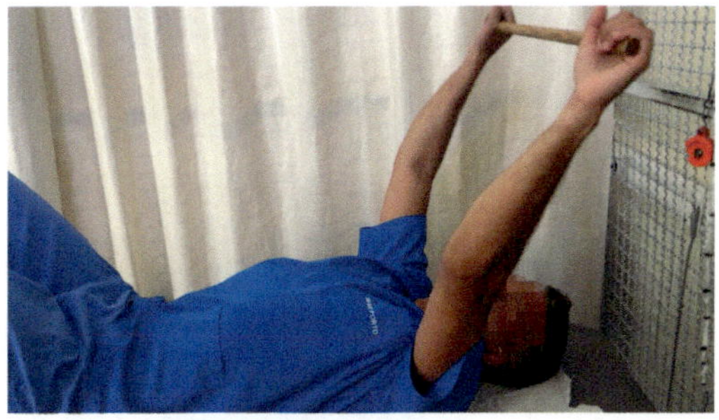

Fig. 22.10 The shoulder pass-through exercise helps to increase joint mobility while still engaging the surrounding muscles of the shoulder

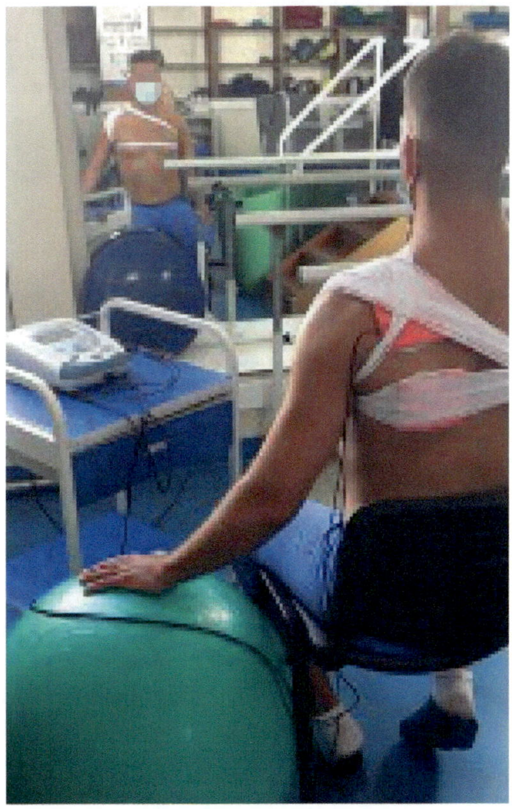

Fig. 22.11 With the use of constant current intensity, in square waves the muscles can work to the maximum of their potential and to tone immediately without creating overload problems. Electrostimulation also avoids subjecting the affected joint to continuous stress, thus eliminating micro-trauma that can be caused by classical physical exercises

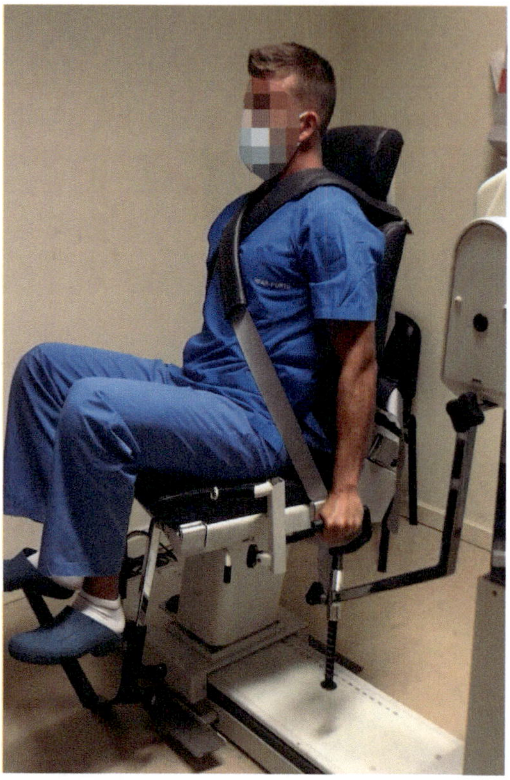

Fig. 22.12 BIODEX evaluation and rehabilitation with the shoulder in flexion

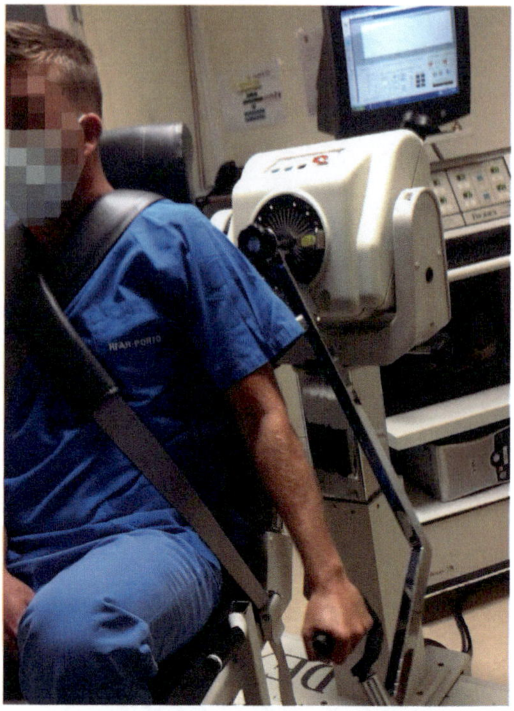

Fig. 22.13 BIODEX evaluation and rehabilitation with the shoulder in abduction and adduction

22.4.2.2 Late Post-operative

- With reference to the data collected by the test during the pre-operative phase, confirmed by the evaluations carried out in the post-operative phase, it is necessary to perform a therapeutic setting at all speeds aimed at strengthening the internal rotator muscles (subscapularis, anterior head of the deltoid and latissimus dorsi muscles) and the external rotator muscles of the left shoulder (teres minor, infraspinatus and posterior head of the deltoid muscles). Work on bilateral strengthening at maximum strength (+ internal rotators), power strength (+ internal rotators) and endurance strength (+ external rotators) should be done. The settings must always take into consideration any limitations of the patient's mobility, inexistent in the presented case.

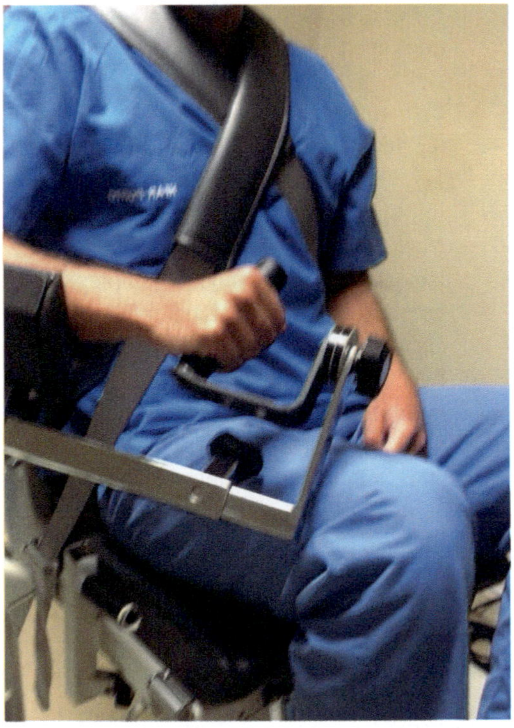

Fig. 22.14 BIODEX evaluation and rehabilitation with the shoulder in internal and external rotation

22.5 Practical Implementation Considerations

- Implementing isokinetic assessment in routine shoulder rehabilitation requires careful attention to both technical and practical factors. The initial equipment investment is substantial, comprehensive Biodex systems typically cost €45,000–80,000 depending on configuration and accessories, which places them beyond reach for many rehabilitation facilities. However, from a health economics perspective, there's an argument that improved precision in return-to-sport timing could reduce re-injury rates; preliminary cost-effectiveness analyses suggest that even a 20–25% reduction in re-injuries may justify the equipment investment in high-volume sports medicine centers [13]. That said, these economic models make numerous assumptions and haven't been validated across different healthcare systems or patient populations.
- Training requirements for clinical staff shouldn't be underestimated. In our experience, achieving competency requires 15–20 supervised testing sessions plus ongoing quality assurance measures (regular equipment calibration, periodic inter-rater reliability checks). Without proper training, measurement error can undermine the precision that makes isokinetic testing valuable in the first place. Some institutions implement certification programs for staff who perform isokinetic assessments, which seems prudent given the technical nature of the procedures.

22.6 Conclusion

- Isokinetic testing and evaluation are a valuable tool for assessing muscle strength and function following shoulder instability surgery. It allows for objective measurement of muscle strength, identification of muscle imbalances and weaknesses, and tracking of progress during rehabilitation. Its use can help ensure a successful recovery and return to normal function following shoulder instability surgery.
- The use of Isokinetic Biodex for the diagnosis and treatment of shoulder instability, in accordance with the literature, was found to be outwardly efficient and reliable both in the pre- and post-operative. The many modes offered by the machine allow you to create a highly specific therapeutic setting for each type of patient.
- The main advantage offered by this method is the ability to work at its maximum load throughout the range of motion, which ensures a faster muscle recovery compared to traditional therapies. In addition, it is possible to carefully select the joint range to safeguard the anatomical structures involved, avoid the appearance of pain and strengthen certain muscle groups.

- However, the need for continuous treatment and the consequent high costs of the machinery do not make it easy to use for every hospital and consequently do not allow, nowadays, to adopt such a system of treatment on a large scale.

Pearls and Pitfalls

Pearls

- *Early Implementation*: Introduce isokinetic exercises early in the post-operative phase, alongside traditional physiotherapy, to promote optimal muscle strengthening.
- *Individualized Protocols*: Use isokinetic testing data to create highly specific therapeutic settings for each patient, addressing their unique deficits and limitations.
- *Focus on Torque Acceleration Energy*: Evaluate torque acceleration energy to assess the patient's ability to generate force quickly, crucial for sports performance.
- *Safe Joint Positioning*: Perform IR/ER testing in the scapular plane to safeguard joint integrity and avoid impingement or apprehension.
- *Bilateral Comparison*: Compare the involved extremity to the uninvolved extremity to identify asymmetries and track progress. Aim for less than 10–15% difference.

Pitfalls

- *Over-reliance on Single Parameters*: Avoid making decisions based solely on one isokinetic parameter (e.g., bilateral comparison). Consider unilateral strength ratios, torque-to-body-weight ratios, and fatigue ratios for a comprehensive assessment.
- *Ignoring Patient Limitations*: Always consider the patient's mobility limitations and pain levels when designing the isokinetic rehabilitation program.
- *Cost and Accessibility*: Be aware that the high cost of isokinetic equipment may limit its accessibility in all clinical settings.
- *Neglecting Traditional Methods*: Isokinetic testing should complement, not replace, traditional methods of muscle testing and clinical examination.
- *Lack of Standardized Protocols*: Be mindful of the variety of testing positions and protocols reported in the literature. Choose a reliable and validated method (e.g., neutral position for IR/ER) and maintain consistency.

References

1. SYSTEM 4 (Advantage BX Software 5.3X) Instructions for use 850-000 840-000 852-000 system 4 [Internet]. Available from: www.biodex.com
2. Ellenbecker TS, George JD. The application of Isokinetics in testing and rehabilitation of the shoulder complex [Internet]. J Athl Train. 2000;35:338. Available from: www.joumalofathletictraining.org
3. Verweij LPE, van den Bekerom MPJ, Kramer S, et al. A modified Delphi study to identify which items should be evaluated in shoulder instability research: a first step in developing a core outcome set. JSES Int. 2023;7(6):2304–10.
4. Moussa MK, El Hariri B, Lefèvre N, et al. Isokinetic strength and balance analyses for predicting return to sports after the Latarjet procedure: a prospective cross-sectional study. Am J Sports Med. 2024;52(12):3086–95.
5. Almeida GPL, Monteiro IL, Marizeiro DF, et al. Reliability of dynamic shoulder strength test battery using multi-joint isokinetic device. Sensors (Basel). 2024;24(11):3568.
6. Gremliza L, Wochatz M, Menn L, et al. Impact of different isokinetic movement patterns on shoulder rehabilitation outcome. Int J Environ Res Public Health. 2022;19(17):10623.
7. Parisini F, Mangone M, Agostini F, et al. Innovative diagnostic framework for shoulder instability: a narrative review on machine learning-enhanced scapular dyskinesis assessment in sports injuries. Sports Med Open. 2025;11(1):42.

8. Knops JE, Meiners TK, Davies GJ. Isokinetic test-retest reliability of the modified neutral shoulder test position. University of LaCrosse; 1998. (unpublished research).
9. Quincy DC, Davies GJ, Kolbeck KJ. Isokinetic exercise: the effects of training specificity on shoulder strength development. J Athl Train. 2000;35(S64)
10. Malavolta EA, Cruz DG, Gracitelli MEC, Assunção JH, Andrade-Silva FB, Andrusaitis FR, et al. Isokinetic evaluation of the shoulder and elbow after Latarjet procedure. Orthop Traumatol Surg Res. 2020;106(6):1079–82.
11. Giovanni Di Giacomo. Trattamento chirurgico dell'instabilità di spalla [Internet]. [cited 2021 Sep 21]. Available from: https://www.spalla.it/trattamento-chirurgico-dellinstabilita-di-spalla/
12. Jan J, Benkalfate T, Rochcongar P. The impact of recurrent dislocation on shoulder rotator muscle balance (a prospective study of 102 male patients). Ann Phys Rehabil Med. 2012;55(6):404–14.
13. Westermann RW, Wolf BR, Elkins JM. Cost-effectiveness analysis of isokinetic testing in sports medicine practice. Health Econ Rev. 2024;14(1):28.

First Time Dislocation in Adolescent Without Bony Lesion

23

Jean Marc Glasson

Keypoints

- First time traumatic dislocation is a common trauma in younger population and more specifically in male athletes.
- The practice of contact sports involving or not the upper limb are predisposing circumstances.
- The recurrence rate is estimated between 50% and 100% depending on age, activities, and constitutional laxity.
- Contrast iconography (CT arthrogram or ContrastMRI) is mandatory in these situations allowing perfect lesions analysis and descriptions.
- Evaluate benefit-risk profile taking account of the very young age of the patient.
- Favor less invasive and risky surgical procedures for these very young patients even if a low recurrence rate may persist.

23.1 Introduction/Background

- Shoulder dislocation is a frequent traumatic condition with a variable prevalence depending on age and sex ratio. With a prevalence rate that hit 100/100000habitants/year in younger male it is more than 4 for time higher than the overall prevalence in the population [1].
- The adolescent population (age < 20 years) is specifically at risk for several and cumulative reasons.

  First of the all the recurrence rate. Prospective studies have evaluated this possible evolution up to 100% [2] with at least 80% in the 12 months following the first episode of dislocation [3]. The recurrence rate increases with the young age, the traumatic or exposed activities (sport or professional) and in male.

  Arthritic evolution after dislocation is well documented. Arthritic evolution increases with the length of follow up and is also more frequent in patient with multiple dislocations (40%) than in patient who only suffered one episode (18%) [4]. Moreover, when considering young patient who ended up having stabilization surgery, as the number of preoperative dislocation episodes raises the amount of postoperative arthritis increases [5].
- Initially reported in 1989 for West Point Cadets [6], the arthroscopic repair of first-time

J. M. Glasson (✉)
Institut Niçois Sport et arthrose (INSA), Nice, France

L. Kovačič et al. (eds.), *Surgical Techniques for Anterior Shoulder Instability*,
https://doi.org/10.1007/978-3-662-73064-5_23

shoulder dislocations in younger athletes was then popularized in multiple publications [7].
- The principle of this indication is mainly linked to the precise evaluation of the balance risk and benefit. This comprises a clear description of the lesions with a contrast iconography.

23.2 Clinical Evaluation

23.2.1 Patient's Background

- Exposed professional or sport activities.
- Sports level (competitor) and wish to pursue.
- Patients interrogation includes: sex, age, arm dominance, delay since the injury, previous shoulder pain, involvement in treatment, understanding of treatment consequences.
- This initial patient evaluation should allow an approximation of the recurrence rate of shoulder dislocation.

23.2.2 Relevant Physical Findings

- First time shoulder "dislocator" visiting in the acute phase are not easily tested clinically because of an understandable apprehension.
- However, evaluation of comparative anteroposterior drawer test in a seating position brings information about possible anterior lesions.
- As for every shoulder dislocation care should be taken to perform accurate axillary nerve testing (motor and sensory).
- General laxity will be evaluated with the Beighton Score or more specifically in comparison with the contralateral upper limb with the exclusion of the shoulder hyper abduction test of course. General or upper limb hyperlaxity increases the recurrence rate whether the patient will be operated or not. The laxity score adds some information for the surgeon in case of arthroscopic repair.

23.2.3 Relevant Imaging

- Xrays are of routine practice with 3 A/P views in different rotations, a Scapular Y view and a glenoid view; preferably the Bloom Obata projection. This latter Xray provides an excellent anterior glenoid margin and posterosuperior head (Hill Sachs) evaluation without any risk of dislocation.
- Xrays will inform about bony lesion on the glenoid or the humeral head. These lesions are excluded in the discussion of this chapter.
- The population considered are teenager, therefore the bone maturation might not be completed. This is very obvious around the shoulder since the inferior glenoid, the coracoid, the acromion and part of the humeral head epiphysis will fuse only at an age around 18 years.
- Identifying dysplasia, or incomplete epiphyseal fusion is important for treatment and surgical techniques strategy.
- Contrast iconography with sectional imaging is mandatory. Unless it is performed in the 3 first weeks (hematoma, inflammation), simple MRI does not have enough sensitivity and specificity to base the surgical indication on it. The CT arthrogram offers a quick and very accurate evaluation of co-occurring bony lesions. Regarding soft tissues injuries, the majority of the patients Arthro CTscan will show a Bankart lesion. Over 95% of the cases according to certain authors [8]. The other lesions encountered are SLAP, IGHL avulsion, capsular rupture, HAGL,….

  The arthroMRI with the injection of Gadolinium brings comparable informations.
- It is only after this complete analysis that the adequate indication and treatment can be issued (Fig. 23.1).

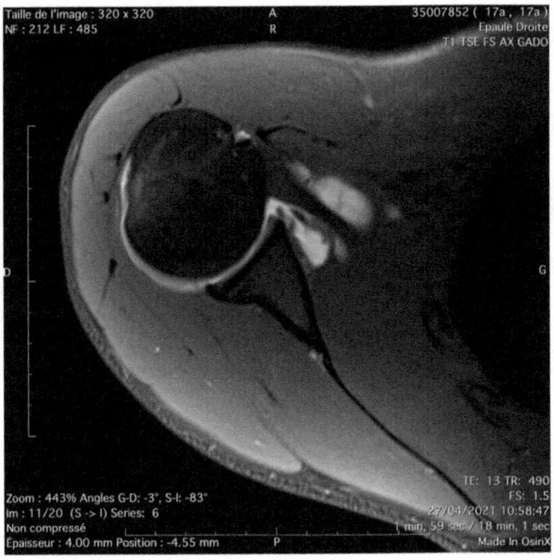

Fig. 23.1 Arthro MRI—17 years, First league football player, dominant arm, promising young player, close to end season. First time traumatic dislocation. Isolated Bankart lesion

23.3 Treatment Options and Indications

- The whole discussion regarding this specific population is the balance of risk and benefit.
- Abstention or sling immobilization with adapted rehabilitation still exposes to a high rate of recurrence. Additionally, in this population, a long term follow-up study [9], emphasizes that for almost 50% of the initially nonoperatively treated patients, a stabilization surgery in the 10 years following will be required.
- With the exclusion of bony lesions, the perspective is to address soft tissue lesions and mostly a Bankart lesion.
- The acute phase after a first shoulder dislocation has been described as in the first 10 days [8]. Nevertheless, the acute phase remains probably eligible in the first post traumatic 3 months. There is no consensus about the delay after a first dislocation which will define the limit of an acute treatment. Capsule distension, fibrotic scaring, and tissue involution may occur with time and undermine the quality of the surgical procedure.
- Arthroscopic direct repair of the lesion is the "Gold standard" in this specific indication. Any "bony" stabilization, modifying the patient anatomy is not recommended here.
- The surgical technic under arthroscopy will target only the lesions encountered. The labrum (Bankart, SLAP) will be reattached with small anchors and if possible, with no knots in contact with the cartilage. The capsule or its humeral insertion might be sutured or reinserted as well. To some extent, the GHLs or the capsule can be tightened while respecting the laxity and the activities performed. The repair has to be securely stabilized for early passive and active mobilization will be authorized.
- Contra indication for surgery or a remote assessment will be necessary in case of associated neurologic symptoms or previously mentioned "Dead arm" syndrome,… (Figs. 23.2 and 23.3).

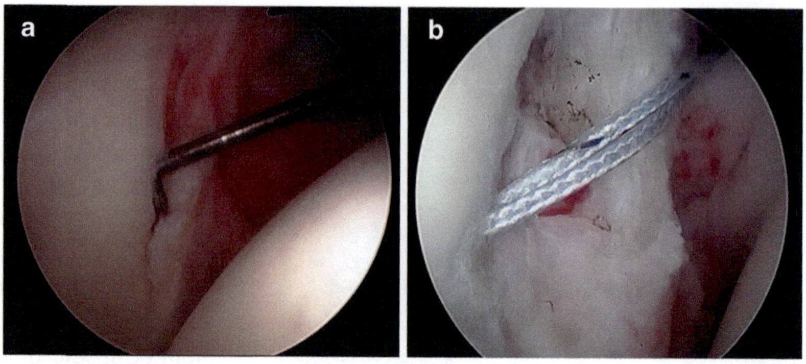

Fig. 23.2 and 23.3 Limited Bankart lesion with direct suture in preparation

23.4 Decision-Making Algorithm

- Young patient under 20 years of age with no bony lesions. Millimetric bony Bankart avulsion, GLAD lesion, or millimetric Hill Sachs are not considered "bony lesions."
- The 2 major factors for arthroscopic indications are age and activities.
- The indication extends from a formal one, based on evidence, in case of a 15 years old male, dominant arm and exposed athletes to a more disputable indication but still validated, in case of a recreative active teenager.
- The iconography prepares the surgical strategy but should not affect the indication for surgery since almost 100% of patients have lesions.
- The arthroscopic surgical treatment should always only be limited to the lesion encountered.
- Post-operative early soft passive and active motion should be advised to avoid capsular retraction.

23.4.1 Outcomes

- In the discussed population the recurrence rate with no surgery is reported to be around 90%. This rate drops at 14% with a follow up of 13 years in case of arthroscopic direct repair [7].
- Complications are rare with this technic but, rare capsulitis, long term bone resorption have been related.

23.4.2 Expert Recommendation

- First time shoulder dislocation in the teenager population exposes to recurrence and with it; higher arthritic long term evolution, extended articular lesions, lower surgical effectiveness, more aggressive surgical technic for stabilization.
- First time dislocation acute phase extends to 6 months if no other instability incidents has occurred in the meantime. The tissue remains of good quality and is easily mobilized.
- Specific arthroscopic technic is necessary with low profile anchors and knots.
- Surgical indications in this population is discussed with fair and clear information.

References

1. Leroux T, Wasserstein D, Veillette C, et al. Epidemiology of primary anterior shoulder dislocation requiring closed reduction in Ontario, Canada. Am J Sports Med. 2014;42(2):442–50. https://doi.org/10.1177/0363546513510391. Epub 2013 Nov 25
2. Rte Slaa RL, Brand R, Marty RK. A prospective arthroscopic study of acute first-time anterior shoulder dislocation in the young: a five-year follow-up study. J Shoulder Elbow Surg. 2003;12(6):529–34. https://doi.org/10.1016/s1058-2746(03)00218-0.
3. Brumet RC, Bach BR, Provencher MT. Arthroscopic stabilization for first-time versus recurrent shoulder instability. Arthroscopy. 2010;26(2):239–48. https://doi.org/10.1016/j.arthro.2009.06.006. Epub 2009 Dec 6.
4. Hovelius L, Saeboe M. Neer award 2008: arthropathy after primary anterior shoulder dislocation–223 shoulders prospectively followed up for twenty-five years. J

Shoulder Elbow Surg. 2009;18(3):339–47. https://doi.org/10.1016/j.jse.2008.11.004. Epub 2009 Feb 28.
5. Buscayret F, Edwards TB, Szabo I, Adeleine P, Coudane H, Walch G. Glenohumeral arthrosis in anterior instability before and after surgical treatment: incidence and contributing factors. Am J Sports Med. 2004;32(5):1165–72. https://doi.org/10.1177/0363546503262686. Epub 2004 May 18.
6. Wheeler JH, Ryan JB, Arciero RA, Mollinari RN. Arthroscopic versus nonoperative treatment of acute shoulder dislocations in young athletes. Arthroscopy. 1989;5(3):213–7. https://doi.org/10.1016/0749-8063(89)90174-6.
7. Arciero RA, Bottoni CR. Arthroscopic repair of primary anterior dislocations of the shoulder. Tech Should Elbow Surg. 2001;2(1):2–16.
8. Taylor DC, Arciero RA. Pathologic changes associated with shoulder dislocations. Arthroscopic and physical examination findings in first time, traumatic anterior dislocations. AJSM. 1997;25(3):306–11. https://doi.org/10.1177/036354659702500306.
9. Hovelius L, et al. Non operative treatment of primary anterior shoulder dislocation in patient forty years of age and younger. A prospective twenty-five-year follow-up. JBJS(A). 2008;90(5):945–52. https://doi.org/10.2106/JBJS.G.00070.

First-Time Dislocation Over 20 Years Without Bony Lesion

24

Edoardo Giovannetti de Sanctis
and Francesco Franceschi

Key Points

- Acute anterior dislocation of the shoulder joint is relatively common with an estimated lifetime incidence of 2% in the general population.
- Traumatic dislocations might damage the soft tissues surrounding the shoulder and sometimes the bony structure of the glenohumeral joint.
- Patients with recurrent shoulder dislocation show a significantly higher degree and prevalence of Bankart and associated previously described lesions than patients with only a first-time shoulder dislocation.
- Age at the time of the initial dislocation is inversely related to the recurrence rate.
- Management strategy for the first-time anterior glenohumeral dislocation remains debated.
- Age, gender, time since dislocation, physical and sport activity level, greater tuberosity fracture and apprehension-relocation test are the main prognostic factors used in decision-making process while treating patients after a first-time shoulder dislocation with no bony lesions.
- Primary surgical stabilization might be preferred in patients with a higher risk for recurrent dislocation based on those characteristics.

E. G. de Sanctis
IULS – Institut Universitaire Locomoteur et Sports, Pasteur 2 Hospital, CHU, Nice, France

F. Franceschi (✉)
Faculty of Medicine and Surgery, Link Campus University, Rome, Italy

Department of Orthopaedic and Trauma Surgery, San Pietro Fatebenefratelli Hospital, Rome, Italy
e-mail: f.franceschi@unilink.it

24.1 Introduction

- Acute anterior dislocation of the shoulder joint is relatively common with an estimated lifetime incidence of 2% in the general population, comprising approximately 50% of all joint dislocations.
- Traumatic dislocations might damage the soft tissues surrounding the shoulder and sometimes the bony structure of the glenohumeral joint. Injury to the dynamic (Rotator Cuff tendons) or static (capsulolabral structures) soft tissue stabilizers of the shoulder may increase the risk of recurrent post-traumatic instability.

L. Kovačič et al. (eds.), *Surgical Techniques for Anterior Shoulder Instability*,
https://doi.org/10.1007/978-3-662-73064-5_24

- The classical Bankart lesion (i.e. antero-inferior detachment of the labrum from the glenoid rim and capsule plastic deformation or tear) could be associated with humeral avulsion of the glenohumeral ligaments (HAGL), extended labral detachment (SLAP and/or isolated posterior labral lesions) and rotator cuff tendon tears (being injured mainly in older patients).
- Patients with recurrent shoulder dislocation show a significantly higher degree and prevalence of Bankart and associated previously described lesions than patients with only a first-time shoulder dislocation (FSD) [1–3]. The increasing episodes of dislocation lead to a progressive and irreversible labral-ligamentous injury and degeneration [4].
- Management strategy for the first-time anterior glenohumeral dislocation is still debated. Traditionally, conservative treatment has been advocated for the majority of patients, leaving the operative treatment reserved only for recurrent dislocators or those involved in high demanding physical activity.
- The high rate of complications, such as recurrent instability, residual pain, and inability to return to sports and unsatisfactory outcomes of non-surgical management, especially in young adults, and less than optimal outcomes of surgical repair of recurrent dislocations have led many authors to search the ideal management and then propose an early arthroscopic Bankart repair after first acute glenohumeral dislocation.
- Arciero et al. first popularized this issue, comparing arthroscopic trans-glenoid repair with nonoperative treatment in militaries with a mean age of 20 years. They had successful and better results with the operative treatment [5].
- Currently, decision between two available options in patients with primary glenohumeral dislocation and age more than 20 years has to be taken. Namely, immediate arthroscopic repair or conservative treatment (with immobilization and rehabilitation). The question which is more appropriate has not been resolved yet [6].

24.2 Relevant Physical Findings

- Initial evaluation after FSD should include patient age, gender and type of instability (unidirectional vs. multidirectional or hyper-laxity). Active range of motion (ROM) using a goniometer, strength, and neurovascular status of both shoulders and upper limbs should be examined.
- Many examination manoeuvres have been described so far such as: the apprehension and relocation test (to assess the stability of the joint in ABER position), the load and shift and anterior-posterior drawer tests (to assess anterior and posterior capsular laxity), the hyper-abduction test described by Gagey (to assess inferior glenohumeral ligament IGHL laxity) and the sulcus sign (to assess Rotator interval laxity).
- Controversial is the ability of those tests in decision making whether treating the patient conservatively or operatively. Safran et al. evaluated the predictivity of the Apprehension test 6 weeks following the FSD and found that a negative test was significantly related to recurrent instability [7]. Redislocations at 2 years follow up occurred in 36.8% and 71.4% of participants with respectively negative and positive apprehension tests.
- Theoretically, patients should be able to be completely pain-free with full active glenohumeral ROM within 6 weeks after the FSD. Additional imaging (whether CT or MRI, based on the age of the patient) is recommended in case of persistent pain, loss of function and if any bony lesion is suspected, approximately 2–6 weeks after the dislocation, as stated within the ESSKA-ESA consensus [6].

24.3 Relevant Imaging

- Radiographic evaluation should include an anteroposterior view in internal and external rotation, a lateral and an axillary view (Fig. 24.1). Magnetic resonance imaging (MRI) is most helpful in evaluating the soft

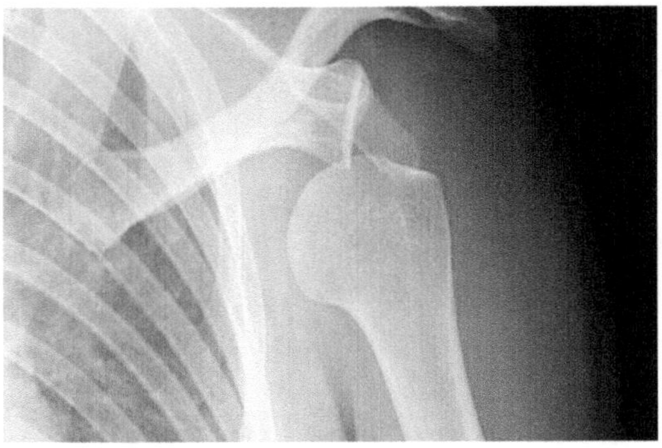

Fig. 24.1 Antero-posterior view shoulder radiograph after a first-time shoulder dislocation

tissue (GH ligaments and the glenoid labrum) injury after a FSD, looking for Bankart and rotator cuff lesions.

- The presence of joint effusion or intraarticular injection of contrast fluid could better detect labro-ligamentous lesions on MR images. It has been reported that 97% of the patients examined with MRI within 10 days after primary traumatic dislocation had joint effusion. If additional imaging needs to be performed after 2 weeks from the FSD, MR arthrography might be another option to be used [1, 7].
- Interestingly, young patients have a significantly lower risk of RC tears compared to older patients (2.9% incidence of RC tears in patients <30 years compared to 53% incidence in patients ≥30 years) [8].

24.4 Treatment Options and Indications

- After the FSD the physician should aim at restoring a fully functional, pain-free and stable shoulder. Both conservative or surgical treatments are usually preceded by closed reduction of glenohumeral joint after the acute dislocation. Different relocation techniques and anaesthetics usage (general anaesthesia or intrarticular injections) have been described while reducing the glenohumeral joint. It has been shown by Hovelius et al. that general anaesthesia during closed reduction is used significantly more frequently in patients with ≥30 years than with ≤22 years [9].
- Conservative management usually requires a period of rest, generally involving immobilization of the arm in a sling, for 3–6 weeks.
- It is still debated whether to immobilize the shoulder in external rotation (ER) and/or abduction instead of adduction and internal rotation. The degree of ER (0–60°) and abduction used by the authors vary significantly. This kind of immobilization might bring the labrum back to a more anatomical position. However, both options might be valid as controversial results in instability recurrence rate have been found related to the reduction method and type or period of immobilization [9–16].
- Operative management incorporates soft-tissue repair (principally arthroscopically Bankart repair) and is usually followed by a supervised physiotherapy programme (Fig. 24.2). In the past several studies suggested arthroscopic washout (AWO), or joint lavage as having therapeutic effects for first-time anterior shoulder dislocation. Yapp et al. showed that arthroscopic bankart repair leads to greater overall shoulder stability and functional outcomes than AWO, in patients with an age < 35 years after an FSD [18].
- Different opinions and controversy exist with regard to patient management after FSD. Reducing the risk of recurrent instability seems to be the main advantage of primary arthroscopic stabilization. However, this treatment exposes patients to the morbidities of surgery.
- Moreover, a non-stable joint could increase the risk of developing shoulder osteoarthritis. It has been shown that operated shoulders did not differ from shoulders with no recurrence with respect to moderate/severe arthropathy at the 25-year follow-up [9, 17].
- Adam et al. in their meta-analysis compared immediate arthroscopic repair with conservative treatment after FSD as well as with arthroscopic reconstruction of recurrent anterior shoulder dislocation in patients with a mean age of 21.3 years [20]. Revision rates

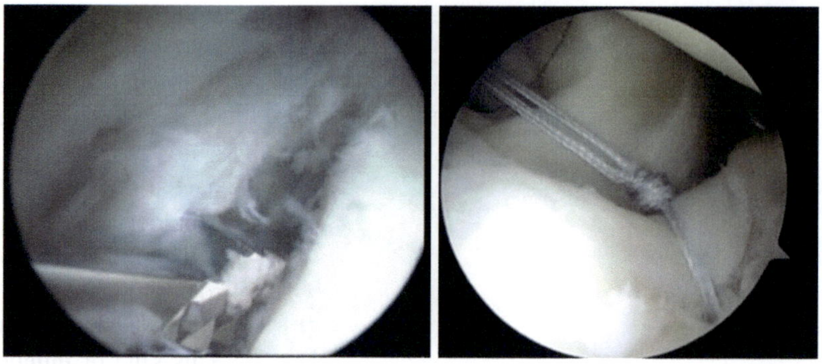

Fig. 24.2 Arthroscopic Bankart repair

were lower in immediate arthroscopic repair of primary shoulder dislocation compared to both conservative treatment and arthroscopic reconstruction of recurrent dislocation.

- In the series of Hovelius et al. [18] the probability of recurrent instability in patients with less than 40 years after a FSD (with no tuberosity fracture) was 54% and 10.9% respectively for nonoperative treatment and primary arthroscopic stabilization [21].
- Kirkley et al. compared immediate arthroscopic stabilization versus immobilization and rehabilitation after FSD in forty patients younger than 30 years [19]. At 3-year follow-up, they found a 47% recurrence in the non-operative group compared with only 16% in the surgical group, recommending that immediate arthroscopic stabilization is the treatment of choice in a subset of patients who are younger than 30 years and are high level athletes.
- Minkus et al. compared immobilization in ER at 60° and ABD versus primary arthroscopic shoulder stabilization for the treatment of FSD in patients with a mean age of 26.2 ± 5.9 years [20]. Despite showing no differences in clinical shoulder scores, they found a significantly higher recurrent instability after nonoperative treatment (19.1% vs. 2.3%; $p = 0.016$).

24.5 Decision-Making Algorithm

- Many risk factors predispose first-time traumatic anterior shoulder dislocations to recurrent instability, that might be helpful to consider during the decision whether treating the patient surgically or not [15]. A predictive model of shoulder instability after a first-time anterior shoulder dislocation has been proposed recently [21]. Surgical stabilization after the first dislocation in patients with those specific characteristics is currently still subject of scientific debate.
- Age at the time of the initial dislocation is inversely related to the recurrence rate. Therefore, young patients have higher risk of recurrent instability compared to older patients [9]. It has been reported a recurrence rate of 72–95% in patients under 20 years of age, 70–82% in patients having between 20 and 30 years, and 14–22% in patients older than 50 years [4]. This may be due to differences in biomechanical properties, collagen fibre type, elasticity of the capsule or changes in activity level with increasing age [15]. Hovelius et al. described the long-term prognosis in 257 FSD treated conservatively (aged 12–40) [10]. At 2 years follow up, patients with age <22 and >30 years showed respectively 31% and 56% of no recurrence rate.
- Extrinsic risk factors of recurrent shoulder instability include occupations which involve using the upper limb above chest height and collision or overhead sports. The failure rate is much higher (up to 68%) in physically active patients. Riccio et al. evaluated 32 participants with first traumatic anterior shoulder dislocation, not involved in sport activity, and not overhead workers, mean aged 27.94 ± 2.23 years [22]. Approach based on rehabilitation seemed to be effective in the

conservative management in adults as none of their patients after 2 years presented a new episode of shoulder dislocation.

- Males and people with hyperlaxity have a greater probability of developing recurrent instability [15].
- The probability of recurrent instability decreased as time from the initial dislocation increased [15]. It is greatest in the first year and decreases up to 5 years after the initial dislocation becoming close to 0.
- Decreased risk of recurrent instability was reported in people with a greater tuberosity fracture (due to a decreased range of external rotation in both abduction and neutral) [9, 15].
- The conservative treatment and a "wait and see" period after FSD before deciding to operate is currently the most widely used method of treating patients with more than 20 years. Interestingly, Berendes et al. [23] stated in their survey amongst Dutch public hospitals that only 2% of the Orthopaedic Surgeons would decide to treat the patient surgically after the FSD. The non-operative treatment has different pros and cons. Its ability of tear healing without the need of surgery was underlined by several authors, indicating that true traumatic ligamentous lesions diagnosed in an early phase after a primary traumatic shoulder dislocation with MRI and/or MRA were likely disappear during the first 3 months [7]. However the patient compliance is fundamental in order to avoid an interruption of the immobilization treatment.
- Age, gender, level or type of physical activity (Sport/job) and time since the dislocation are important issues to be considered in decision-making of operative treatment (Fig. 24.3). There is no yet a clear consensus on cut-off values to be used while looking at this parameters and no scores used worldwide available helping the physician in decision-making after a FSD, usually not associated with bone defects. The ISIS score [24], for example, was designed as a guide to help the surgeon identifying patients at a higher risk of instability recurrence after an arthroscopic Bankart procedure, therefore better treated by an open operation.
- It might be considered to treat surgically patients with one or more of the prognostic factors, due to their higher recurrence rate (Fig. 24.3). Younger age, male gender and demanding job with the elevated arms or sports activity are main characteristics in the treatment decision-making of the first-time dislocator. Other prognostic factors suggesting and leading to an operative procedure are

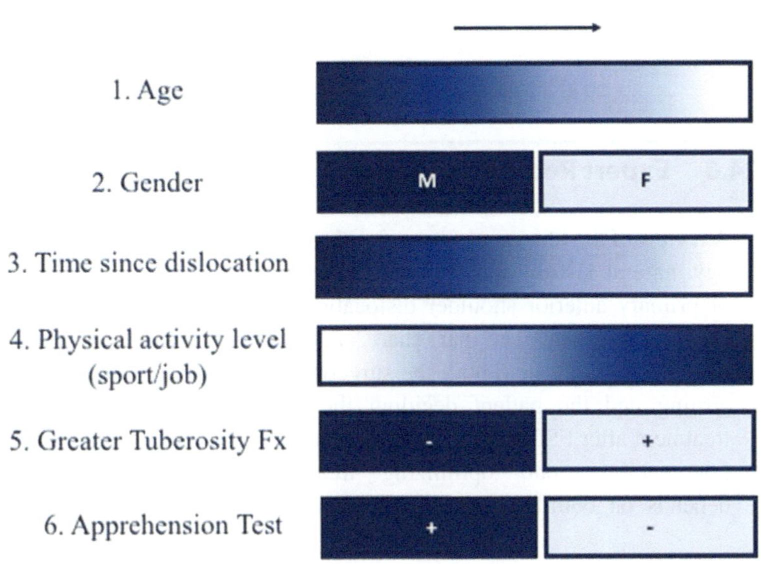

Fig. 24.3 Recurrence rate predictive factors. It allows physicians to accurately predict the expected outcome of treatment and risk of recurrence. It is helpful tool in informed decision-making. The darkest the blue the highest the risk of recurrence; M Male, F Female; "–" Negative; "+" Positive; The arrow indicates the direction of an increasing value

continued positive apprehension test and failure to return to work or sport. However, there is no significant evidence to justify the repair of every patient after a FSD rather than waiting for recurrent dislocation to occur. In different scenarios, such as a FSD in middle-aged or elderly patients, the risk of recurrence is lower and nonoperative treatment would be the first choice leading to optimal outcomes.

- Hovelius et al. confirmed the importance of patient's age in treatment decision-making [9]. They stated that at the 10-year follow-up, subjects aged ≤25 years had had surgery earlier (≤5 years after the first dislocation) and subjects aged ≥26 years later (between 5 and 10 years after the first dislocation, $p < 0.02$).

Pearls and Pitfalls

- Understanding the type of instability that the patient is experiencing and obtaining. A thorough history is critical for the success of the treatment
- A complete physical examination is essential to making the correct diagnosis
- The successful management of patients with anterior shoulder instability can be a significant challenge
- Active and younger patients treated with a physical therapy program might be associated with a higher recurrence rates

24.6 Expert Recommendation

- A review of the literature concerning the etiology, natural history and treatment outcomes of primary anterior shoulder dislocation has been carried out. The bar chart presented (Fig. 24.3) might help both the surgeon suggesting and the patient deciding the right treatment after FSD with no bony defects.
- For each patient, optimizing treatment depends on both outcome probabilities and personal preferences. Treatment has to be "à la carte", i.e. adapted to each specific patient. Each treatment strategy could not be proper for every patient. Shared decision-making, where both the physician and the patient discuss case-specific clinical outcome likelihoods is fundamental to optimize the results. A clear example are in-season athletes willing to risk additional dislocations in order to avoid being out of field. Therefore, patients with a strong aversion to surgery may be best treated nonoperatively.
- There is significant evidence to consider surgery as the best treatment for patients at high risk of recurrent instability with conservative strategy. Patients requiring a full return to a high performance level to properly execute their jobs (such as professional athletes and military cadets), as well as those with an increased risk of reinjury should undergo operative stabilization. However, treating all patients surgically is almost certainly overtreatment.
- As previously mentioned, patients over 40 years are tipicalluy managed non operatively, due to the low recurrence rate. However, this population has often associated injuries such as rotator cuff tears that need to be faced, changing the treatment of choice. If a RC tear is diagnosed after a FSD and the operative treatment has been chosen, we prefer to perform the arthroscopic repair within 3 weeks from the injury, in order to have still optimal tissue conditions.
- We would suggest and encourage non-operative treatment first in cases with a low risk of recurrent instability or with a complex condition of the shoulder, such as: in patients older than 25 years, younger but not actively engaged in overhead activities and with no other negative prognostic factors and patients with multi-directional instability or soft-tissue laxity. In those cases a "wait and see" approach with a strict surveillance and immediate re-evaluation in case of recurrence are the best options in deciding whether to perform surgery or not.

Take Home Message

- Age, gender, time since dislocation, physical activity level, greater tuberosity fracture and apprehension-relocation test are the main prognostic factors used in decision-making process while treating patients after a FSD with no bony lesions.
- Primary conservative treatment should be preferred in nondemanding population.
- Primary surgical stabilization might be preferred in patients with a high risk for recurrent dislocation based on those characteristics.
- RC tears in patients over 40 needs to be ruled out.

References

1. Kim DS, Yoon YS, Yi CH. Prevalence comparison of accompanying lesions between primary and recurrent anterior dislocation in the shoulder. Am J Sports Med. 2010;38(10):2071–6.
2. Rugg CM, Hettrich CM, Ortiz S, Wolf BR, Group MSI, Zhang AL. Surgical stabilization for first-time shoulder dislocators: a multicenter analysis. J Shoulder Elbow Surg. 2018;27(4):674–85.
3. Gutierrez V, Monckeberg JE, Pinedo M, Radice F. Arthroscopically determined degree of injury after shoulder dislocation relates to recurrence rate. Clin Orthop Relat Res. 2012;470(4):961–4.
4. Boone JL, Arciero RA. First-time anterior shoulder dislocations: has the standard changed? Br J Sports Med. 2010;44(5):355–60.
5. Arciero RA, Wheeler JH, Ryan JB, McBride JT. Arthroscopic Bankart repair versus nonoperative treatment for acute, initial anterior shoulder dislocations. Am J Sports Med. 1994;22(5):589–94.
6. Age and time specific management of traumatic anterior shoulder instability – The ESSKA-ESA formal consensus.
7. Liavaag S, Stiris MG, Svenningsen S, Enger M, Pripp AH, Brox JI. Capsular lesions with glenohumeral ligament injuries in patients with primary shoulder dislocation: magnetic resonance imaging and magnetic resonance arthrography evaluation. Scand J Med Sci Sports. 2011;21(6):e291–7.
8. Antonio GE, Griffith JF, Yu AB, Yung PS, Chan KM, Ahuja AT. First-time shoulder dislocation: high prevalence of labral injury and age-related differences revealed by MR arthrography. J Magn Reson Imaging. 2007;26(4):983–91.
9. Hovelius L, Rahme H. Primary anterior dislocation of the shoulder: long-term prognosis at the age of 40 years or younger. Knee Surg Sports Traumatol Arthrosc. 2016;24(2):330–42.
10. Itoi E, Hatakeyama Y, Sato T, Kido T, Minagawa H, Yamamoto N, et al. Immobilization in external rotation after shoulder dislocation reduces the risk of recurrence. A randomized controlled trial. J Bone Joint Surg Am. 2007;89(10):2124–31.
11. Konigshausen M, Schliemann B, Schildhauer TA, Seybold D. Evaluation of immobilization in external rotation after primary traumatic anterior shoulder dislocation: 5-year results. Musculoskelet Surg. 2014;98(2):143–51.
12. Heidari K, Asadollahi S, Vafaee R, Barfehei A, Kamalifar H, Chaboksavar ZA, et al. Immobilization in external rotation combined with abduction reduces the risk of recurrence after primary anterior shoulder dislocation. J Shoulder Elb Surg. 2014;23(6):759–66.
13. Chan SK, Bentick KR, Kuiper JH, Kelly CP. External rotation bracing for first-time anterior dislocation of the shoulder: a discontinued randomised controlled trial comparing external rotation bracing with conventional sling. Shoulder Elbow. 2019;11(4):256–64.
14. Hurley ET, Fried JW, Alaia MJ, Strauss EJ, Jazrawi LM, Matache BA. Immobilisation in external rotation after first-time traumatic anterior shoulder instability reduces recurrent instability: a meta-analysis. J ISAKOS. 2021;6(1):22–7.
15. Olds M, Ellis R, Donaldson K, Parmar P, Kersten P. Risk factors which predispose first-time traumatic anterior shoulder dislocations to recurrent instability in adults: a systematic review and meta-analysis. Br J Sports Med. 2015;49(14):913–22.
16. Liavaag S, Brox JI, Pripp AH, Enger M, Soldal LA, Svenningsen S. Immobilization in external rotation after primary shoulder dislocation did not reduce the risk of recurrence: a randomized controlled trial. J Bone Joint Surg Am. 2011;93(10):897–904.
17. Godin J, Sekiya JK. Systematic review of rehabilitation versus operative stabilization for the treatment of first-time anterior shoulder dislocations. Sports Health. 2010;2(2):156–65.
18. Hovelius L, Olofsson A, Sandstrom B, Augustini BG, Krantz L, Fredin H, et al. Nonoperative treatment of primary anterior shoulder dislocation in patients forty years of age and younger. A prospective twenty-five-year follow-up. J Bone Joint Surg Am. 2008;90(5):945–52.
19. Kirkley A, Werstine R, Ratjek A, Griffin S. Prospe ctive randomized clinical trial comparing the effectiveness of immediate arthroscopic stabilization versus immobilization and rehabilitation in first traumatic anterior dislocations of the shoulder: long-term evaluation. Arthroscopy. 2005;21(1):55–63.
20. Minkus M, Konigshausen M, Maier D, Mauch F, Stein T, Greiner S, et al. Immobilization in external rota-

tion and abduction versus arthroscopic stabilization after first-time anterior shoulder dislocation: a multi-center randomized controlled trial. Am J Sports Med. 2021;49(4):857–65.
21. Mather RC 3rd, Orlando LA, Henderson RA, Lawrence JT, Taylor DC. A predictive model of shoulder instability after a first-time anterior shoulder dislocation. J Shoulder Elb Surg. 2011;20(2):259–66.
22. Riccio I, de Sire A, Latte C, Pascarella F, Gimigliano F. Conservative treatment of traumatic shoulder instability: a case series study. Musculoskelet Surg. 2015;99(2):133–7.
23. Berendes TD, Pilot P, Nagels J, Vochteloo AJ, Nelissen RG. Survey on the management of acute first-time anterior shoulder dislocation amongst Dutch public hospitals. Arch Orthop Trauma Surg. 2015;135(4):447–54.
24. Balg F, Boileau P. The instability severity index score. A simple pre-operative score to select patients for arthroscopic or open shoulder stabilisation. J Bone Joint Surg Br. 2007;89(11):1470–7.

25 First-Time Dislocation with On-Track Hill-Sachs Lesion and Subcritical Glenoid Bone Loss

Olaf Lorbach and Matthias Brockmeyer

25.1 Case Presentation

- 26 year old male patient, who suffered from a bicycle accident with traumatic anterior luxation of the right shoulder. He has high functional demand on his shoulder and is not able to perform sports anymore due to the subjectively highly unstable shoulder.
- Imaging shows minor anterior bone loss of the glenoid with a medialized Bankart lesion as well as a Hill-Sachs-impression (Fig. 25.1a–d).
- A shoulder arthroscopy was planned in order to stabilize the shoulder by performing a bankart repair with capsular plication and additional remplissage.

Supplementary Information The online version contains supplementary material available at https://doi.org/10.1007/978-3-662-73064-5_25.

O. Lorbach (✉)
Schoen-Clinic Lorsch, Department of Shoulder Surgery and Sports Traumatology, Lorsch, Germany
e-mail: olaf.lorbach@uks.eu

M. Brockmeyer
Department of Orthopaedic Surgery, Saarland University, Homburg (Saar), Germany

L. Kovačič et al. (eds.), *Surgical Techniques for Anterior Shoulder Instability*,
https://doi.org/10.1007/978-3-662-73064-5_25

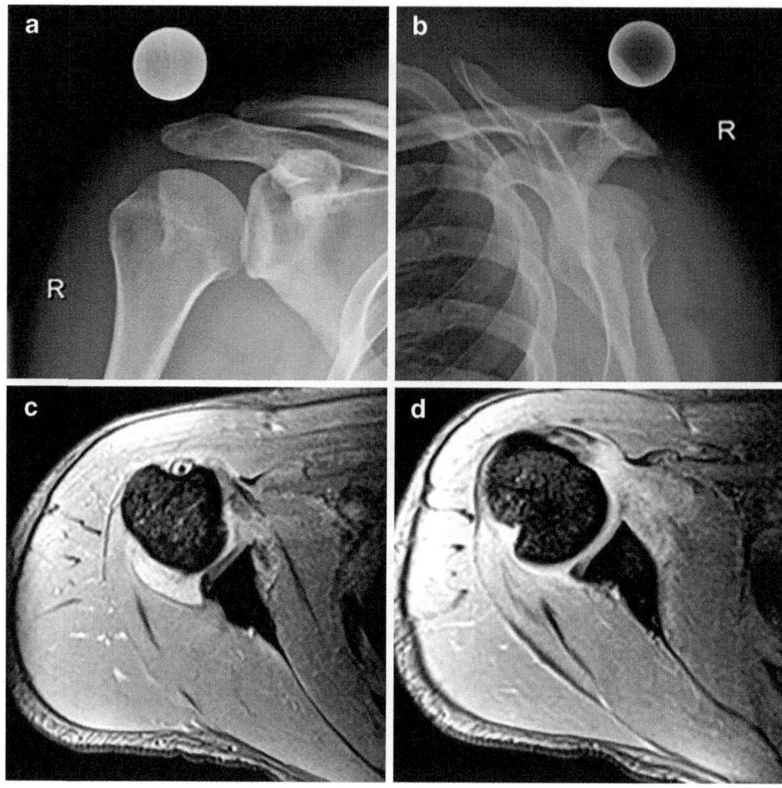

Fig. 25.1 (a–d) Imaging show minor anterior bone loss of the glenoid with a medialized Bankart lesion as well as a Hill-Sachs-impression

25.2 Surgical Technique

- Surgery was performed in lateral decubitus position. After the diagnostic round in order to rule out concomitant pathologies, an anterior and anterolateral portal was established, and the arthroscope was switched to the anterolateral portal.
- The present case showed a labral lesion with an unstable labral rag and concomitant Hill-Sachs lesion with multiple free chondral and bony fragments (Figs. 25.2a, b and 25.3).
- The anterolateral labrum was mobilized and the bone debrided (Fig. 25.4).
- A suture lasso was used to penetrate the anteroinferior capsule and labrum to shuttle a high strength suture (Fiberwire, Arthrex, Naples, USA) through the capsule-labrum complex (Fig. 25.5).
- Then a drill hole was made at the bone edge (5 o'clock position) of the anteroinferior glenoid in order to re-attach the labrum to the bone with additional re-tensioning of the anteroinferior capsule using a pressfit anchor (2.9 mm Bio-PushLock, Arthrex, Naples, USA).
- Two more high strength sutures were submitted through the capsule and labrum at the 4 and 3 o'clock position and the capsule-labrum-complex was further re-attached by two additional pressfit anchors. Figure 25.6 demonstrates the final fixation of the capsule-labrum-complex.
- Due to the complex labral damage with concomitant Hill-Sachs-Lesion, an additional remplissage procedure was performed.
- The bony surface of the Hill-Sachs impression was debrided by an arthroscopic burr and a

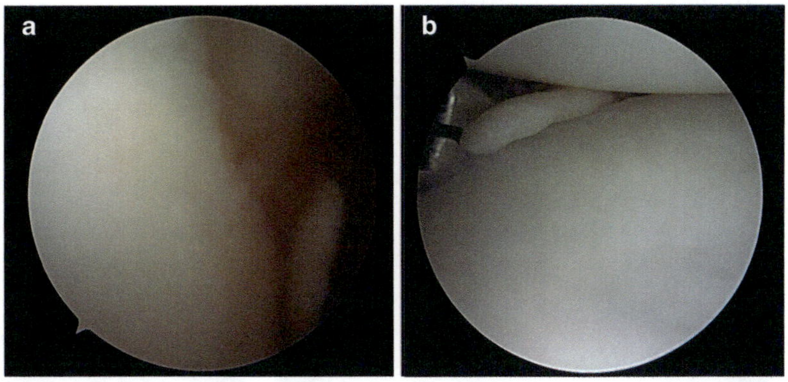

Fig. 25.2 (**a**, **b**) View from the posterior and anterolateral portal—the labral lesion with an instable labral rag is visible

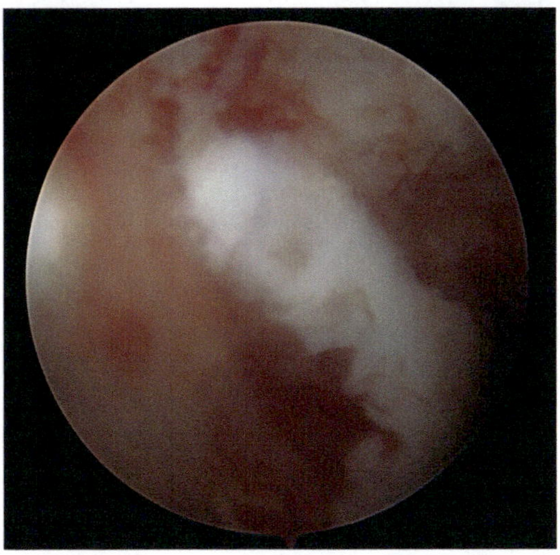

Fig. 25.3 View from the posterior portal showing the Hill-Sachs lesion with multiple instable chondral and bony pieces

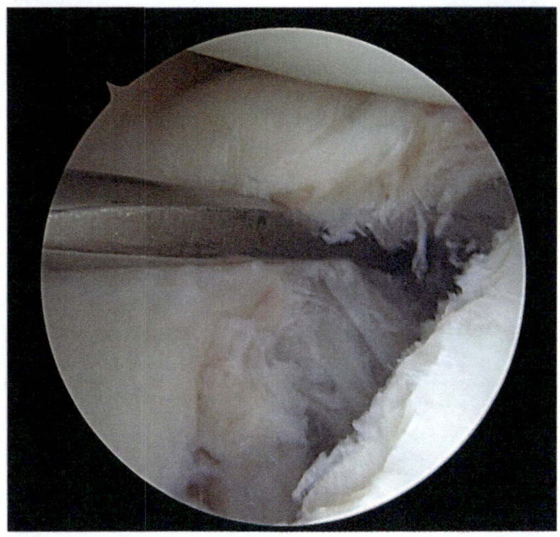

Fig. 25.4 View from the anterolateral portal—the labrum and the glenoid rim is debrided and the labrum is sufficiently mobilized

double-loaded suture anchor was inserted in the defect (Fig. 25.7). Special care was taken concerning the position of the anchor, which should not be inserted to medial in order to avoid restriction of external rotation.

- The sutures were submitted through the infraspinatus tendon and posterior capsule by a piercing instrument in a mattress stitch configuration (Rhino, Arthrex, Naples, USA) (Fig. 25.8).
- The sutures were knotted by several half-stiches (Fig. 25.9). If no cannula is used, it is recommended to switch the arthroscope to the subacromial space in order to avoid accidental tightening of the delta muscle within the knots.

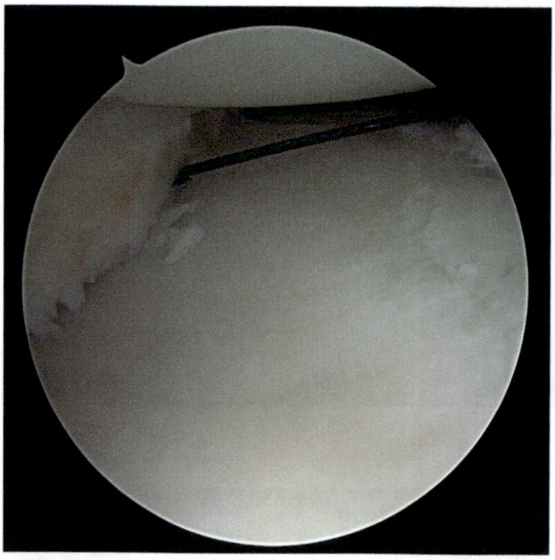

Fig. 25.5 The labrum and inferior capsule is penetrated by a suture lasso in order to shuttle a high strength suture (Fiberwire, Arthrex, Naples, USA) through the capsule-labrum-complex

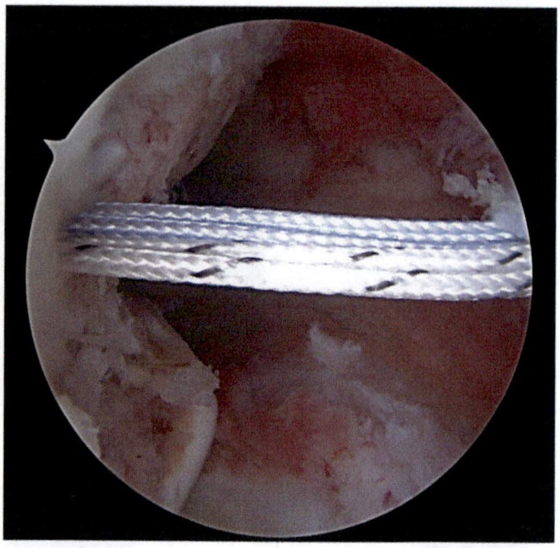

Fig. 25.7 After debridement of the Hill-Sachs defect, a bio-absorbable suture anchor (Bio-5.5 mm Bio-Corkscrew, Arthrex, Naples, USA) is inserted in the defect and the sutures are shuttled through the infraspinatus tendon and posterior capsule by a sharp piercing instrument (Rhino, Arthrex, Naples, USA)

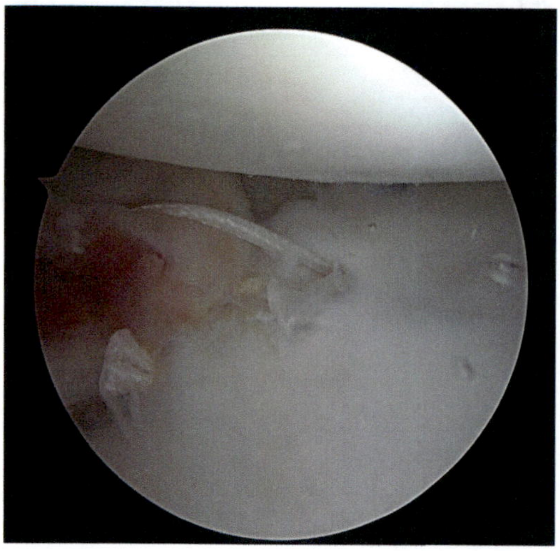

Fig. 25.6 The labrum is reattached to the glenoid by high strength sutures and three pressfit anchors (2.9 mm Bio-PushLock, Arthrex, Naples, USA)

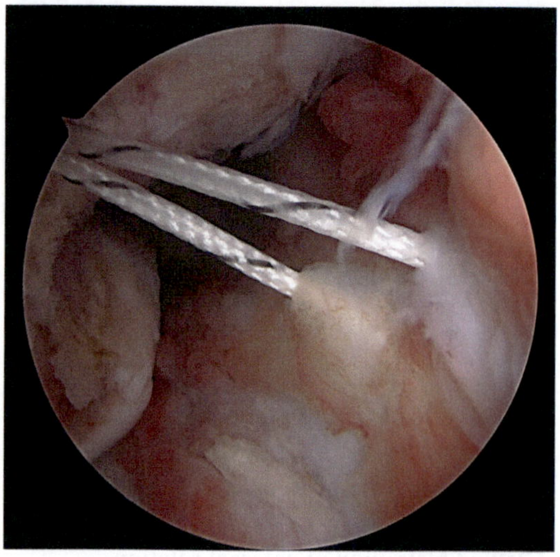

Fig. 25.8 The suture is submitted in a mattress stitch configuration and the sutures are tied by several half-stitches

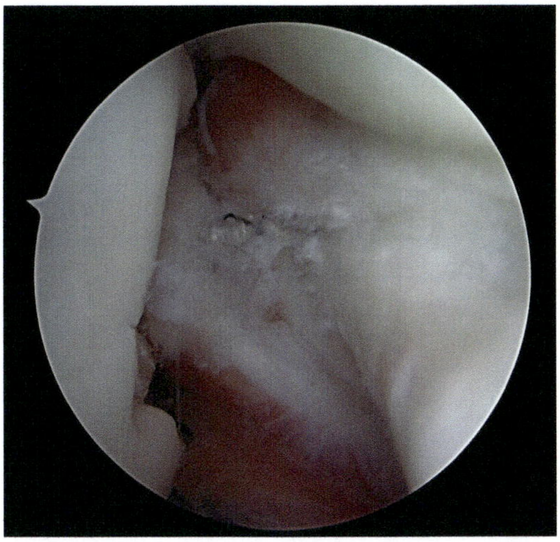

Fig. 25.9 Final fixation of the infraspinatus tendon and the posterior capsule into the Hill-Sachs defect

25.3 Postoperative Rehabilitation

- Immobilisation for 48 hours with shoulder abduction pillow with the arm in neutral rotation,
- Isometrics, lymphatic drainage, no mobilisation.

25.4 First–Third Postoperative Week

- Pendulum exercises out of the abduction pillow
- Mobilisation of the adjacent joints
- Scapulothoracic rhythm

25.5 Third–Sixth Postoperative Week

- Passive mobilisation to a maximum of 60° of flexion und abduction, avoid external rotation.
- No resistance.
- Work in pain-free range of motion.

25.6 From the Seventh Postoperative Week

- Removal of the shoulder abduction pillow, work on free range of motion.
- Work out in pain-free area/motion.
- Exercise bath und aqua-jogging.
- Strengthening of the rotator cuff and the deltoid muscle as well as concomitant stabilisers of the shoulder joint.
- Co-ordination training.

25.7 From the 12th Postoperative Week

- Sport specific exercises.
- Return to sport after consultation with the treating surgeon/physical therapist.

Pearls for Success and Pitfalls

- Adequate mobilisation of the labrum—the subscapularis fibers should be seen between the labrum and the glenoid.
- Piercing of the capsule inferior to the glenoid in order to perform a superior capsule shift.
- low positioning of the inferior anchor at the five o'clock position.
- Correct tensioning of the sutures by knots or pressfit anchors—avoid over tensioning, when using pressfit anchors and position knots anterior to the labrum in suture anchors.
- Correct positioning and angle of the anchor in the Hill-Sachs defect—avoid too medial and too lateral positioning of the anchor.
- Avoid strangulation of the delta muscle/fascia within the remplissage by using a posterior cannula. If no cannula is used, switching of the arthroscopy to the subacromial space is recommended, before tying the knot in order to determine free passage of the sutures, especially if more suture strands are used.

Take Home Message

- Adding a remplissage to the reattachment of the anteroinferior capsule—labrum—complex is a viable additional soft tissue procedure in patients with small to subcritical bone defects of the glenoid and/or concomitant humeral defects (Hill-Sachs lesions) as well as in patients with revision Bankart repair and/or bad tissue quality of the labrum.
- The presented technique significantly increases stability of the construct with a low complication rate, especially compared to any additional bony procedures.

Part IV

Complex and Revision Problems

Instability and Epilepsy

26

Michael Hantes and George A. Komnos

Key Points

- Seizures can result in shoulder dislocation producing large bony abnormalities of the humeral head and/or the glenoid, and persistent instability.
- Existing epilepsy along with the other comorbidities make management of this patients extremely challenging. Severe bone loss in the glenoid and the humeral head and repetitive trauma from frequent conclusive episodes are essential parts of the issue.
- Pain and limitation of the range of motion are the predominant symptoms following dislocation due to seizures.
- Surgical treatment methods mainly include soft tissue procedures and bone augmentation procedures depending on the amount of bone defects of the glenoid and humerus.
- In cases with osteoarthritis, arthroplasty is also an option, while glenohumeral arthrodesis is used as a salvage procedure.

26.1 Introduction

- Shoulder instability can occur following seizures. Initial shoulder dislocation often results in large bony abnormalities of the humeral head and/or the glenoid, which are difficult to diagnose and cope with.
- Not scarce, these injuries remain undiagnosed with severe subsequent instability.
- The underlying disease along with the other comorbidities make the diagnosis and management extremely challenging.
- Seizure-related shoulder instability comprises a spectrum of disorders including initial dislocation, recurrent instability, fracture-dislocation and chronic-locked dislocation [1].
- Musculoskeletal injuries can occur in up to 30% of patients with uncontrolled epilepsy [2]. Epilepsy tends to provoke repetitive seizures increasing the risk for shoulder dislocation and instability. Primary epilepsy has been reported to have a prevalence of 0.5%, while the lifetime risk of a single seizure is 5% [1].

Supplementary Information The online version contains supplementary material available at https://doi.org/10.1007/978-3-662-73064-5_26.

M. Hantes (✉) · G. A. Komnos
Faculty of Medicine, School of Health Sciences, University of Thessaly, Department of Orthopaedics, Larisa, Greece
e-mail: hantesmi@otenet.gr

L. Kovačič et al. (eds.), *Surgical Techniques for Anterior Shoulder Instability*,
https://doi.org/10.1007/978-3-662-73064-5_26

Although it is harsh to estimate the true incidence of dislocation caused by seizures, considering the high amount of those being misdiagnosed, this is demonstrated to be around 0.6% [3]. Instability, anterior and posterior, is commonly established after dislocation in these patients [4]. Epilepsy is the main reason associated with seizure-related instability and mainly affects men between 20 and 45 years old [5, 6].

- It is well known that anterior dislocation and instability are much more frequent than posterior one. Nevertheless, there is a predominance of posterior instability related to seizures [4]. The mechanism lying behind the dislocation consists of forceful, and imbalanced muscle contraction during the seizure. This muscle contraction results in a shoulder position of adduction, internal rotation and flexion. Pectoralis muscles and latissimus dorsi overweight the external rotators and displace the humeral head superiorly and posteriorly. However, recent published data have highlighted that these patients may principally suffer from anterior instability [7, 8].
- The main risk factors predisposing to shoulder instability are severe bone loss in the glenoid and the humeral head and repetitive trauma from frequent conclusive episodes. Bone loss is the consequence of consecutive dislocations and reduced bone mineral density that is correlated with anti-epileptic drugs [9].

26.2 Physical Findings

- As aforementioned, misdiagnosis or delay in diagnosis is common. Due to socioeconomic factors and the fact that the patients usually give priority to the management of epilepsy and seizures, a high proportion of them present to the orthopedic surgeon quite late.
- Pain and limitation of the range of motion are the predominant symptoms following dislocation due to seizures.
- The frequency of the episodes should be investigated.
- Initial clinical evaluation includes assessment of the range of motion, rotator cuff function, neurovascular status and exclusion of fracture.
- Evaluation of the instability with apprehension and load and shift tests are of paramount importance. Provocative tests should be performed in an attempt to define the directions and extent of instability [10].
- In posterior instability, the main clinical sign is the painful loss of passive external rotation.
- Locked dislocations can be also established, with the patients having limited pain, but a remarkable loss of motion.

26.3 Relevant Imaging

- Severe bone loss from the glenoid and humeral head is the hallmark of seizure-related instability [11].
- Plain radiographs with standard anteroposterior and axillary views are the initial diagnosing tool. Dislocation and fracture can be evaluated through them. However, these are often unreliable in diagnosing posterior dislocations.
- If bony lesions are apparent on radiographs, or if there is doubt or suspicion for posterior dislocation then 3D (three-dimensional) Computed Tomography (CT) should be performed to set the diagnosis or fully define the extent of the osseous injury and bone loss.
- Magnetic Resonance Arthrography (MRA) may be useful in capturing soft-tissue lesions.

26.4 Treatment Options and Indications

- The management of this type of injuries and patients requires a multidisciplinary approach. The underlying disease (epilepsy) should always be initially addressed, and the patients should be counseled to receive the appropriate medication. When a surgical approach is proposed, the significance of medication is even greater, since the risk of perioperative seizures is high. Psychological assessment may also be essential.

- Conservative treatment is suggested in patients with slight bone loss, older patients, patients with limited demands, and those who are not compliant with the medications. This mainly consists of physiotherapy and activity modification.
- Surgical management includes various soft tissue procedures (Putti-Platt, MacLaughlin, Bankart repair), bone augmentation procedures (coracoid transfer, glenoid neck/humeral osteotomy) and arthrodesis [12].
- There is a paucity of data about the treatment of dislocations and instability in epileptic patients and most of the available knowledge comes from general management of these conditions, and not from particular evidence in the specific populations.
- The main cause for the instability is bone loss. Subsequently, most surgical strategies focalize on bone augmentation [6, 13]. The use of bony augmentation procedures may have improved the outcomes after surgical intervention, but currently there is no evidence-based consensus to guide treatment.
- Noteworthy, soft tissue procedures can be applied in selected cases.
- In seizure-related anterior instability, initial management consists of closed reduction and immobilization for 2–3 weeks.
- Some studies suggest surgical repair mainly in young, active patients [1]. Some general indications for primary surgery that could apply to this population include a large bony Bankart lesion, a displaced greater tuberosity fracture, or an acute rotator cuff tear [14, 15].
- If the defect covers the 1/4 of the glenoid surface and consists of less than 20% of its surface area, a soft tissue procedure can be performed [16]. Soft tissue procedures (either open or arthroscopic) have satisfying outcomes when the loss of the glenoid bone is less than 20% [6].
- In most cases, and especially when bone loss is greater than 20%, then bone augmentation procedures are preferred. Latarjet procedure and its modifications is the preferred means of treatment in these cases [17, 18].
- Latarjet procedure is widely applied in epileptic patients with satisfactory functional improvement. Outcomes after this procedure have been demonstrated to be equal to those applied to non-epileptic patients with anterior shoulder instability [19]. Khater et al. reported a satisfactory rate of 95% at midterm follow-up [20]. In conclusion, the Latarjet procedure is a suitable technique for those patients since it addresses both glenoid and humeral head bone defects.
- In seizure-related posterior instability, closed reduction under anesthesia is initially attempted, with special caution for preventing a humerus head fracture. This mostly applies in dislocations less than 3 weeks old and with minor humeral head bony defect. On the contrary, closed reduction is ineffective in dislocations established for more than 3 weeks [21].
- When the shoulder is unstable in neutral internal rotation, then primary surgical treatment is advanced. Reconstruction of the humeral head defect is the main surgical treatment. Depending on the size of the defect, autogenous bone grafts, or allografts may be utilized. Augmentation with allograft to fit the lesion or posterior bone-block augmentation of the glenoid can be performed [22, 23]. Nonetheless, the McLaughlin procedure and arthroscopic reduction of established posterior shoulder instability with remplissage of the subscapularis tendon in humeral head defects of <30% has shown satisfactory clinical outcomes with a relatively low rate of complications [21, 24].
- In cases that osteoarthritis is present, or in end-stage cases, arthroplasty is also an option, with no long-term survivorship data about epileptic patients, though. Fixed-fulcrum fully constrained reverse shoulder arthroplasty has been proposed for the treatment of recurrent shoulder instability in patients with epilepsy [25].
- Locked dislocation may be also established. On such occasions, "skillful neglect" could be considered in older patients with remarkable

bone defects, to achieve a painless shoulder with function similar to arthrodesis. In young patients with small bone defects and a recent history of fewer than 3 months an effort for closed reduction can be done, while open reduction is necessary in large defects, or more neglected cases. If persistent instability is diagnosed then reconstruction of the defect is required.

- Glenohumeral arthrodesis is used as a salvage procedure, without consistent data for its effectiveness in epileptic patients. Thangarajah et al. reported a series of six patients (out of a total cohort of 179 epileptic patients with shoulder instability) who underwent arthrodesis [26]. They found arthrodesis effective in eliminating perceived instability, with a low rate of complications and improvement of the functional scores. Of note, they applied this technique mainly in patients with multiple prior surgeries.

26.5 Decision-Making Algorithm

- Several factors related to the patient and the injury can guide the treatment decision.
- Regarding the patient, age, expectations and activity level are the most essential ones.
- In terms of the injury, the extent of the glenoid bone loss and degenerative changes should always be taken into consideration.
- In established posterior dislocations the chronicity of the injury will guide to a closed or open reduction. Dislocation less than 3 weeks ago can be reduced by close means, but open reduction is preferred in more neglected cases.
- As mentioned above, quantification of the glenoid bone loss is the element that will guide the decision for a soft tissue or a bone augmentation procedure. The applied margin is 20% of the glenoid surface area, with lower than that leading to soft tissue procedures and higher to bone block procedures. On the contrary, defects extending into 2 or more quadrants of the glenoid are a risk factor for failure of bone block procedures, leading to the choice of arthrodesis. The role of arthroplasty is not clearly established yet in this group of patients.

26.6 Clinical Case/Example/ Preferred Treatment Option

- We present a 64-years old male with a history of seizures and neglected chronic posterior shoulder dislocation.
- He was diagnosed with epilepsy 5 years ago as a result of a brain injury. He received medications as advised. These included levetiracetam and zolpidem.
- He had at least three incidents of posterior dislocation of his left shoulder in the last 4 years before his admission to our department. He was treated elsewhere for all these incidents.
- At his admission, he underwent plain radiographs and computed tomography, which revealed a locked posterior dislocation and a reverse Hill Sachs lesion (Fig. 26.1). This type of lesion, the reverse Hill Sachs lesion, is quite often in posterior dislocation with a reported incidence of 40–90% [27].
- Due to the findings and the quite intact glenoid, a soft tissue procedure could be decided.
- The chronicity of the dislocation (more than 3 weeks) led us to the decision for an open reduction.

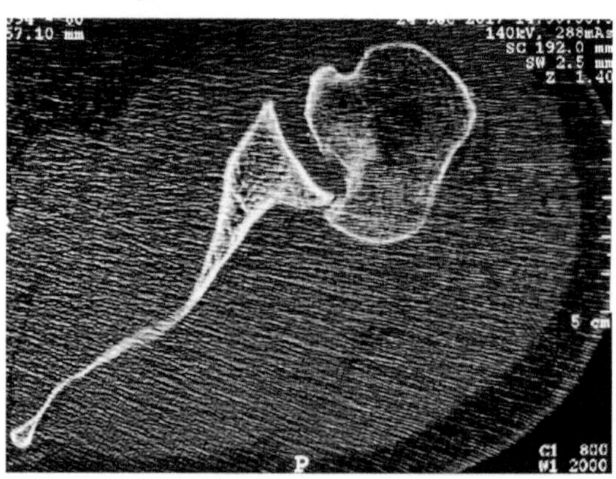

Fig. 26.1 CT images revealing reverse Hill Sachs lesion, without severe glenoid bone loss

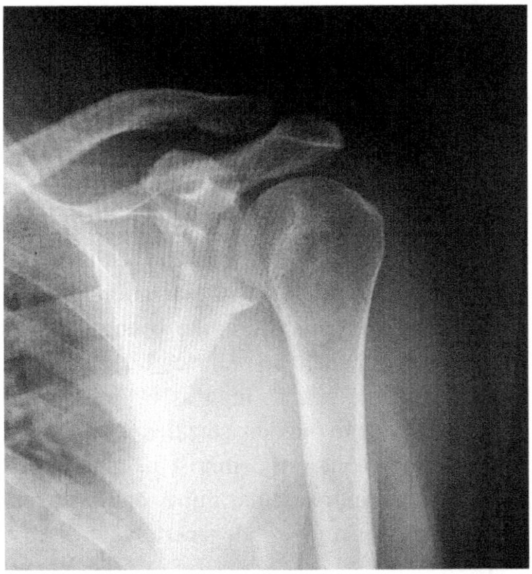

Fig. 26.2 Last follow-up radiographs with no signs of remarkable osteoarthritis

- Under general anesthesia, open reduction of the shoulder with gradual soft tissue release and a McLaughlin procedure with remplissage of the subscapularis tendon was performed (Fig. 26.2a, b). Two anchors were utilized.
- Post-operative course was uneventful. At 3 years follow-up the patient has not experienced no further dislocation with satisfying range of motion and use of his arm (Video 26.1).
- Last radiographs did not reveal any signs of remarkable osteoarthritis (Fig. 26.3).
- MRI at last follow-up revealed full incorporation of the subscapularis tendon with full coverage of the defect (Fig. 26.3).

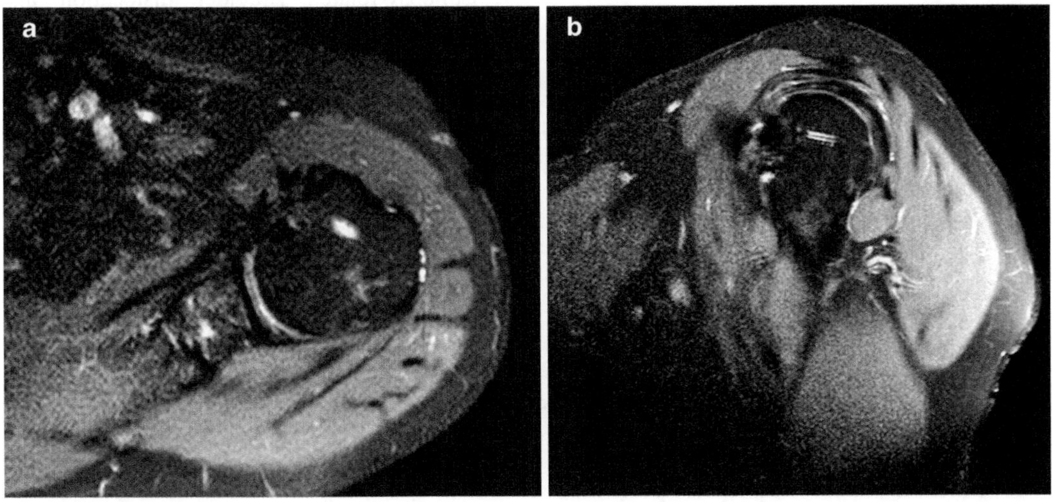

Fig. 26.3 (**a, b**) MRI images at last follow-up revealed full incorporation of the subscapularis tendon with full coverage of the defect (the 2 anchors are also shown)

Pearls and Pitfalls

- Management of seizure-related shoulder instability is extremely challenging and should always be individualized.
- Treatment should address both the underlying disease and the shoulder injury.
- Control of the seizures with medication is necessary, while bony augmentation procedures are the cornerstone of surgical management for recurrent instability.
- Neurologic evaluation is mandatory preoperatively and compliance with anticonvulsive medication is of paramount significance.
- All patients following episodes of seizures should be in depth evaluated for potent dislocation.
- High forces developing during the seizures that result in the shoulder dislocation should be taken into consideration for the primary repair.
- In young and active patients, soft tissue, bone preservation procedures are an option, but with the increased risk for recurrent dislocations. Bone loss of the glenoid less than 20% of total surface seems to be a prognostic factor for satisfactory results.
- The Latarjet procedure along with control of the epilepsy is the recommended treatment in young patients with seizure-related anterior shoulder instability.
- McLaughlin procedure leads to optimized outcomes and low rate of complications in patients with chronic posterior dislocation.
- Dislocations in this group of patients are mostly high-energy injuries that can provoke large fractures of the glenoid rim or the humeral head. These fractures should always be addressed during the surgery since they constitute a negative risk factor for persistent instability.

26.7 Potential Complications

- Unfortunately, complications are quite common in these patients. The most frequent one is recurrent instability.
- The recurrence rate in the epileptic population is remarkably higher (69% vs. 10% in non-epileptic patients) [28]. This can be the consequence of further seizures, failure of the reconstructive procedure, the young patient's age or poor patient compliance [6].
- A recurrence rate as high as 69% has been reported due to ongoing seizures [28].
- Other complications comprise pain, stiffness, infection, neurovascular injury and posttraumatic/postoperative degenerative disease [29].

26.8 Expert Recommendation

- Epilepsy-related shoulder dislocation and instability pose an essential challenge to the orthopedic surgeon.
- The cornerstones of treatment consist of seizure control, and individualized patient management with selecting the proper procedure depending on the lesion.
- Patient's characteristics, the chronicity or establishment of the dislocation and the amount of glenoid bone loss are the main factors defining the treatment.

Take Home Message

- Careful and in-depth evaluation of the patient is of paramount importance.
- Pre-operative planning for selecting the appropriate procedure is essential.
- Compliance of the patient to the medication for eliminating seizures can ultimately result in satisfying outcomes.

References

1. Goudie EB, Murray IR, Robinson CM. Instability of the shoulder following seizures. J Bone Joint Surg Br B. 2012;94 B:721–8. [cited 2021 May 25]. Available from: https://pubmed.ncbi.nlm.nih.gov/22628584/
2. Mattson RH, Gidal BE. Fractures, epilepsy, and antiepileptic drugs. Epilepsy Behav. 2004;5(SUPPL. 2) [cited 2021 Jun 1]. Available from: https://pubmed.ncbi.nlm.nih.gov/15123010/
3. DeToledo JC, Lowe MR. Seizures, lateral decubitus, aspiration, and shoulder dislocation: time to change the guidelines? Neurology (Lippincott Williams and Wilkins). 2001;56:290–1. [cited 2021 May 25]. Available from: https://pubmed.ncbi.nlm.nih.gov/11235662/
4. Robinson CM, Seah M, Akhtar MA. The epidemiology, risk of recurrence, and functional outcome after an acute traumatic posterior dislocation of the shoulder. J Bone Joint Surg – Ser A. 2011;93(17):1605–13. [cited 2021 May 25]. Available from: https://pubmed.ncbi.nlm.nih.gov/21915575/
5. Hawkins RJ, Neer CS, Pianta RM, Mendoza FX. Locked posterior dislocation of the shoulder. J Bone Joint Surg – Ser A. 1987;69(1):9–18. [cited 2021 May 25]. Available from: https://pubmed.ncbi.nlm.nih.gov/3805075/
6. Bühler M, Gerber C. Shoulder instability related to epileptic seizures. J Shoulder Elbow Surg. 2002;11(4):339–44. [cited 2021 May 25]. Available from: https://pubmed.ncbi.nlm.nih.gov/12195251/
7. Thangarajah T, Lambert S. The management of recurrent shoulder instability in patients with epilepsy: a 15-year experience. J Shoulder Elbow Surg. 2015;24(11):1723–7. [cited 2021 May 28]. Available from: https://pubmed.ncbi.nlm.nih.gov/26119633/
8. Raiss P, Lin A, Mizuno N, Melis B, Walch G. Results of the Latarjet procedure for recurrent anterior dislocation of the shoulder in patients with epilepsy. J Bone Joint Surg – Ser B. 2012;94 B(9):1260–4. [cited 2021 Jun 7]. Available from: https://pubmed.ncbi.nlm.nih.gov/22933500/
9. Petty SJ, O'Brien TJ, Wark JD. Anti-epileptic medication and bone health. Osteoporos Int. 2007;18:129–42. [cited 2021 May 26]. Available from: https://pubmed.ncbi.nlm.nih.gov/17091219/
10. Johnson SM, Robinson CM. Shoulder instability in patients with joint hyperlaxity. J Bone Joint Surg – Ser A. 2010;92(6):1545–57. [cited 2021 May 26]. Available from: https://pubmed.ncbi.nlm.nih.gov/20516333/
11. Provencher MT, McCormick F, Dewing C, McIntire S, Solomon D. A prospective analysis of 179 type 2 superior labrum anterior and posterior repairs: outcomes and factors associated with success and failure. Am J Sports Med. 2013;41:880.
12. Thangarajah T, Lambert SM. Management of recurrent shoulder instability in patients with epilepsy. J Shoulder Elbow Surg (Mosby Inc). 2016;25:1376–84. [cited 2021 Jun 1]. Available from: https://pubmed.ncbi.nlm.nih.gov/27288273/
13. Bone buttress operation for recurrent anterior shoulder dislocation in epilepsy – PubMed [cited 2021 May 31]. Available from: https://pubmed.ncbi.nlm.nih.gov/7593109/
14. Dimakopoulos P, Panagopoulos A, Kasimatis G, Syggelos SA, Lambiris E. Anterior traumatic shoulder dislocation associated with displaced greater tuberosity fracture: the necessity of operative treatment. J Orthop Trauma. 2007;21(2):104–12. [cited 2021 May 27]. Available from: https://pubmed.ncbi.nlm.nih.gov/17304065/
15. Porcellini G, Campi F, Paladini P. Arthroscopic approach to acute bony Bankart lesion. Arthroscopy. 2002;18(7):764–9. [cited 2021 May 27]. Available from: https://pubmed.ncbi.nlm.nih.gov/12209435/
16. Itoi E, Lee SB, Berglund LJ, Berge LL, An KN. The effect of a glenoid defect on anteroinferior stability of the shoulder after Bankart repair: a cadaveric study. J Bone Joint Surg – Ser A. 2000;82(1):35–46. [cited 2021 May 31]. Available from: https://pubmed.ncbi.nlm.nih.gov/10653082/
17. Burkhart SS, de Beer JF, Barth JRH, Criswell T, Roberts C, Richards DP. Results of modified Latarjet reconstruction in patients with Anteroinferior instability and significant bone loss. Arthroscopy. 2007;23(10):1033–41. [cited 2021 May 28]. Available from: https://pubmed.ncbi.nlm.nih.gov/17916467/
18. Young AA, Maia R, Berhouet J, Walch G. Open Latarjet procedure for management of bone loss in anterior instability of the glenohumeral joint. J Shoulder Elb Surg. 2011;20(2):S61–9. [cited 2021 May 28]. Available from: https://pubmed.ncbi.nlm.nih.gov/21145262/
19. Erşen A, Bayram S, Birişik F, Atalar AC, Demirhan M. The effectiveness of the Latarjet procedure for shoulder instability in patients with epilepsy. Orthop Traumatol Surg Res. 2017;103(8):1277–82. [cited 2021 Jun 4]. Available from: https://pubmed.ncbi.nlm.nih.gov/28987528/
20. Khater AH, Sobhy MH, Said HG, Kandil A, Reda W, Seifeldin AF, et al. Latarjet procedure for anterior shoulder instability due to tramadol-induced seizures. Am J Sports Med. 2016;44(4):957–62. [cited 2021 Jun 7]. Available from: https://pubmed.ncbi.nlm.nih.gov/26818452/
21. Romano AM, Edwards TB, Nastrucci G, Casillo P, di Giunta A, Zappia M, et al. Arthroscopic reduction and subscapularis remplissage (ARR) of chronic posterior locked shoulder dislocation leads to optimized outcomes and low rate of complications. Knee Surg Sports Traumatol Arthrosc. 2020; [cited 2021 Jun 7]. Available from: https://pubmed.ncbi.nlm.nih.gov/33074421/
22. Servien E, Walch G, Cortes ZE, Edwards TB, O'Connor DP. Posterior bone block procedure for

posterior shoulder instability. Knee Surg Sports Traumatol Arthrosc. 2007;15(9):1130–6. [cited 2021 May 28]. Available from: https://pubmed.ncbi.nlm.nih.gov/17370061/
23. Gerber C, Lambert SM. Allograft reconstruction of segmental defects of the humeral head for the treatment of chronic locked posterior dislocation of the shoulder. J Bone Joint Surg – Ser A. 1996;78(3):376–82. [cited 2021 May 28]. Available from: https://pubmed.ncbi.nlm.nih.gov/8613444/
24. Delcogliano A, Caporaso A, Chiossi S, Menghi A, Cillo M, Delcogliano M. Surgical management of chronic, unreduced posterior dislocation of the shoulder. Knee Surg Sports Traumatol Arthrosc. 2005;13(2):151–5. [cited 2021 Jun 7]. Available from: https://pubmed.ncbi.nlm.nih.gov/15756620/
25. Thangarajah T, Higgs D, Bayley JIL, Lambert SM. Constrained fixed-fulcrum reverse shoulder arthroplasty improves functional outcome in epileptic patients with recurrent shoulder instability. World J Orthop. 2016;7(7):434–41. [cited 2021 Jun 1]. Available from: https://pubmed.ncbi.nlm.nih.gov/27458554/
26. Thangarajah T, Alexander S, Bayley I, Lambert SM. Glenohumeral arthrodesis for the treatment of recurrent shoulder instability in epileptic patients. Bone Joint J. 2014;96B(11):1525–9. [cited 2021 Jun 1]. Available from: https://pubmed.ncbi.nlm.nih.gov/25371468/
27. Shams A, El-Sayed M, Gamal O, ElSawy M, Azzam W. Modified technique for reconstructing reverse Hill–Sachs lesion in locked chronic posterior shoulder dislocation. Eur J Orthop Surg Traumatol. 2016;26(8):843–9. [cited 2021 Jun 7]. Available from: https://pubmed.ncbi.nlm.nih.gov/27541313/
28. Thangarajah T, Lambert S. The management of recurrent shoulder instability in patients with epilepsy: a 15-year experience. J Shoulder Elbow Surg. 2015;24(11):1723–7. [cited 2021 May 31]. Available from: https://pubmed.ncbi.nlm.nih.gov/26119633/
29. Robinson CM, Aderinto J. Current concepts review: posterior shoulder dislocations and fracture-dislocations. J Bone Joint Surg Am. 2005;87:639–50. [cited 2021 May 28] Available from: https://pubmed.ncbi.nlm.nih.gov/15741636/

How to Address Massive Bone Defects

27

Giuseppe Bertoni, Luca Prasciolu, Maristella F. Saccomanno, and Giuseppe Milano

Key Points
- Massive bone defects are defined by the presence of a critical glenoid bone loss associated to a medium-to-large Hill-Sachs.
- A positive bony apprehension test can raise the suspicious of a bony-mediated instability.
- 3D VRT CT scan is the gold standard for quantification of bipolar bone defects
- 3D printed technology could improve the planning and facilitate the shaping of the graft intraoperatively
- Anatomic reconstruction of bipolar bone defects should be always attempted.

G. Bertoni · L. Prasciolu
Department of Medical and Surgical Specialties, Radiological Sciences, and Public Health, University of Brescia, Brescia, Italy

M. F. Saccomanno (✉)
Department of Bone and Joint Surgery, Spedali Civili, Brescia, Italy

Department of Orthopedics, Fondazione Policlinico Univarsitario A Gemelli IRCSS, Rome, Italy

G. Milano
Department of Medical and Surgical Specialties, Radiological Sciences, and Public Health, University of Brescia, Brescia, Italy

Department of Bone and Joint Surgery, Spedali Civili, Brescia, Italy
e-mail: giuseppe.milano@unibs.it

27.1 Introduction

- The glenohumeral joint is the most frequently dislocated large joint in the human body, with the majority of instability events occurring anteriorly [32].
- The presence of bipolar bone loss plays an important role in the success of stabilization procedures. Particularly, soft tissue procedures are surely contraindicated, due to high risk of recurrency [4].
- Multiple treatment algorithms for managing subcritical and critical bone loss in recurrent anterior shoulder instability have been proposed [9, 10, 34, 36], however massive bone loss remains a challenge.
- Massive bone defects can be defined as a critical glenoid bone loss associated to a medium-to-large Hill-Sachs lesion. They are the results of:
  - A long history of instability
  - Chronic locked dislocations
  - Failed instability surgery

27.2 Relevant Physical Findings

- Clinical history may raise a high suspicion of glenohumeral bone deficiency [42, 46] The most relevant predictors are:
  - Traumatic onset
  - Young age

L. Kovačič et al. (eds.), *Surgical Techniques for Anterior Shoulder Instability*,
https://doi.org/10.1007/978-3-662-73064-5_27

- High number of dislocations
- Contact/collision sport activities

- A complete physical examination remains paramount even when a bony-mediated instability is suspected to rule out signs of joint hyperlaxity, multidirectional instability, or concomitant rotator cuff tears.
- Bony apprehension test: Apprehension is perceived by the patient at 45° abduction and 45° external rotation [7]. It depends on the lack of osseous contour, which is the main stabilizer at the mid-range of motion [19, 20].

27.3 Relevant Imaging

- *Conventional radiology*: Several x-rays views have been described. They showed high specificity and sensitivity in *identification* of glenohumeral bone defect, but they are not useful in *quantification* of the bone defect [38, 47].
- *Computed tomography (CT)*: Three-dimensional volume rendering technique (3D-VRT) is the gold standard for the quantification of bipolar bone defects.
  - *Glenoid bone loss*: Burkhart et al. [5] first described the term *inverted pear-glenoid* as the result of a large anterior glenoid bone defect that changes the shape of the glenoid from normal pear-shaped to inverted. Since then, several measurement methods have been described [45], albeit recent literature claimed that most of those methods are inaccurate [48]:
    - *Diameter-based methods*: overestimates true glenoid bone loss [3]
    - *Digital surface area methods*: led to impreciseness of scapula positioning for creation of an *en-face* view, which significantly alter glenoid defect size measurement results [22, 30]
  - *Humeral head bone loss*: Several studies tried to clearly visualize and detect Hill-Sachs lesions, [23] however, no consistent method of measurement has been accepted so far. The Hill-Sachs lesion is usually described at least by three characteristics: *location, width and depth* [21, 37]
  - *Bipolar bone loss*: In case of massive bone defects, the application of the on-track/off track method [9] will surely show an off-track lesion. It is helpful in the identification of critical bone loss, but not in its quantification.
- *3D-printing technology*: Few studies documented the use of 3D-printing technology for assessment and treatment planning of anterior shoulder instability [40, 49]. Main proposed advantages in complex cases, such as massive bone defects, are:
  - Enhancing the understanding of depth and size of bony lesions, thus allowing a volumetric reconstruction of the defects (Fig. 27.1)

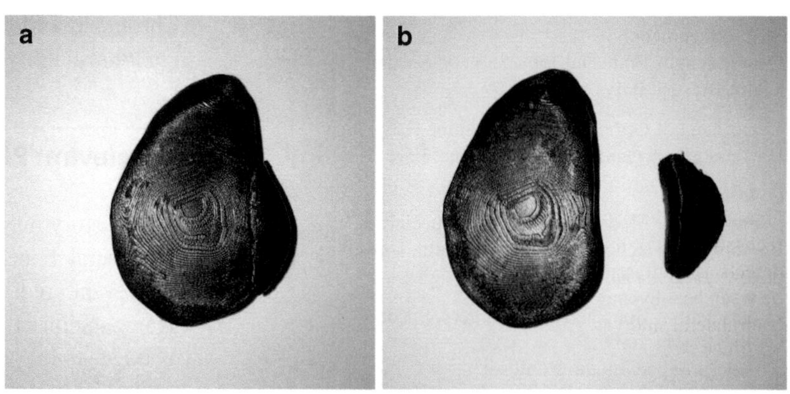

Fig. 27.1 Volumetric reconstruction of a glenoid bone defect using 3D-printing technology (**a**). The reconstructed missing bone and the glenoid shows perfect matching (**b**)

  - Potentially reducing intraoperative complications related to impreciseness of standard preoperative CT-based planning
  - Allowing the production of personalized implants/template to restore substantial glenoid or humeral head bone loss, glenohumeral morphology and stability

27.4 Treatment Options and Indications

Although massive bone defects are usually addressed in an open fashion, the arthroscopic approach has also been described at least for managing glenoid bone loss [41]. Treatment options are mainly related to bone loss quantification. The most frequent clinical scenarios are:

- *Critical glenoid bone loss and medium size Hill-Sachs lesion*
  - Open or arthroscopic Latarjet is the first line option in case of glenoid defects between 13 and 25–30% of glenoid area [9, 19, 39]
  - Congruent arc modification [6] can be helpful in larger glenoid defects to increase the bone block effect and improve the radius of curvature [8]
  - Medium size Hill-Sachs lesion can be usually addressed by a *remplissage* procedure [9, 19, 39]
- *Glenoid bone loss exceeding 25–30% of glenoid area and large Hill Sachs lesion*
  - Auto- or allograft are needed to address glenoid bone loss exceeding classic or modified Latarjet capacity as well as large Hill-Sachs lesion. The most commonly used grafts are:
    - Auto or allograft iliac crest [15, 26, 33, 43, 44, 51]
    - Distal tibial allograft [2, 50]
    - Femoral head allograft [52]
    - Talus allograft [1, 14]
    - Humeral head allograft [17, 25, 41, 52]

27.5 Decision-Making Algorithm

No standardized decision-making algorithms have been developed for the management of massive bone defects. It's authors preference to follow this path:

- Accurate clinical and physical examination, taking into consideration major predictors of bony-mediated instability [7, 29].
- 3D-VRT CT reconstruction of both glenoid and humeral head.
- A dedicated software [11] is used to apply a rigid surface matching between the 3D models of affected and health glenoid as well as humeral head, thus obtaining a volumetric reconstruction of bone defects as a difference between healthy and contralateral side (Fig. 27.2).
- A distal tibial allograft is usually preferred to reconstruct the glenoid side, as well as

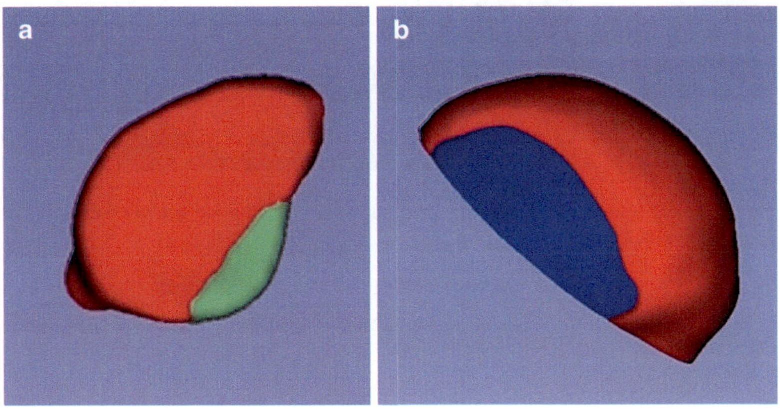

Fig. 27.2 A dedicated software is used to create 3D models of affected and health glenoid (**a**) as well as humeral head (**b**), thus obtaining a volumetric reconstruction of bone defects as a difference between healthy and contralateral side

humeral head allograft is used on the humeral side.
- When anterior soft tissues are seriously damaged (e.g. revision cases or long history of instability), an Achilles tendon allograft with its calcaneus is used to reconstruct the glenoid side and the anterior capsule (Fig. 27.3).

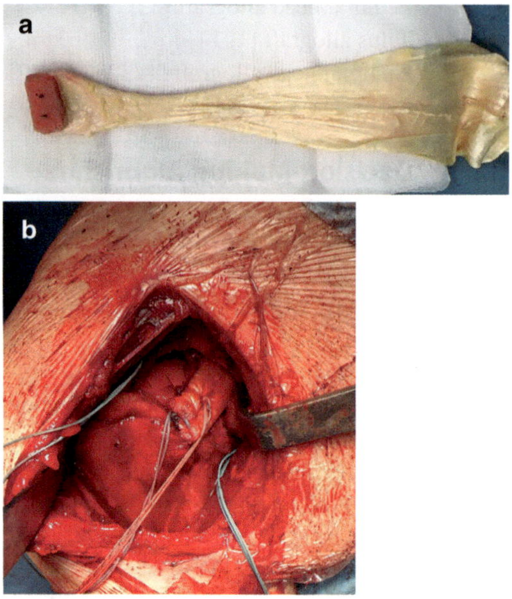

Fig. 27.3 Achilles bone-tendon allograft (**a**) is used to reconstruct the glenoid bone and the anterior capsule (**b**)

27.6 Clinical Case

A 23-year-old right-handed male presented to the outpatient clinic with a history of anterior glenohumeral instability in his left shoulder (non-dominant side) due to seizures. He accounted for more than ten episodes of dislocation in the last 5 years. He attended recreational non over-head sport activities.

At the physical examination, he presented a positive bony apprehension test with no sign of shoulder hyperlaxity (add-ER <85°, negative Gagey test) or generalized joint laxity (Beighton score = 3). No signs of posterior instability could be found either.

A 3D-CT scan was performed. Bipolar bone defects were deemed as off-track injury pattern. A volumetric reconstruction of glenoid and humeral head defects was attempted, as above mentioned, thus showing a critical glenoid bone loss associated to a large Hill-Sachs lesion (Fig. 27.4). An Achilles tendon allograft with its calcaneus was used to reconstruct the glenoid side and the anterior capsule, severely damaged by the long history of instability (Fig. 27.5). Part of the calcaneus bone was used to reconstruct the Hill-Sachs defect (Fig. 27.6). After surgery, the arm was immobilized in a sling with an abduction pillow for

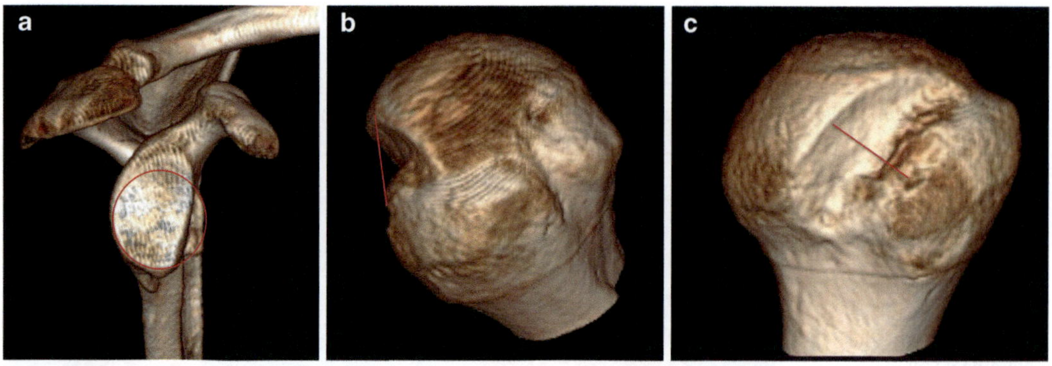

Fig. 27.4 3D-CT scan of a right shoulder showing critical bone defect of the glenoid (**a**) associated to a large Hill-Sachs lesion (**b, c**)

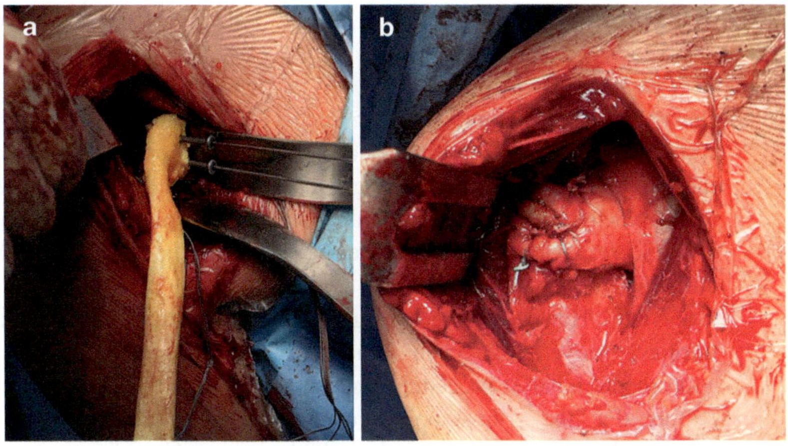

Fig. 27.5 An Achilles tendon allograft with its calcaneus was used to reconstruct the glenoid side (**a**) and the anterior capsule (**b**)

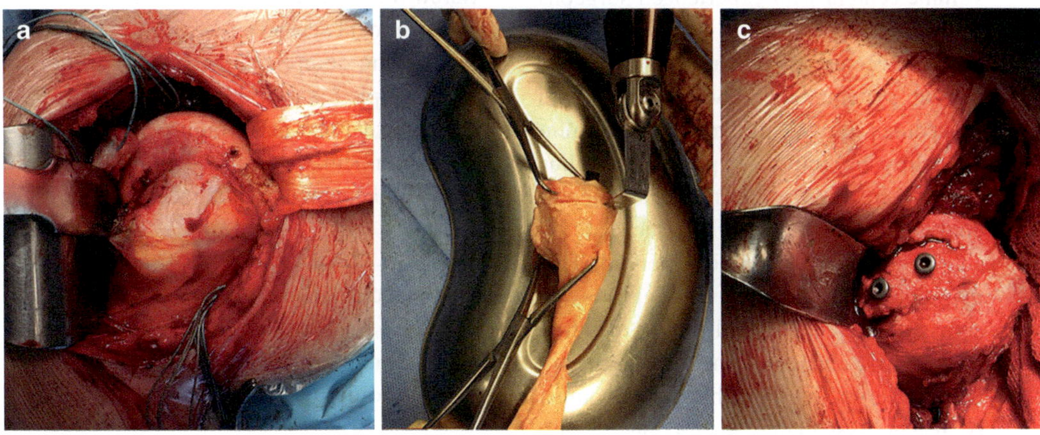

Fig. 27.6 Treatment of large Hill-Sachs lesion (**a**). Part of the calcaneus bone was used to reconstruct the Hill-Sachs defect (**b**). The graft was fixed with 2 4 mm cannulated screws (**c**)

4 weeks. After sling removal, 8 weeks of rehabilitation program started. At 6 months follow-up, the patient presented a full range of motion with no pain and no sign of residual instability.

Pearls and Pitfalls

- 3D-VRT CT reconstruction is fundamental to visualize and quantify the defects.
- The intraoperative use of a 3D-printed template is particularly useful, especially in the treatment of the glenoid side.
- Soft tissue quality must be taken into account even if the main problem is the bone loss.
- Open surgery allows a better visualization and placement of both grafts.
- Inaccurate preoperative quantification (underestimation) of bone loss can lead to a failure.

27.7 Outcomes

- *Critical glenoid bone loss*
  - Open versus arthroscopic Latarjet: Recent systematic reviews and meta-analysis showed that both resulted in significant improvements in patient function and outcome scores, with low rates of recurrent instability (about 2%) and similar complication rates. However, there is a significant learning curve associated with the arthroscopic Latarjet procedure, thus suggesting that the arthroscopic procedure may be advisable to perform only in high-volume centers with experienced surgeons [18, 24].
  - Classic versus congruent arc Latarjet: Recent systematic reviews deemed both procedures equivalent in terms of recurrent instability and return to sport [27]. Radius of curvature of the inferior face of the coracoid graft (used with the congruent arc) is similar to that of the native glenoid. This may potentially decrease contact pressure across the glenohumeral joint, avoiding degenerative changes in the long term [36].
  - Latarjet versus free-bone block procedures: A recent systematic review and meta-analysis showed no significant differences between the procedures in rates of recurrent instability, other complications, osteoarthritis progression, and return to sports [12].
  - Autograft versus allograft free bone block: no significant differences in recurrency and complications were reported by a recent meta-analysis [13].
- *Humeral head bone loss*
  - Several techniques have been described to fill a large Hill-Sachs lesion mainly using the following allograft: femoral head, [31] humeral head [16] and talus [35]. Further studies are needed to report the outcomes of abovementioned surgical techniques.

27.8 Potential Complications/Difficulties

Main surgical difficulty is usually related to graft placement for glenoid reconstruction. A proud graft could be painful and speed the osteoarthritic development [28]. A medialized graft won't perform the bone block effect.

- Postoperative graft related complications [18, 27]: <4%
  - Nonunion
  - Graft migration
  - Graft fracture
- Screw related complications [18, 27]: < 2%
  - Prominent screws
- Neurologic complications (reported only for arthroscopic Latarjet) [18]: 1%
  - Suprascapular nerve injury
  - Musculocutaneous nerve injury
  - Medial cutaneous antebrachial nerve injury

27.9 Expert Recommendation

Some relevant questions remain open. In the near future we should focus on:

- A standardized method to quantify massive bipolar bone loss
- A standardized decision-making algorithm
- The role of soft tissue in bony-mediated instability

Take Home Message

- Patient selection is always the key to success
- A careful clinical examination and an accurate preoperative planning are paramount
- The goal of the surgery should always be an anatomic reconstruction

References

1. Aman ZS, Peebles LA, Johnson DW, Hanson JA, Provencher MT. Multidirectional shoulder instability with circumferential labral tear and bony reverse hill Sachs: treatment with 270° labral repair and fresh talus Osteochondral allograft to the humeral head. Arthrosc Tech. 2021;10:e781–7.
2. Amar E, Konstantinidis G, Coady C, Wong IH. Arthroscopic treatment of shoulder instability with glenoid bone loss using distal Tibial allograft augmentation: safety profile and short-term radiological outcomes. Orthop J Sports Med. 2018;6:2325967118774507.
3. Bhatia S, Saigal A, Frank RM, Bach BR, Cole BJ, Romeo AA, Verma NN. Glenoid diameter is an inaccurate method for percent glenoid bone loss quantification: analysis and techniques for improved accuracy. Arthroscopy. 2015;31:608–614.e1.
4. Bois AJ, Mayer MJ, Fening SD, Jones MH, Miniaci A. Management of bone loss in recurrent traumatic anterior shoulder instability: a survey of North American surgeons. JSES Int. 2020;4:574–83.
5. Burkhart SS, De Beer JF. Traumatic glenohumeral bone defects and their relationship to failure of arthroscopic Bankart repairs: significance of the inverted-pear glenoid and the humeral engaging Hill-Sachs lesion. Arthroscopy. 2000;16:677–94.
6. Burkhart SS, De Beer JF, Barth JRH, Cresswell T, Criswell T, Roberts C, Richards DP. Results of modified Latarjet reconstruction in patients with anteroinferior instability and significant bone loss. Arthroscopy. 2007;23:1033–41.
7. Bushnell BD, Creighton RA, Herring MM. Bony instability of the shoulder. Arthroscopy. 2008;24:1061–73.
8. de Beer JF, Roberts C. Glenoid bone defects–open latarjet with congruent arc modification. Orthop Clin North Am. 2010;41:407–15.
9. Di Giacomo G, Itoi E, Burkhart SS. Evolving concept of bipolar bone loss and the Hill-Sachs lesion: from "engaging/non-engaging" lesion to "on-track/off-track" lesion. Arthroscopy. 2014;30:90–8.
10. Di Giacomo G, Peebles LA, Pugliese M, Dekker TJ, Golijanin P, Sanchez A, Provencher MT. Glenoid track instability management score: radiographic modification of the instability severity index score. Arthroscopy. 2020;36:56–67.
11. Fedorov A, Beichel R, Kalpathy-Cramer J, Finet J, Fillion-Robin J-C, Pujol S, Bauer C, Jennings D, Fennessy F, Sonka M, Buatti J, Aylward S, Miller JV, Pieper S, Kikinis R. 3D slicer as an image computing platform for the quantitative imaging network. Magn Reson Imaging. 2012;30:1323–41.
12. Gilat R, Haunschild ED, Lavoie-Gagne OZ, Tauro TM, Knapik DM, Fu MC, Cole BJ. Outcomes of the Latarjet procedure versus free bone block procedures for anterior shoulder instability: a systematic review and meta-analysis. Am J Sports Med. 2021;49:805–16.
13. Gilat R, Wong SE, Lavoie-Gagne O, Haunschild ED, Knapik DM, Fu MC, Chahla J, Forsythe B, Cole BJ. Outcomes are comparable using free bone block autografts versus allografts for the management of anterior shoulder instability with glenoid bone loss: a systematic review and meta-analysis of "The Non-Latarjet". Knee Surg Sports Traumatol Arthrosc. 2021;29:2159–74.
14. Griswold BG, Paré DW, Herzwurm ZP, Murphy CS, Morpeth BG, Provencher MT, Parada SA. Utility of allograft talus as a source for grafting of concurrent humeral and glenoid defects associated with anterior Glenohumeral instability: an anthropometric analysis. Arthroscopy. 2021;37:845–51.
15. Gürsan O, Eroğlu ON, Türemiş C, Akdoğan EK, Şevik K, Hapa O. Autologous free iliac crest bone grafting of glenoid through the rotator interval using double-barrelled cannula. Eur J Orthop Surg Traumatol. 2021;32:279.
16. Haber DB, Sanchez A, Sanchez G, Ferrari MB, Ferdousian S, Provencher MT. Bipolar bone loss of the shoulder joint due to recurrent instability: use of fresh Osteochondral distal tibia and humeral head allografts. Arthrosc Tech. 2017;6:e893–9.
17. Hart R, Okál F, Komzák M. Transhumeral head plasty and massive osteocartilaginous allograft transplantation for the management of large hill-sachs lesions. Acta Chir Orthop Traumatol Cechoslov. 2010;77:402–10.
18. Hurley ET, Lim Fat D, Farrington SK, Mullett H. Open versus arthroscopic Latarjet procedure for anterior shoulder instability: a systematic review and meta-analysis. Am J Sports Med. 2019;47:1248–53.
19. Itoi E. "On-track" and "off-track" shoulder lesions. EFORT Open Rev. 2017;2:343–51.
20. Kawakami J, Yamamoto N, Etoh T, Hatta T, Mineta M, Itoi E, Isawa R. In vivo glenoid track width can be better predicted with the use of shoulder horizontal extension angle. Am J Sports Med. 2019;47:922–7.
21. Kurokawa D, Yamamoto N, Nagamoto H, Omori Y, Tanaka M, Sano H, Itoi E. The prevalence of a large hill-Sachs lesion that needs to be treated. J Shoulder Elb Surg. 2013;22:1285–9.
22. Lacheta L, Herbst E, Voss A, Braun S, Jungmann P, Millett PJ, Imhoff A, Martetschläger F. Insufficient consensus regarding circle size and bone loss width using the ratio-"best fit circle"-method even with three-dimensional computed tomography. Knee Surg Sports Traumatol Arthrosc. 2019;27:3222–9.
23. Maio M, Sarmento M, Moura N, Cartucho A. How to measure a Hill-Sachs lesion: a systematic review. EFORT Open Rev. 2019;4:151–7.

24. Malahias M-A, Fandridis E, Chytas D, Chronopulos E, Brilakis E, Antonogiannakis E. Arthroscopic versus open Latarjet: a step-by-step comprehensive and systematic review. Eur J Orthop Surg Traumatol. 2019;29:957–66.
25. Marcheggiani Muccioli GM, Rinaldi VG, Lullini G, Ritali A, Mosca M, Romagnoli M, Guerra E, Zaffagnini S. Mid-Term outcomes following fresh-frozen humeral head osteochondral allograft reconstruction for reverse Hill Sachs lesion: a case series. BMC Musculoskelet Disord. 2021;22:768.
26. Martinez-Catalan N, Werthel J-D, Kazum E, Valenti P. Failed Latarjet treated with full arthroscopic Eden-Hybinette procedure using two cortical suture buttons leads to satisfactory clinical outcomes and low recurrence rate. Arthroscopy. 2021; https://doi.org/10.1016/j.arthro.2021.10.026.
27. Mengers SRP, Knapik DM, Kaufman MW, Edwards G, Voos JE, Gillespie RJ, Karns MR. Clinical outcomes of the traditional Latarjet versus the congruent arc modification for the treatment of recurrent anterior shoulder instability: a meta-analysis. Orthop J Sports Med. 2021;9:23259671211030204.
28. Menon A, Fossati C, Magnani M, Boveri S, Compagnoni R, Randelli PS. Low grade of osteoarthritis development after Latarjet procedure with a minimum 5 years of follow-up: a systematic review and pooled analysis. Knee Surg Sports Traumatol Arthrosc. 2021;30:2074.
29. Milano G, Grasso A, Russo A, Magarelli N, Santagada DA, Deriu L, Baudi P, Bonomo L, Fabbriciani C. Analysis of risk factors for glenoid bone defect in anterior shoulder instability. Am J Sports Med. 2011;39:1870–6.
30. Moroder P, Plachel F, Huettner A, Ernstbrunner L, Minkus M, Boehm E, Gerhardt C, Scheibel M. The effect of scapula tilt and best-fit circle placement when measuring glenoid bone loss in shoulder instability patients. Arthroscopy. 2018;34:398–404.
31. Murphy LE, Tucker A, Charlwood AP. Fresh frozen femoral head osteochondral allograft reconstruction of the humeral head reverse hill sachs lesion. J Orthop. 2018;15:772–5.
32. Pak T, Kim AM. Anterior Glenohumeral joint dislocation. In: StatPearls. Treasure Island (FL): StatPearls Publishing; 2021.
33. Pauzenberger L, Dyrna F, Obopilwe E, Heuberer PR, Arciero RA, Anderl W, Mazzocca AD. Biomechanical evaluation of glenoid reconstruction with an implant-free J-bone graft for anterior glenoid bone loss. Am J Sports Med. 2017;45:2849–57.
34. Prada C, Al-Mohrej OA, Patel A, Flood B, Leroux T, Khan M. Managing bone loss in shoulder instability-techniques and outcomes: a scoping review. Curr Rev Musculoskelet Med. 2021;14:447.
35. Provencher MT, Sanchez G, Schantz K, Ferrari M, Sanchez A, Frangiamore S, Mannava S. Anatomic humeral head reconstruction with fresh Osteochondral talus allograft for recurrent Glenohumeral instability with reverse hill-Sachs lesion. Arthrosc Tech. 2017;6:e255–61.
36. Rossi LA, Frank RM, Wilke D, Provencher CMT, Millet PJ, Romeo A, Walch G, Lo I, Yamamoto N, Bokor D, Di Giacomo G, Tokish J, Lech O, Itoi E, Garrigues G, Scheibel M, Boileau P, Calvo E, Arce G, Toro F, Sugaya H, Ranalletta M, Parada S, Savoie F, Verma NN, Chahla J. Evaluation and management of glenohumeral Instability with associated bone loss: an expert consensus statement using the modified Delphi technique. Arthroscopy. 2021;37:1719–28.
37. Saito H, Itoi E, Minagawa H, Yamamoto N, Tuoheti Y, Seki N. Location of the Hill-Sachs lesion in shoulders with recurrent anterior dislocation. Arch Orthop Trauma Surg. 2009;129:1327–34.
38. Saliken DJ, Bornes TD, Bouliane MJ, Sheps DM, Beaupre LA. Imaging methods for quantifying glenoid and Hill-Sachs bone loss in traumatic instability of the shoulder: a scoping review. BMC Musculoskelet Disord. 2015;16:164.
39. Shaha JS, Cook JB, Song DJ, Rowles DJ, Bottoni CR, Shaha SH, Tokish JM. Redefining "critical" bone loss in shoulder instability: functional outcomes worsen with "subcritical" bone loss. Am J Sports Med. 2015;43:1719–25.
40. Sheth U, Theodoropoulos J, Abouali J. Use of 3-dimensional printing for preoperative planning in the treatment of recurrent anterior shoulder instability. Arthrosc Tech. 2015;4:e311–6.
41. Tang J, Xu C, Zhao J. Arthroscopic bone grafting of the humeral head for treatment of a Deep Hill-Sachs lesion. Arthrosc Tech. 2017;6:e1653–9.
42. Trasolini NA, Dandu N, Azua EN, Garrigues GE, Verma NN, Yanke AB. Inconsistencies in controlling for risk factors for recurrent shoulder instability after primary arthroscopic Bankart repair: a systematic review. Am J Sports Med. 2021;50:3705.
43. Ueda Y, Sugaya H, Takahashi N, Matsuki K, Tokai M, Morioka T, Hoshika S. Arthroscopic iliac bone grafting for traumatic anterior shoulder instability with significant glenoid bone loss yields low recurrence and good outcome at a minimum of five-year follow-up. Arthroscopy. 2021;37:2399–408.
44. Valenti P, Martinez-Catalan N, Werthel J-D, Kazum E. Full arthroscopic Eden-Hybinette procedure using 2 cortical suture buttons for the reconstruction of Anteroinferior glenoid defects. Tech Hand Up Extrem Surg. 2021; https://doi.org/10.1097/BTH.0000000000000348.
45. Verweij LPE, Schuit AA, Kerkhoffs GMMJ, Blankevoort L, van den Bekerom MPJ, van Deurzen DFP. Accuracy of currently available methods in quantifying anterior glenoid bone loss: controversy regarding gold standard-a systematic review. Arthroscopy. 2020;36:2295–2313.e1.
46. Verweij LPE, van Spanning SH, Grillo A, Kerkhoffs GMMJ, Priester-Vink S, van Deurzen DFP, van den Bekerom MPJ. Age, participation in competitive sports, bony lesions, ALPSA lesions, >1 preoperative

dislocations, surgical delay and ISIS score>3 are risk factors for recurrence following arthroscopic Bankart repair: a systematic review and meta-analysis of 4584 shoulders. Knee Surg Sports Traumatol Arthrosc. 2021;29:4004.

47. Vopat ML, Peebles LA, McBride T, Cirone I, Rider D, Provencher CMT. Accuracy and reliability of imaging modalities for the diagnosis and quantification of hill-Sachs lesions: a systematic review. Arthroscopy. 2021;37:391–401.
48. Weil S, Arnander M, Pearse Y, Tennent D. Reporting of glenoid bone loss measurement in clinical studies and the need for standardization : a systematic review. Bone Joint J. 2022;104-B:12–8.
49. Willemsen K, Berendes TD, Geurkink T, Bleys RLAW, Leeflang MA, Weinans H, Castelein RM, Nelissen RGHH, van der Wal BCH. A novel treatment for anterior shoulder instability: a biomechanical comparison between a patient-specific implant and the Latarjet procedure. J Bone Joint Surg Am. 2019;101:e68.
50. Wong I, John R, Ma J, Coady CM. Arthroscopic anatomic glenoid reconstruction using distal Tibial allograft for recurrent anterior shoulder instability: clinical and radiographic outcomes. Am J Sports Med. 2020;48:3316–21.
51. Zhao L, Lu M, He L, Xing J, Xu T, Wang C. Arthroscopic autologous iliac crest bone grafting for reconstruction of the glenoid: a nonrigid fixation technique. Arthrosc Tech. 2021;10:e2597–605.
52. Zhuo H, Xu Y, Zhu F, Pan L, Li J. Osteochondral allograft transplantation for large Hill-Sachs lesions: a retrospective case series with a minimum 2-year follow-up. J Orthop Surg Res. 2019;14:344.

Avoiding and Dealing with Iatrogenic Lesions

28

Emre Koraman, Ismail Turkmen, and Mustafa Karahan

Key Points

- Understanding the pathoanatomy and the patient
- Management of the bone loss
- Surgical indications and techniques

28.1 Introduction

- Shoulder instability is a frequent condition in the general population with a rate of 1.7% and 14.8% in young athletic population [1].
- Young age, male sex, contact sports and bone loss are generally identified as a risk factors for recurrent instability [2]. These risk factors should be considered in order to avoid recurrent surgeries and iatrogenic lesions.
- The most favorable treatment of recurrent shoulder instability remains a controversial issue with a wide range of surgical techniques being developed in progress of time [3]. Surgical techniques are imperative to consider when evaluating the causes of a failed shoulder instability repair [4].
- In this section, some of tips and tricks about anterior shoulder instability surgery are discussed to avoid recurrent instability and iatrogenic lesions.

28.2 Relevant Physical Findings

- The first step in a patient with shoulder instability should be to learn the degree of the patient's discomfort, the number of dislocation, neurological disorders, and the prior treatments [5, 6]. Besides, other shoulder pathologies such as cuff tears, tendinopathy/tendinitis, arthritis should be rule out.
- Assessment of the shoulder should include an evaluation of injured and the contralateral shoulder.
- Provocative tests such as apprehension and/or relocation test, which focuses on the level of instability in the shoulder joint should be performed [4]. Furthermore, the other critical test is the load and shift test in physical findings,

Supplementary Information The online version contains supplementary material available at https://doi.org/10.1007/978-3-662-73064-5_28.

E. Koraman
Tuzla State Hospital Department of Orthopaedics and Traumatology, Istanbul, Turkey

I. Turkmen
Goztepe City Hospital Department of Orthopaedics and Traumatology, Istanbul, Turkey

M. Karahan (✉)
Acibadem Mehmet Ali Aydinlar University School of Medicine Department of Orthopaedics and Traumatology, Istanbul, Turkey

L. Kovačič et al. (eds.), *Surgical Techniques for Anterior Shoulder Instability*, https://doi.org/10.1007/978-3-662-73064-5_28

because it tests the adequacy of the glenohumeral motion [6].

- The Gagey test for the evaluation of the laxity of the inferior glenohumeral ligament (IGHL) is also important for the assessment of postoperative instability [4]. Additionally, the sulcus sign must be examined for evaluating capsular laxity [4].
- Also, multidirectional instability, neuromuscular deficit and dyskinesis should be evaluated [4].

28.3 Relevant Imaging

- Different imaging options exist to diagnose shoulder instability. These include plain radiography, computerized tomography (CT), magnetic resonance imaging (MRI), and ultrasonography (USG) [6].
- Initial radiologic assessment should begin with plain radiographies [4]. It is essential to use the basic views (axillary, anteroposterior, lateral) and other views such as Stryker notch and West Point views to demonstrate glenohumeral reduction, and loss of glenoid contour or humeral head lesions [4]. Besides, Grashey view can best visualize the Hill- Sachs lesion [5].
- Advanced imaging with MRI or CT leads to evaluate of previous anchor placement, humeral head and/or glenoid bone loss, and additional soft tissue pathologies [4].
- 3D CT imaging has become the gold standard when determining the severity of bone loss.
- MRI may be useful for anchor placement and soft tissue evaluation [4, 6]. In previous studies it has been shown that MRI is useful of quantifying bone loss, but there has been no evidence that it should be preferred over 3D-CT [6].
- 3D-MRI has been demonstrated that it may be a proper modality of assessing humeral head and glenoid bone loss [7]. It has been demonstrated that 3D-CT osseous reconstructions had similar results to 3D-MRI osseous reconstructions, and there was no statistical significance in the measurement differences of bone loss [7].
- MR arthrogram (MRA) is more sensitive and specific for pan-labral lesions such as Perthes and SLAP lesions than MRI [7].
- USG is another useful technique in quantifying bone loss of humeral head [6].

28.4 Treatment Options and Indications

28.4.1 Arthroscopic Bankart Repair

- Arthroscopic Bankart repair, also known as initial repair for first-time dislocation and recurrent instability, is currently the treatment of choice according to studies [2, 3]. Arthroscopic Bankart repair is indicated in patients with Bankart lesion confirmed by MRI in high demand athletes, athlete younger than 25 years of age, recurrent subluxation/dislocation after nonoperative treatment, <20–25% glenoid bone loss [3–5].
- In a recent study, the long-term results of arthroscopic Bankart repair and arthroscopic washout in the first-time anterior dislocation have been compared [2]. It was suggested that the risk of recurrence is higher in patients underwent arthroscopic washout than arthroscopic Bankart repair [2].
- Additionally, it was stated that the presence of glenoid bone loss, hyperlaxity, engaging Hill-Sachs lesion, the number and placement of anchors utilized in the repair are identified as potential risk factors for failure of arthroscopic Bankart repair previously [5].
- Also, restoration of the soft tissue tension of the IGHL in addition to repairing the labrum to ensure an anatomic soft tissue bumper are necessary for the effectiveness of Bankart repair [5].
- Generally, this procedure requires a minimum of 3 anchors to achieve their aims [4, 5]. However, it must be careful that arthroscopic Bankart repairs can cause glenoid fractures

through the anchor holes, resulting in recurrent instabilities [3, 5].

- It has also been advocated that patient positioning affects arthroscopic treatment outcomes. Lower recurrence was observed in patients treated in the lateral decubitus compared to beach chair position [8]. It has been suggested that the lateral decubitus position allows for better visualization [8].

28.4.2 Remplisagge

- Humeral head lesions are considered as a major risk factor for recurrence, after an inadequate "soft tissue" reconstruction procedure. Therefore, remplissage procedure should be added to Bankart repair if glenoid bone loss is not excessive in engaged, off-track Hill-Sachs lesions [5].
- The success of the remplissage procedure depends on its ability to reduce the predisposition or humeral head excursion for engagement and recurrent subluxations [5].
- To perform Bankart repair plus remplissage procedure, remplissage procedure should be completed before labral repair [5].

28.4.3 Open Bankart Repair

- Open Bankart repair can be performed in revision cases after failed arthroscopic Bankart repair, and in HAGL lesions however it is technically challenging [4, 5].
- Recently, it has been demonstrated that open Bankart repair plus capsular shift for capsular tightening has lower incidence of recurrent instability [5].

28.4.4 Latarjet/Bone Block Procedures

- In the management of anterior shoulder instability, studies have focused on glenoid bone loss in the last 2 decades while investigating the causes of surgical failure [9].
- It has been shown that Latarjet and free bone block procedures may be used in case of critical glenoid deficiency (inverted pear deformity to glenoid) [4].
- The Latarjet is also the first-line treatment method in the setting of failed primary repair as a salvage procedure [3].
- Glenoid reconstruction with free bone block has been suggested as an alternative for the Latarjet or as a revision after failed Latarjet procedure [10].
- Autografts such as iliac crest, distal clavicle, and free partial-thickness coracoid; allografts such as distal tibia, proximal tibia, distal femur, iliac crest may be used for free bone block procedures [10].
- Outcomes of the Latarjet and free bone block procedures have been demonstrated to be similar [10].

28.5 Decision-Making Algorithm

- When determining a surgical technique, there is a multiple factors that surgeons must consider beyond the aforementioned. However, which procedure serves the lowest recurrence rates and most consistent improvements in objective outcomes remains unclear.
- Recent studies showed higher recurrent instability with isolated arthroscopic Bankart repair especially in the setting of young contact athletes with the Hill-Sachs lesions or subcritical/critical glenoid bone loss [9]. The majority of Hill-Sachs defects requiring surgery is due to their size and/or engagement [11].
- Additionally, in case of glenoid bone loss, bone block procedures should be performed to avoid revision surgeries [11].
- Recent literature offers an update on the notion that glenoid bone loss of 25% requires the bone block procedure, because there is increasing evidence suggesting that the amount of glenoid bone loss to indicate bone block procedures may be lower than previously thought [11]. Furthermore, the concept of what is the critical amount of glenoid bone

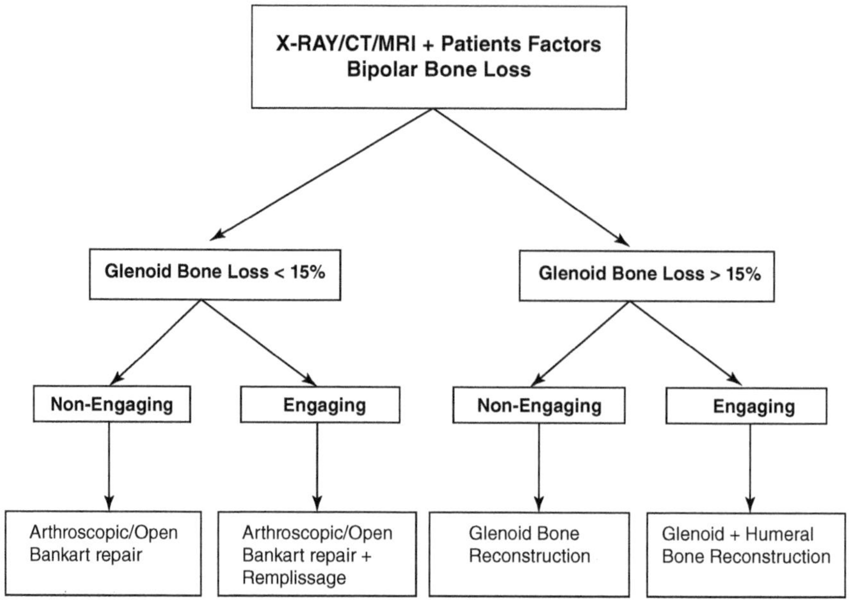

Fig. 28.1 Treatment algorithm for bipolar bone loss in anterior shoulder instability

loss has been questioned, and thresholds as low as 13.5–17% were suggested to necessitate additional procedures above and beyond isolated Bankart repair [11].

- This debate has not been resolved yet with no clear guidelines. On the other hand, an algorithm has been created to facilitate decision making in the treatment (Fig. 28.1) [12]

28.6 Clinical Case

- A 45-year-old man underwent Bankart repair for recurrent anterior shoulder dislocation 7 years ago. Cartilage damage and arthrosis have consisted of improper anchors' locations and directions (Fig. 28.2, Video 28.1).

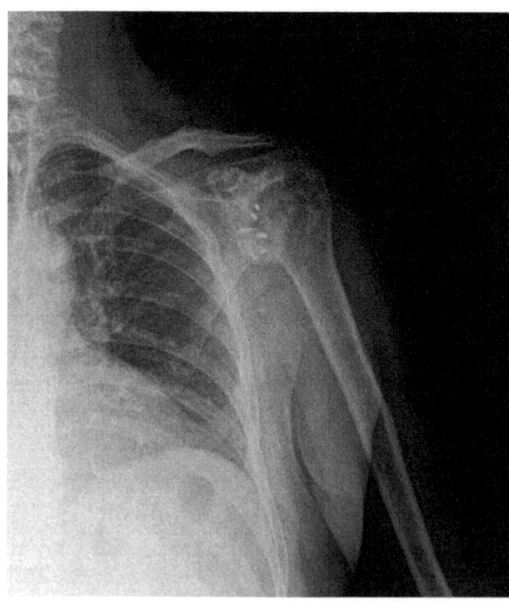

Fig. 28.2 Glenohumeral arthrosis after failed Bankart repair

Pearls and Pitfalls

Preoperative Evaluation

- Young patient, male sex, contact athlete, military personnel at risk of recurrence.
- Avoid surgery if there is uncontrolled epilepsy.
- Evaluate patients' voluntary instability before surgery.
- Evaluate hyperlaxity.
- Evaluate glenoid and/or humeral bone loss.
- Evaluate concomitant anatomic lesions (ALPSA, HAGL, etc.).

Arthroscopic/Open Bankart Repair

- Avoid improper anchor placement.
- Take care of the importance of a minimum three anhor repair.
- Improper anchor directions and prominent metal anchors cause cartilage damage.
- Mobilize the labrum through the glenoid well from the 6 o'clock position (Fig. 28.3).
- Insufficient mobilization of the labrum causes medialized repair.
- Take care of failure to achieve concentric restoration of the capsulolabral bump.
- Decorticate the glenoid rim to the cancellous bone for good healing.
- Use stable knot techniques.
- Presence of symptomatic sulcus sign indicates that requirement of inferior capsular shift (Open Bankart repair).
- Horizontal capsulotomy instead of vertical along the glenoid rim may prevent excessive tightening of the capsule medially and consequently restriction of external rotation (Open Bankart repair).

Remplissage

- "Doublepulley" suture technique has been described to broaden the footprint of the repair and avoid infraspinatus muscle strangulation. Tie the sutures over tendon rather than muscle.

Latarjet/Bone Block Procedures

- Perform the osteotomy perpendicularly to the coracoid in order to avoid iatrogenic glenoid fracture.
- Take care to protect medial aspect of the conjoint tendon not to disturb the blood supply to the graft.
- Minimize releasing the soft tissue and pectoralis minor to avoid devascularization of the graft.
- With an oscillating saw, decorticate the posterior aspect of the coracoid along the long axis to expose a broad, flat cancellous bed to optimize graft healing to the glenoid margin.
- The optimal position lies between 3-and 5 o clock on the glenoid flush to or just medial (1–2 mm) to the native glenoid with the posterior surface.
- The graft can be rotated and the medial surface affixed to the native glenoid (congruent arc technique). The coracoid is typically wider in horizontal plane. Congruent arc technique can better restore the glenoid width in cases of severe bone loss. However, the trade-off is that the area of screw placement is decreased and fracture of the coracoid or loss of fixation can occur, particularly in cases where the coracoid is very small.
- The graft should lie parallel to the anterior border of the glenoid.
- Use "two-finger technique" to tighten screws to avoid iatrogenic coracoid fracture
- Screws must cross both cortices
- Avoid excessive decortication of the graft, which can result in iatrogenic fracture. The holes should be far apart while drilling of the graft.

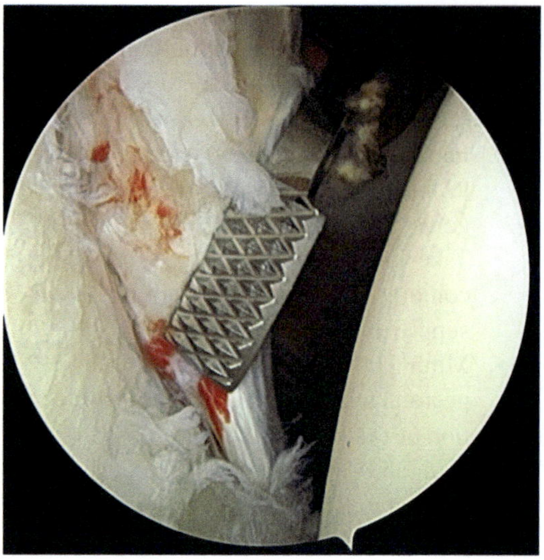

Fig. 28.3 Mobilization of the labrum in arthroscopic Bankart repair

28.7 Outcomes

- In the literature, recurrence of shoulder dislocations when managed nonoperatively has been detailed to be between 38% and 80% [5].
- Isolated Bankart repair increases the risk of recurrence in the presence of Hill-Sachs lesions [12].
- Latarjet procedure has been demonstrated superior outcomes compared to the Bankart repair in recurrent cases [13].
- In another study, the recurrence of instability among patients with bipolar bone loss was reported as 19.5% in Bankart repairs, 8.7% in Latarjet procedures, and 4.4% in arthroscopic remplissage with Bankart repair [12].
- It has been shown that glenoid reconstruction with using free bone block had similar outcomes to Latarjet [10].

28.8 Potential Complications/ Difficulties

- Recurrence is the most common complication in the management of anterior shoulder instability that can be often due to unrecognized bone loss and/or pan-labral tear, poor surgical technique, neglected preoperative risk factors [14].
- Arthroscopic techniques can avoid many of the complications associated with open procedures such as subscapularis weakness and ruptures, limited range of motion, infection, and arthrofibrosis [14]. However, anchor pull-out is one of the disadvantages arthroscopic surgery because of improper anchor placement [14]. Also, biceps tendinitis is a complication related to arthroscopic soft tissue procedures, particularly remplissage [15]. Remplissage can also cause stiffness, particularly in external rotation [15].
- Moreover, Latarjet is a technically challenging procedure with complications such as graft, screw complications, postoperative limited range of motion, potential neurovascular injury [10]. Graft complications include non-union/malunion, osteolysis, fracture and migration [16]. The frequency of graft osteolysis has been demonstrated that significantly more prominent around the proximal screw than the distal screw [15]. Also, screw complications are related to screw misplaced, length or failure [3]. Additionally, performing subscapularis tenotomy for the Latarjet, which can serve as a source of instability, recurrence, stiffness, or weakness if it is not repaired anatomically [1]. Eventually, the extra-anatomic nature of Latarjet with released pectoralis minor, transposition of the conjoined tendons, and a permenant split of the subscapularis might lead to scapular dyskinesis and make revision more complicated [17].

28.9 Expert Recommendation

- The most common and most important complication of anterior shoulder instability is recurrence. There are factors related to the patient and the surgery in its etiology. These are age, ligamentous laxity, anchor location, number of anchors, lesion type, contact sports, and bone loss. To avoid iatrogenic lesions surgeon should take care of these factors and should have standard checklists for surgery.

Take Home Message

- Patient assessment should be done appropriately.
- Soft tissues and bone loss should be well evaluated.
- The appropriate surgical indication should be determined and the surgeries should be performed in standard steps.

References

1. Lau BC, Johnston TR, Gregory BP, Bejarano Pineda L, Wu M, Fletcher AN, et al. Outcomes after revision anterior shoulder stabilization: a systematic review. Orthop J Sports Med. 2020;8(5):2325967120922571.
2. Yapp LZ, Nicholson JA, Robinson CM. Primary arthroscopic stabilization for a first-time anterior dislocation of the shoulder: long-term follow-up of a randomized, double-blinded trial. J Bone Joint Surg Am. 2020;102(6):460–7.
3. An VVG, Sivakumar BS, Phan K, Trantalis J. A systematic review and meta-analysis of clinical and patient-reported outcomes following two procedures for recurrent traumatic anterior instability of the shoulder: Latarjet procedure vs. Bankart repair. J Shoulder Elb Surg. 2016;25(5):853–63.
4. Donohue MA, Mauntel TC, Dickens JF. Recurrent shoulder instability after primary Bankart repair. Sports Med Arthrosc. 2017;25(3):123–30.
5. White AE, Patel NK, Hadley CJ, Dodson CC. An algorithmic approach to the management of shoulder instability. J Am Acad Orthop Surg Glob Res Rev. 2019;3(12)
6. Provencher MT, Frank RM, Leclere LE, Metzger PD, Ryu JJ, Bernhardson A, et al. The Hill-Sachs lesion: diagnosis, classification, and management. J Am Acad Orthop Surg. 2012;20(4):242–52.
7. Stillwater L, Koenig J, Maycher B, Davidson M. 3D-MR vs. 3D-CT of the shoulder in patients with glenohumeral instability. Skeletal Radiol. 2017;46(3):325–31.
8. Frank RM, Saccomanno MF, McDonald LS, Moric M, Romeo AA, Provencher MT. Outcomes of arthroscopic anterior shoulder instability in the beach chair versus lateral decubitus position: a systematic review and meta-regression analysis. Arthroscopy. 2014;30(10):1349–65.
9. Di Giacomo G, de Gasperis N, Scarso P. Bipolar bone defect in the shoulder anterior dislocation. Knee Surg Sports Traumatol Arthrosc. 2016;24(2):479–88.
10. Gilat R, Haunschild ED, Lavoie-Gagne OZ, Tauro TM, Knapik DM, Fu MC, et al. Outcomes of the Latarjet procedure versus free bone block procedures for anterior shoulder instability: a systematic review and meta-analysis. Am J Sports Med. 2021;49(3):805–16.
11. Haroun HK, Sobhy MH, Abdelrahman AA. Arthroscopic Bankart repair with remplissage versus Latarjet procedure for management of engaging Hill-Sachs lesions with subcritical glenoid bone loss in traumatic anterior shoulder instability: a systematic review and meta-analysis. J Shoulder Elb Surg. 2020;29(10):2163–74.
12. Gowd AK, Liu JN, Cabarcas BC, Garcia GH, Cvetanovich GL, Provencher MT, et al. Management of recurrent anterior shoulder instability with bipolar bone loss: a systematic review to assess critical bone loss amounts. Am J Sports Med. 2019;47(10):2484–93.
13. Imam MA, Shehata MSA, Martin A, Attia H, Sinokrot M, Bahbah EI, et al. Repair versus Latarjet procedure for recurrent anterior shoulder instability: a systematic review and meta-analysis of 3275 shoulders. Am J Sports Med. 2020:363546520962082.
14. Hohmann E, Tetsworth K, Glatt V. Open versus arthroscopic surgical treatment for anterior shoulder dislocation: a comparative systematic review and meta-analysis over the past 20 years. J Shoulder Elb Surg. 2017;26(10):1873–80.
15. Williams HLM, Evans JP, Furness ND, Smith CD. It's not all about redislocation: a systematic review of complications after anterior shoulder stabilization surgery. Am J Sports Med. 2019;47(13):3277–83.
16. Hurley ET, Lim Fat D, Farrington SK, Mullett H. Open versus arthroscopic Latarjet procedure for anterior shoulder instability: a systematic review and meta-analysis. Am J Sports Med. 2019;47(5):1248–53.
17. Moroder P, Schulz E, Wierer G, Auffarth A, Habermeyer P, Resch H, et al. Neer award 2019: Latarjet procedure vs. iliac crest bone graft transfer for treatment of anterior shoulder instability with glenoid bone loss: a prospective randomized trial. J Shoulder Elb Surg. 2019;28(7):1298–307.

Management of Instability with Subscapularis Tear

29

Bruno Toussaint

Key Points

- Cuff tears modify strategy and management of shoulder instability. Because the cuff contributes to the stability of the gleno-humeral joint.
- It is important to diagnose the association of the two lesions. And that the precise diagnosis of the lesion of the cuff is made at the same time as the assessment of capsulo-labral and bone damage.
- The cuff tear may be concomitant with or pre-existing the dislocation. Both situations will influence repair and stabilization techniques.
- The therapeutic strategy will depend mainly on the age and type and reparability of the lesion of the cuff.
- The results will be based on the ability to restore anatomy closest to normal anatomy.

29.1 Introduction

- First, we must review the role of the cuff in the stability of the gleno-humeral joint. Itoi [7] reports very interesting work of Saha [9] on the role of the cuff in stabilizing glenohumeral joint. The glenohumeral ligaments, which prevent excessive translation of the humeral head in the end-range of motion, remain tension-free until glenohumeral motion approaches its terminal range. In the mid-range of motion, during which there is no increase in capsular tension, dynamic glenohumeral stability must be provided by active muscle contraction.
- Lee [8] in a cadaveric study showed that the subscapularis and supraspinatus provided significantly greater dynamic stability in the anterior direction than did the posterior cuff muscles. Conversely, in the end-range of motion, the dynamic stability index revealed that the subscapularis, infraspinatus, and teres minor provided significantly greater stability than did the supraspinatus.
- Trillat [11] describes, in first, the anterior functional belt consisting of extensible elements (capsule and synovia), inextensible elements (labrum and gleno-humeral ligaments) and subscapularis muscle. For him, the Bankart lesion puts in, more or less distant, on the anterior face of the scapula the insertion of the belt, and she can no longer fulfil her role in external rotation. It explains the recurrent dislocation because the humeral head, deprived of previous counter-support, will present two successive movements. A rotation movement then an earlier translation movement as soon as the stability limit is reached (this limit

B. Toussaint (✉)
Teomera, Le Grand Saconnex, Switzerland

L. Kovačič et al. (eds.), *Surgical Techniques for Anterior Shoulder Instability*,
https://doi.org/10.1007/978-3-662-73064-5_29

depends on the degree of lesions of the anterior functional belt). He joins Saha [9] in describing neuro-muscular imbalance.

- Under these conditions any damage of the subscapularis can only aggravate the instability of the gleno-humeral joint. The role of the subscapularis muscle is therefore different and superior to the role that other rotator cuff muscles can play. Subscapularis muscle damage is always more severe. But it depends on the severity of the lesion.
- To appreciate and quantify the rupture of muscle subscapularis the French Arthroscopy Society classification [10] is the most suitable of the existing classifications. Because it evaluates the rupture in the cranio-caudal and A-P planes. And it takes also into consideration the long head of the biceps, the coraco-humeral ligament and the superior gleno-humeral ligament.

29.2 Relevant Physical Findings

- Clinical signs include specific signs of subscapularis muscle involvement and signs of instability. They are sometimes difficult to separate. They also depend on the severity of the lesion.
- The Bear Hug test described by Burkhart [1, 2] is one of the best signs of damage to the muscle subscapularis, and it is little disturbed by the signs of suffering of the anterior bulge of the anterior functional belt.
- The clinical examination is complete by looking for the lift off sign and the evaluation of muscle strength of subscapularis.
- Other cuff tests are less accurate and less important to look for.
- Instability tests are less important, diagnosis is based on the notion of recurrence and positive anterior apprehension in external rotation and abduction.
- The limitation of mobility is a factor of severity because it is related to an extension of the subscapularis lesion.
- It is important to clarify if there were signs of rotator cuff pain prior to first dislocation, the number of dislocations and subluxations is important as well.

29.3 Relevant Imaging

- The imaging, after eliminating bone damage on simple X-rays, will rely on the arthro MRI which allows the simultaneous study of the labrum and the capsulo-ligament complex and the rotator cuff.
- Bankart lesion is not always very important. On the other hand, it is necessary to be very attentive to the signs of damage of the muscle subscapularis, but also of the long head of the biceps and the coraco-humeral ligament and superior gleno-humeral ligament.
- Other rotator cuff muscles may also be affected.
- A complete degloving of the rotator cuff is possible and associated with a dislocation, difficult to reduce, with sometimes a posterior dislocation of the long head of the biceps.
- When the rupture of the subscapularis muscle is caused by the dislocation, it is very often a complete avulsion of the tendon, with a rapid retraction of the tendon.
- It is difficult to identify the avulsion of the lower third of the muscle which inserts directly on the humerus without tendon. The best landmark is the tendon of the pectoralis major or latissimus dorsi for an assessment of inferior subscapularis muscle avulsion.
- Evaluation of the reparability of the subscapularis tendon is based on the muscle volume and fatty infiltration of the muscle. Loss of volume is the best sign of an already old rupture with an increased risk of difficulties to reduce the tendon in good position onto the less tuberosity.
- Kobayashi described the reverse comma sign as the most sensitive and specific sign to evaluate subscapularis tear and muscle atrophy of the two superior third.

29.4 Treatment Options and Indications

- There are different options that depend primarily on the patient's age and the age of rotator cuff tear.
- Even if young patients very rarely have rotator cuff tears during dislocations, it is important to quickly make the diagnosis when recovery after the first dislocation is abnormal.
- Repair of the subscapularis must be as fast as possible to prevent muscle atrophy and muscle fatty infiltration and especially the difficulties of tendon reduction on the lesser tuberosity.
- Chronic lesions of subscapularis are difficult problems to solve in the young patients.
- In young patients, the most important thing is to repair the rotator cuff tear. Often this single repair is sufficient and restores the stability of the gleno-humeral joint, especially if the quality of the tendon and muscle is of sufficient quality. The Bankart lesion is minimal and can heal without additional gesture.
- Gomberawalla [6] reported in a systematic review that rotator cuff repair alone is sufficient for the majority of cases. But sometimes, in view of the extent of the Bankart lesion it is necessary to repair at the same time the capsulo-ligamentary complex [5].
- Very rarely, there is a bone defect large enough to require a bone graft. In these cases the technique of Eden-Hybbinette is indicated, because the simultaneous realization of a Latarjet procedure or a Trillat procedure and a subscapularis repair are inadequate.
- Trillat procedure is not a good indication in anterior or anterior-superior rotator cuff ruptures associated with recurrent shoulder dislocation. Because the Sling effect is ineffective or totally ineffective if the subscapularis is irreparable.
- In elderly, treatment options are multiple and depend on age and consequences of rotator cuff tear on shoulder function.
- In the younger population of elderly, if the shoulder mobility is good and the posterior cuff is healthy, the theory of Saha [9] can be used. But the transfer of the latissimus dorsi muscle, proposed by him, is based on our experience too complicated and too aggressive.
- Hill-Sachs lesion is very often found as damage to the humeral head in dislocations and the engaging Hill-Sachs lesion is an aggravating factor in the recurrence of the dislocation of the gleno-humeral joint and its association with the weakness of the anterior functional belt further increases this risk.
- Reducing the Hill-Sachs lesion may reduce the risk of dislocation despite the weakness of the anterior functional belt and even for non-engaging Hill-Sachs lesions. Because it can have the same effect of pulling back as the latissimus dorsi muscle transfer proposed by Saha [9]. This is what Connolly [4] did when he proposed, for Bankart repair failures, a teno-capsulodesis of the infraspinatus in the lesion of Hill-Sachs to prevent the dislocation. By reducing the volume of the notch, it decreases the dislocating effect of Hill-Sachs lesion. Wolff described the arthroscopic technique of this procedure by associating it with an arthroscopic Bankart repair. In case of old and retracted and irreparable tear of the subscapularis muscle, this technique allows to treat the instability without necessity to do a reverse total shoulder arthroplasty (RTSA) (Fig. 29.1).
- After 75-years or when the rupture of the muscle subscapularis is totally irreparable and is pseudo-paralysis, with a massive loss of range of motion, the solution is the establishment of a reverse total shoulder arthroplasty (RTSA).
- Another case for indication of RTSA is associated fracture of the anterior edge of the glenoid. Often the humeral head is anteriorly subluxated. This explains the loss of range of motion and pseudoparalysis.

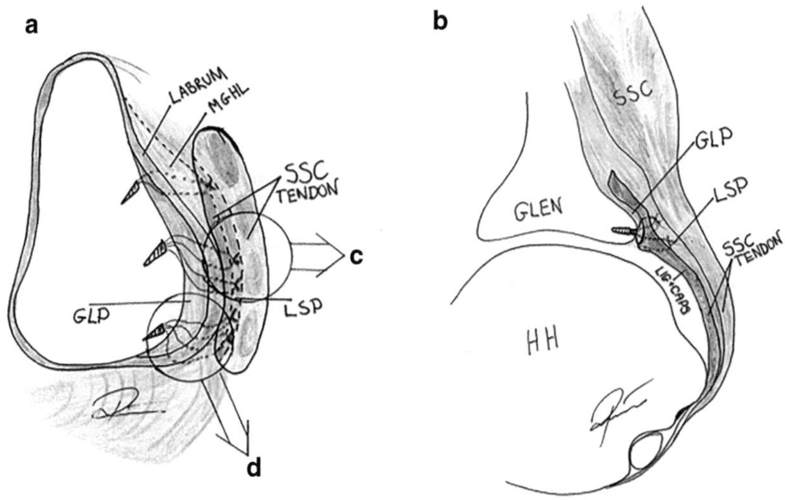

Fig. 29.1 The concept of 2 separate intervals for arthroscopic Bankart repair, the Glenoid-Labrum Pouch (GLP) and Labrum- Subscapularis Pouch (LSP), is introduced. Arthroscopic knots are kept away from the articular surface by virtue of being tied from the LSP (**a** and **b**), and visualization of this space for knot tying is accomplished through the anterolateral portal (**c** and **d**). MGHL indicates middle glenohumeral ligament, HH humeral head. (Courtesy R. BRZOSKA)

- The Reverse total shoulder arthroplasty, which is a semi-constrained prosthesis, stabilizes the gleno-humeral joint and restores shoulder mobility with high reliability.
- Difficulties in RTSA implanting are directly related to the glenoid bone stock.
- At both ends, surgical indications are easy. In the younger ones, repair of the muscle subscapularis is necessary and should be as anatomical as possible and does not always require repair of associated Bankart lesion. And there is no indication for Latarjet or Trillat procedures. In the elderly, RTSA is the easiest solution that guarantees the best results in the absence of complications.
- The indications and decisions are more complicated between 45 and 60 years and especially when there is atrophy or fatty infiltration of the muscle subscapularis which makes repair of the muscle subscapularis questionable.
  - For the younger ones, a muscle transfer is probably the best option to reinforce the subscapularis muscle. Latissimus dorsi transfer onto the lesser tuberosity could be the best.
  - And for the older ones, the "remplissage" technique significantly reduces the risk of recurrence of dislocation. RTSA could be next stage or salvage procedure.

29.5 Decision-Making Algorithm

- Under 40 years:
  - Subscapularis tear without atrophy or fatty infiltration: subscapularis repair associated with Bankart repair depending on capsular lesions.
  - Subscapularis tear with atrophy and/or fatty infiltration: subscapularis repair if it is possible with Bankart repair and possible subscapularis reinforcement by latissimus dorsi transfer [9].
- Between 40 and 70 years:
  - In general, subscapularis repair whenever possible if there sufficient muscle tendon quality
  - For the youngest in the age group, if the repair is partially possible: subscapularis repair with possible reinforcement with muscle transfer.

- For others:
  - "remplissage" technique to delay RTSA as long as possible.
- After 70 years:
  - RTSA salvage surgery in case of subluxation and pseudo-paralysis.

Pearls and Pitfalls

- For the subscapularis muscle repair, the release of the tendon must be careful not to damage the vascularization of the upper third.
- Sometimes the axillary nerve can be adherent to the anterior side of the subscapularis and can be stretched during tendon reduction and fixation on the lesser tuberosity.
- Fixation of the tendon must be without tension.
- Probably double row fixation is safer than single row.
- Long head of biceps tenodesis is necessary to improve tendon healing.
- If a Bankart repair is necessary, the BLS technique described by Brzoska [3] allows the separation of the capsular plane and the muscular plane. And Bankart repair could be easier.
- For the "remplissage" technique, the use of two anchors in the humeral head is the minimum to be respected to be strong enough.
- For the RTSA the Macenzie approach is probably the best option, because in the absence of being able to repair the subscapularis, it reduces the risk of dislocation of the prosthesis which is the complication to be feared the most.

29.6 Outcomes

- Outcomes are complex, because the cuff repair requires an early passive mobilization and stabilization on the other hand a relative immobilization at the beginning. This contradiction must be twisted in favour of the subscapularis repair in young patients.
- Management of instability with subscapularis tear is always more difficult than a simple cuff repair or a simple repair of Bankart. It requires a minimum of experience for an arthroscopic repair and is more time consuming.

Take-Home Messages

- It is necessary to have a complete and precise diagnostic approach since the symptomatology is atypical after an episode of recurrent dislocation.
- It is necessary to look for the cuff tear and more particularly of the subscapularis like all the other complications of recurrent dislocations.
- After diagnosis, the important points are, is the tear cuff repairable, and what is the best solution depending on the patient's age. Choosing the right treatment is already the first step to a good end result.

References

1. Barth J, Audebert S, Toussaint B, Charousset C, Godeneche A, Graveleau N, Joudet T, Lefebvre Y, Nove-Josserand L, Petroff E, Solignac N, Szymanski C, Pitermann M, Thelu C-E, French Arthroscopy Society. Diagnosis of subscapularis tendon tears: are available diagnostic tests pertinent for a positive diagnosis? Orthop Traumatol Surg Res. 2012;98(8 Suppl):S178–85.
2. Barth J, Burkhart S, De Beer JF. The bear-hug test: a new and sensitive test for diagnosing a subscapularis tear. Arthroscopy. 2006;22(10):1076–84.
3. Brzoska R, Blasiak A, Hldaki W, Streit J, Toussaint B, Solecki W. Arthroscopic bankart repair using extracapsular suture between the glenohumeral ligaments and subscapularis tendon (BLS technique): a technical note. Tech Should Elbow Surg. 2012;13(2):45–100.
4. Connolly JF. Humeral head defects associated with shoulder dislocation—their diagnostic and surgical significance. Instr Course Lect. 1972;21:42–54.

5. Goldberg JA, Chan KY, Best JP, Bruce WJM, Walsh W, Parry W. Surgical management of large rotator cuff tears combined with instability in elite rugby football players. Br J Sports Med. 2003;37:179–81.
6. Gomberawalla MM, Sekiya JK. Rotator cuff tear and glenohumeral instability a systematic review. Clin Orthop Relat Res. 2014;472:2448–56.
7. Itoi E, Tabata S. Rotator cuff tears in anterior dislocation of the shoulder. Int Orthopaed (SICOT). 1992;16:240–4.
8. Lee S-B, Kim K-J, O'driscoll S. W, Morrey B F, And An K-N : Dynamic glenohumeral stability provided by the rotator cuff muscles in the mid-range and end-range of motion JBJS 82-A, 6, 849–857. 2000.
9. Saha AK. Dynamic stability of the glenohumeral joint. Acta Orthop Scandinavica. 1971;42:491–505.
10. Toussaint B, Barth J, Charousset C, Godeneche A, Joudet T, Lefebvre Y, Nove-Josserand L, Petroff E, Solignac N, Hardy P, Szymanski C, Maynou C, Thelu C-E, Boileau P, Graveleau N, Audebert S, The French Arthroscopy Society (SFA). New endoscopic classification for subscapularis lesions. Orthop Traumatol Surg Res. 2012;98(8 Suppl):S186–92.
11. Trillat A, Leclerc-Chalvet F. Luxation récidivante de l'épaule (Recurrent shoulder dislocation) in French Masson and Cie Paris Ed; 1973. pp. 32–55.

Shoulder Instablity and Nerve Injury

30

Roger Hackney and Grainne Bourke

Key Points

- Shoulder dislocation can be a potential cause of nerve injury.
- The axillary nerve is particularly at risk.
- Brachial plexus, predominantly the infraclavicular part, can be injured as well.
- Careful neurological assessment and documentation is important.
- Poorly managed nerve injuries lead to avoidable long-term disability.
- There is a trend towards earlier surgical intervention.
- With high grade injuries a more aggressive treatment approach is required.

Supplementary Information The online version contains supplementary material available at https://doi.org/10.1007/978-3-662-73064-5_30.

R. Hackney (✉) · G. Bourke
Spire Hospital Leeds, Leeds, UK
e-mail: roger.hackney@nhs.net;
grainnebourke@nhs.net

30.1 Introduction

- Shoulder dislocation is known to be a potential cause of nerve injury. Every medical student is taught about the risk to the axillary nerve and the need to examine the 'regimental badge' area for numbness with a dislocation of the glenohumeral joint. Despite this, nerve injuries associated with shoulder dislocation are missed and/or poorly managed leading to avoidable long-term disability.
- In a long term prospective study the incidence of neurological deficit with shoulder dislocation was 13.5% [1]. If electromyograph (EMG) studies are used the incidence can rise to 48% [2].
- The axillary nerve is the nerve most commonly injured, but the brachial plexus, predominantly the infraclavicular part, can be injured [3].
- The axillary nerve is particularly at risk because of it's anatomy. As it passes through the quadrilateral space it sits adjacent to the inferior capsule of the shoulder and the surgical neck of the humerus.
- A significant cohort, (six out of ten cases with nerve injury in a UK study) will have a global infraclavicular brachial plexus injury. Pan plexus injuries are more common than expected and the recovery from these injuries is very mixed.

L. Kovačič et al. (eds.), *Surgical Techniques for Anterior Shoulder Instability*,
https://doi.org/10.1007/978-3-662-73064-5_30

Table 30.1 Risk Factors for nerve injury and glenohumeral dislocation

Primary dislocation
Delayed reduction beyond 12 hours.
High energy dislocation
Increasing age of patient
Co-existing vascular injury
Neuropathic pain associated with axillary nerve injury
Fracture of humerus of scapula (doubles the risk)
Rotator cuff injury
Greater tuberosity fracture
Male

- Delay in referral to specialist centres for rehabilitation combined with neuropathic pain and older age group contribute to poor functional outcome in these cases.
- Associated suprascapular nerve deficit is more difficult to define clinically due to concomitant rotator cuff injury or tear.
- Risk factors that should increase the index of suspicion for nerve injury are found in Table 30.1.

30.2 Relevant Physical Findings

- Careful neurological assessment and documentation is important at the time of presentation to the emergency department both pre and post reduction. Those patients with neurological deficit should be referred to an acute shoulder clinic with access to specialists in peripheral nerve surgery and therapy.
- Whilst most nerve injuries are low grade it is important to detect any neurological deficit, as prediction of which injury may recover and which may not is unreliable at an early stage.
- The axillary nerve is the most frequently affected nerve, followed by the ulnar nerve. There is significant risk that there will be no real recovery of ulnar nerve function in low energy dislocations. This is due to a combination of the age of the cohort and the distance from the injury site to the hand for intrinsic re-innervation.
- Unfortunately, sensation in the classic regimental badge area is not a fully reliable guide to the presence of an axillary nerve injury. This is because the anterior branch with the cutaneous element may leave the axillary nerve proximal to the injury, and may be preserved in over 50% of cases severe enough to require surgery [4].
- Persisting deltoid weakness at a week following injury, once the initial pain and swelling have settled, is diagnostic. The presence of a massive rotator cuff tear in an older patient may give a confusing, clinical picture but palpation of the deltoid during an attempted contraction will distinguish an axillary nerve injury [2].
- Clinical tests have been described to isolate deltoid function [5–7], but can give false positives, and in the acute setting and in the presence of fractures may be difficult to apply.
- Cutaneous sensory recovery is poor which leads to functional impairments of hand function. Poor cutaneous sensory recovery is seen in all age groups and all mechanisms of injury. This is supported by previous experimental evidence of greater early loss of sensory neurons in the Dorsal root ganglia with severe peripheral nerve injury thus impairing the possibility for regeneration and recovery.
- A high index of suspicion of a nerve injury should lead to early referral for urgent EMG studies.

30.3 Electromyelographic Studies

- The incidence of nerve injuries is much higher when EMG studies are performed compared with clinical examination alone.
- Once an injury is suspected clinically, EMG studies are necessary to determine the grade of injury.
  - Grade 1, neuropraxia, demyelination
  - Grade 2, axonotmesis, axonal disruption
  - Grade 3 neurotmesis, disruption of the nerve continuity.
- A compound muscle action potential (CMAP) of less than 10% of the contralateral side, absent motor units on EMG and a significant

reduction in motor unit action potential (MUAP) are all indicators of poor prognosis [8].

- Early EMGs can distinguish low- and high-grade injuries, even as early as 2 weeks following injury.
- However, EMG cannot distinguish between severe axonotmesis and neurotmesis.
- A series of EMG studies may be necessary to determine whether reinnervation is taking place, and any absence or delay in reinnervation should prompt surgical exploration.

30.4 Treatment Options and Indications

- The majority of nerve injuries will improve with time and achieve return to function. Grade 1, neurapraxia, will recover by 3 months and grade 2, axonotmesis, 6–7 months.
- Recovery can be monitored with clinical examination and serial EMG studies. If recovery is slower than anticipated, or if there is a grade-3 injury then surgical options need exploring.
- Early recognition of a high grade injury allows early referral to a peripheral nerve injury unit where specialised care can be implemented. There is a trend towards earlier surgical intervention.
- If a high-grade injury is suspected early, then MRI neurography should be requested, if available. This can demonstrate nerve discontinuity, and the position of the injury and large haematomas which can be evacuated to reduce subsequent fibrosis.
- The timing of surgical intervention is crucial to avoid long term disability. Delay in surgery for repair or grafting beyond 6 months leads to a poorer outcome [9]. This is likely to be due in part to a loss of the motor end plate at the neuromuscular junction, which is irreversible, although the precise timeframe is humans is unknown [10].
- Urgent nerve exploration is indicated in cases with high energy injury where nerve rupture or severe traction and attenuation is suspected. These are often younger patients with real potential for recovery with reconstruction.
- Radiological imaging such as ultrasound and MRI may be value in supporting the diagnosis but if there is clinical suspicion of nerve rupture then exploration to assess the nerve is warranted with immediate reconstruction if indicated.
- Surgical exploration allows the site of the damage to be identified (Fig. 30.1). The nerve can then be freed from any surrounding scar tissue and a neurolysis performed. An interfascicular neurolysis may be necessary. Neurolysis removes constricting scar tissue which can improve nerve conduction. This may be all that is necessary for a poorly recovering low grade injury.
- With high grade injuries a more aggressive approach is required, with nerve grafting or nerve transfer.
- Nerve reconstruction with nerve transfers or nerve grafting can yield good functional outcomes particularly for isolated axillary nerve injury.
  - Transfers using the nerve to either the long head of triceps [11] or the medial head of triceps [12] have been described and are used regularly with good outcomes.
  - Nerve grafting can result in very good outcomes in young patients with Medical Research Council muscle power grade 4 or 5.

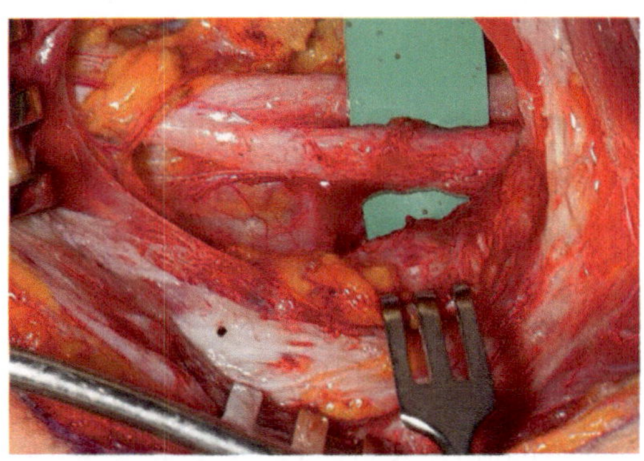

Fig. 30.1 Neurolysis of the musculocutaneous nerve involved in scar tissue following a Latarjet procedure

- Multidisciplinary team working in a specialised centre is the key for this patient population with combined early nerve and shoulder surgery for exploration and reconstruction being optimal when feasible.

30.5 Clinical Case

- An 18 year old male (JD), presented in late 2020 for a second opinion to a routine outpatient clinic, with a complex history of shoulder instability. He was in his final year at school. His sport was motocross, following his father's sport.
- Motocross is a form of off-road motorcycle racing held on enclosed off-road circuits. Studies consistently rank motocross among the most physically demanding sports. During a typical race day, a professional motocross rider wrestles with a 200-plus-pound bike for 30 or more minutes in each of two events. Speeds vary depending on the track, but you can expect to see competitors going in excess of 60 mph at a typical supercross race. Riders soar as far as 70 feet in distance, while flying as high as a three-story building off jumps called "triples" (Fig. 30.2).
- Patient JD suffered his first dislocation falling off his motocross bike aged nine. His and his parent's recollection of how he was managed at the time was vague, but it was noted at the time that he had axillary nerve damage and he subsequently noted significant muscle wasting. He was not investigated at the time, nor referred for specialist opinion. Unfortunately, he only made a partial recovery.
- Despite this JD was able to return to his sport and compete at National level with some success but was struggling with loss of power from deltoid. His parents were in the process of seeking help in 2016 when he came off his bike again and suffered a tear of his rotator cuff. This was repaired arthroscopically, and he returned to competing only to suffer a fracture dislocation.

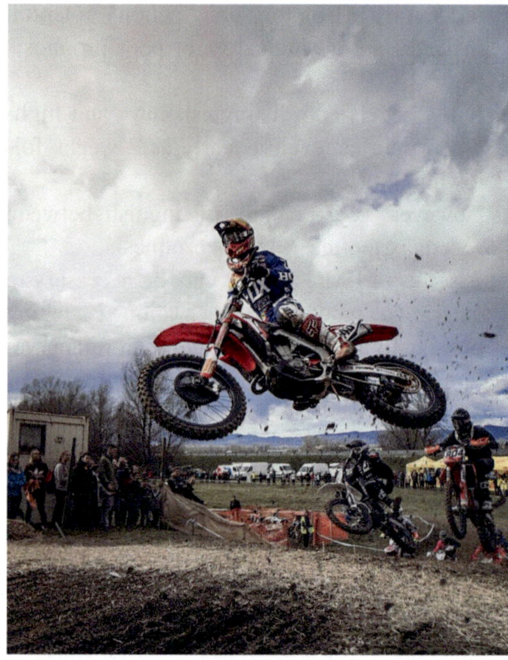

Fig. 30.2 Rider of motocross while flying jumps

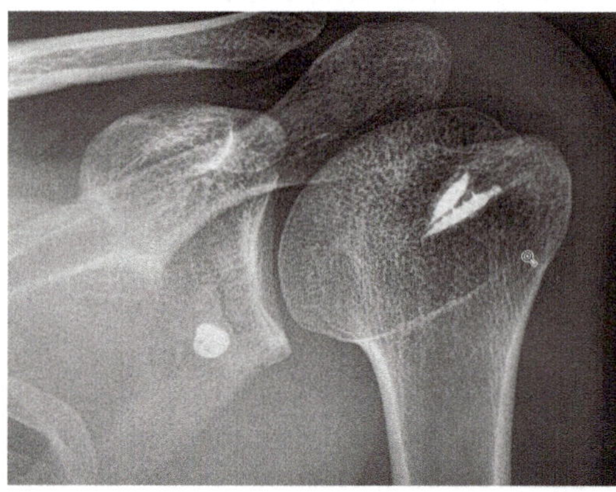

Fig. 30.3 Radiograph of the glenoid fracture following fixation and previous rotator cuff repair

- Dislocation of shoulder with glenoid fracture was repaired via an open approach with a single screw (Fig. 30.3), but rather medial, and after returning to competing, his arm jolted and his shoulder dislocated once more (Fig. 30.4).
- Examination in the clinic revealed significant wasting of deltoid with reduced power (Fig. 30.5). Sensation over the regimental badge area was present. There was considerable apprehension in the classic position for assessing glenohumeral instability.

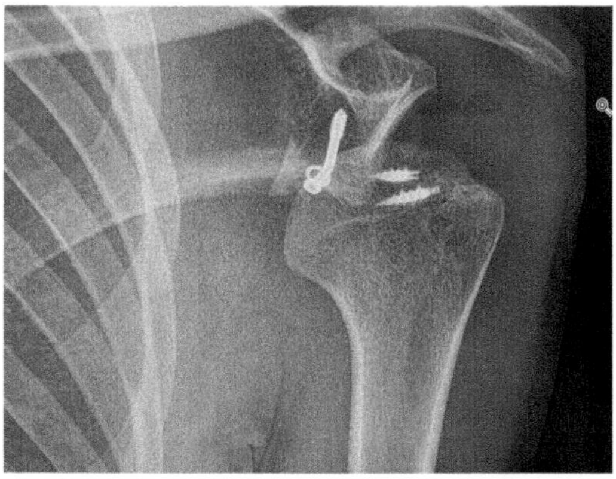

Fig. 30.4 Radiograph showing shoulder dislocation with bent screw from previous glenoid fracture fixation

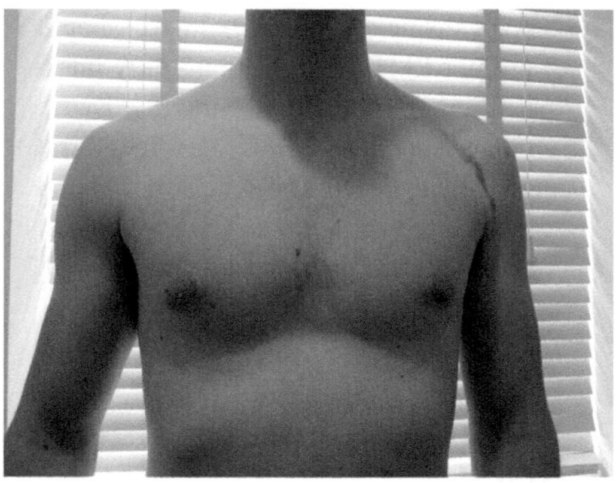

Fig. 30.5 Patient with the deltoid muscle wasting following axillary nerve injury and scar from previous surgery

- Patient JD was hoping to compete at European level the following year and this required a stable shoulder. He had been advised by his previous surgeon that this would require a Latarjet procedure, but this would be risky in terms of the surgery and that a return to motocross was not advisable.
- From our side, he was advised that Latarjet was the procedure of choice, the previous screw would require removal and the bony fragment assessed at the time. He was advised concerning the risks to the musculocutaneous nerve.
- At the time of surgery, the following month an open Latarjet procedure was performed. This was performed under general anaesthetic with an interscalene nerve block. The musculocutaneous nerve was found to have a distal insertion into the conjoined tendon. The coracoid process was harvested and mobilised. Subscapularis was split. The whole area was very scarred. The screw was located and removed. The bony Bankart fracture/repair was un-united and medial. The coracoid transfer was placed with two screws.
- At the 2 week review he was found to have suffered a musculocutaneous nerve palsy. Urgent EMG studies were requested. These were reported as showing that the "functional deficit is disproportionally more than the neurophysiological abnormality found on the EMGs, suggesting this lesion is predominantly neuropraxic with very little axonal loss. The nerve is in anatomical continuity and he should improve, over a period of time."
- At the 3 months review, good biceps contraction had been restored although sensation in the forearm was still to fully return.
- This case illustrates the risk of nerve injury associated with shoulder dislocation. JD first dislocated his shoulder aged nine and suffered an injury to the axillary nerve. Although such an injury is highly unusual it was not managed according to the recommendations detailed in this chapter. Urgent nerve exploration is indicated in cases with high energy injury where nerve rupture or severe traction and attenuation is suspected. These are often younger patients with real potential for recovery with reconstruction. Radiological imaging such as ultrasound and MRI may be value in supporting the diagnosis but if there is clinical suspicion of nerve rupture then exploration to assess the nerve is warranted with immediate reconstruction if indicated.
- The opinion of a peripheral nerve surgeon was sought around the time of his second shoulder injury, at 5 years following the initial dislocation. This was such an unusual case that the opinion of surgeons from the USA and UK was sought via the internet on the DocMatter forum. Nerve transfer was not favoured and neurolysis was not thought likely to be beneficial. It was simply too late following the initial injury.

- A second nerve injury was sustained during surgery. This was detected early and an appropriated investigation was requested. This demonstrated that the nerve was in continuity and predominantly a neuropraxic injury with the expectation of recovery.

Pearls and Pitfalls
- A high index of suspicion of a nerve injury associated with shoulder dislocation is required in each patient.
- Sensation in the classic regimental badge area is not a fully reliable guide to the presence of an axillary nerve injury.
- Which injury may recover and which may not is unreliable at an early stage.
- Urgent nerve exploration is indicated in cases with high energy injury where nerve rupture or severe traction and attenuation is suspected.
- Delay in surgery for repair or grafting beyond 6 months leads to a poorer outcome.

30.6 Outcomes

- The best results are undoubtedly with early intervention.
- There is a trend towards better outcomes with intervention before 4 to 6 months following injury [4, 13, 14].
- Significantly poorer results are caused by a delay of 9–12 months [15, 16].
- A number of risk factors for poor outcome following surgical intervention (Table 30.2).

Table 30.2 Risk factors for poor outcome following nerve injury and surgical intervention

Delay in intervention of 9–12 months
Poorer outcome over the age of 30, even worse over 50 [15, 16]
High BMI [15]
Associated tears of the rotator cuff [16]
Neurolysis alone gives a better outcome, although this is related to the severity of the injury.
Graft length may be worse with nerve grafts, although this is unclear [8].

Take-Home Message
- The incidence of nerve injury with glenohumeral dislocation is high when EMG studies are used to confirm the pathology.
- The majority of injuries occur to the axillary nerve, although pan plexus injuries do occur.
- A number of risk factors for severity of injury have been recognised, and the presence of one or more of these should prompt a more vigorous examination.
- Loss of sensation over the regimental badge area can be present with a significant axillary nerve injury.
- Any suspicion of nerve injury should prompt EMG investigation. Early intervention for high grade injury gives a better outcome. Therefore, early referral to a specialist centre with a peripheral nerve surgeon and team gives the best hope for a better outcome for the patient.

References

1. Robinson CM, Shur N, Sharpe T, Ray A, Murray IR. Injuries associated with traumatic anterior glenohumeral dislocations. J Bone Joint Surg Am. 2012;94:18–26.
2. Visser CP, Coene LN, Brand R, Tavy DL. The incidence of nerve injury in anterior dislocation of the shoulder and its influence on functional recovery. A prospective clinical and EMG study. J Bone Joint Surg (Br). 1999;81:679–85.
3. Gutkowska O, Martynkiewicz J, Urban M, et al. Brachial plexus injury after shoulder dislocation: a literature review. Neurosurg Rev. 2020;43:407–23.
4. Wehbe J, Maalouf G, Habanbo J, et al. Surgical treatment of traumatic lesions of the axillary nerve. A retrospective study of 33 cases. Acta Orthop Belg. 2004;70:11–8.
5. Hertel R, Lambert SM, Ballmer FT. The deltoid extension lag sign for diagnosis and grading of axillary nerve palsy. J Shoulder Elb Surg. 1998;7:97–9.
6. Nishijma N, Yamamuro T, Fujio K, Ohba M. The swallow-tail sign: a test of deltoid function. J Bone Joint Surg (Br). 1995;77:152–3.
7. Bertelli JA, Ghizoni MF. Abduction in internal rotation: a test for the diagnosis of axillary nerve palsy. J Hand Surg [Am]. 2011;36:2017–23.

8. Avis D, Power D. Axillary nerve injury associated with glenohumeral joint dislocation. A review and algorithm for management. EFORT Open Rev. 2018;3:70–7.
9. Bentolila V, Nizard R, Bizot P, Sedel L. Complete traumatic brachial plexus palsy. Treatment and outcome after repair. J Bone Joint Surg Am. 1999;81(1):20–8.
10. Gupta R, Chan JP, Uong J, Palipsis WA, Wright DJ, Shah SB, Ward SR, Lee TQ, Steward O. Human motor endplate remodelling after traumatic nerve injury. J Neurosurg. 2020;
11. Leechavengvongs S, Witoonchart K, Uerpariojkit C, Thuvasethakul. Nerve transfer to deltoid using the nerve to the long head of the triceps, part II: a report of 7 cases. JHSAm. 2003;28(4):633–8.
12. Colbert S, Mackinnon S. Posterior approach for double nerve transfer for restoration of shoulder function in upper brachial plexus palsy. Hand. 2006;1(2):71–7.
13. Mikami Y, Nagano A, Ochiai N, Yamamoto S. Results of nerve grafting for injuries of the axillary and suprascapular nerves. J Bone Joint Surg (Br). 1997;79:527–31.
14. Terzis JK, Kokkalis ZT. Shoulder function following primary axillary nerve reconstruction in obstetrical brachial plexus patients. Plast Reconstr Surg. 2008;122:1457–69.
15. Fu SY, Gordon T. Contributing factors to poor functional recovery after delayed nerve repair: prolonged denervation. J Neurosci. 1995;15:3886–95.
16. Degeorges R, Lebellec Y, Alnot JY. Facteurs pronostiques de la chirurgie du nerf axillaire. Rev Chir Orthop Repar Appar Mot. 2004;90:103–10.

Revision of Soft Tissue Repair Failure

31

Marco-Christopher Rupp, Jonas Pogorzelski, and Andreas B. Imhoff

31.1 Introduction/Background

- Surgical shoulder stabilization has been reported to provide an absolute risk reduction of 80% for recurrence of subsequent episodes of glenohumeral instability.
- Heterogenous rates of failure after soft tissue repair have been reported between 0% and 60% [12], with an average rate of 13% when pooling contemporary high-quality trials [7].
- Reasons for the incidence of recurrent instability after Bankart repair are multifactorial and include patient specific risk behavioral factors, technical inadequacy at index stabilization as well as a variety of anatomical soft-tissue mediated as well as bone mediated glenoidal and humeral risk factors.
- In the presence of a substantial symptomatic burden at the individual level and to mitigate the secondary risk of subsequent instability arthropathy, proactive management is indicated for recurrent instability in the situation of soft tissue repair failure.
- While lacking a gold standard in the literature, a differentiated approach in diagnosis and surgical management is suggested to reproduce the encouraging results reported in the literature.

31.2 Relevant Physical Findings

- Patient history: Essential to differentiate patient specific risk factors associated with the failure of soft tissue repair and should focus on the following aspects:
  - Type of primary instability: direction of dislocation, type and mechanism of event at onset of instability, number of previous dislocations, potential concomitant muscular disbalances or generalized joint hyperlaxity.
  - Onset of recurrence: differentiation of the adequacy of the mechanism leading to the onset of recurrent instability.
  - Type and severity recurrence of instability: differentiation between subluxation or dislocation, onset of symptoms already during activities of daily life, sleep or in midrange motion, potentially indicating severe instability.
  - Demographic risk factors: Age < 20 years [25] and male sex [17].

Supplementary Information The online version contains supplementary material available at https://doi.org/10.1007/978-3-662-73064-5_31.

M.-C. Rupp · J. Pogorzelski · A. B. Imhoff (✉)
Department of Orthopaedic Sports Medicine, Technical University of Munich, Munich, Germany
e-mail: marco.rupp@tum.de; jonas.pogorzelski@tum.de; imhoff@tum.de

L. Kovačič et al. (eds.), *Surgical Techniques for Anterior Shoulder Instability*,
https://doi.org/10.1007/978-3-662-73064-5_31

  - Behavioral risk factors: Involvement in contact sports or a heavy physical occupation.
- Physical examination: essential to assess the type, direction and severity of instability as well additional risk factors and concomitant pathologies in the situation of soft tissue failure and should focus on:
  - Instability tests: critical to determine direction (uni–/bi–/multidirectional) and severity of instability:
    - Antero-inferior instability: anterior apprehension test (including documentation of abduction and external rotation), relocation release test, anterior load and shift tests (grade 0–3).
    - Posterior instability: Jerk-test, Kim-test, posterior Load and Shift test (grade 0–3).
  - Hyperlaxity: Hyperabduction Test (HAT) according to Gagey, Sulcus sign in internal (IR) and external rotation (ER) (grade 0–2), Beighton score (>3 indicates generalized hyperlaxity) [8], external rotation.
  - An assessment of active stabilizers should be performed to uncover a potential functional component of the instability and concomitant glenohumeral injuries such as an long head of the biceps (LHB) pathology or rotator cuff injury or affection of the axillary nerve should be excluded.
- Surgical history: to determine technical risk factors potentially associated with failure of soft tissue repair, a review of surgical documents relevant for the index shoulder stabilization should include available preoperative imaging, surgical reports and possibly arthroscopic footage:
  - Imaging prior to index stabilization: should be assessed to exclude any risk factors such as glenoid bone loss, prevalence of a special labral tear configuration (anterior labroligamentous periosteal sleeve avulsion (APLSA)/humeral avulsion glenohumeral ligament (HAGL)/superior labrum anterior posterior (SLAP)/glenolabral articular disruption (GLAD)/Perthes lesion), increased capsular volume indicative of joint hyperlaxity or a dysplastic labrum, that were potentially overlooked at index surgery.
  - Soft tissue fixation material: determination of number, type and positioning of anchors inserted at index stabilization, clarification if a sufficient capsular plication was performed.
  - Compliance in rehabilitation after index stabilization.

31.3 Relevant Imaging

- An X-ray in three planes should be routinely performed to assess for potential static dislocation, bony Bankart lesions, fractures of the tubercle or inferior subluxation of the humeral head indicative of axillary nerve damage.
- A computed tomography (CT) is the gold standard to assess for bone-mediated risk factors for instability.
  - Various methods employing 2D or 3D reconstructions and digital subtraction of the humeral head have been proposed to assess for anteroinferior glenoid bone loss (GLB). In the setting of a failed Bankart repair, conservative thresholds ranging around 15% as suggested in the current literature should guide decision making, rather than historically propagated thresholds of 20% [22].
  - In the setting of a bipolar defect, composed of GLB and a Hill-Sachs lesion (HSL), the glenoid track (GT) concept has proven its validity in risk stratification. [GT = 0.84D (diameter anteroinferior glenoid)—d (GLB); HSI (Hill Sachs interval) = HS (width of the HSL) + BB (bone bridge between lateral margin of the HSL and the insertion of the infraspinatus muscle)]. In case of an HSI greater than the GT, an “off-track” situation requires a bone-based reconstruction or more complex arthroscopic adjunct procedures.
  - The glenoidal positioning of the anchors can be appreciated, both sagittal in their positioning on the glenoid clockface, as

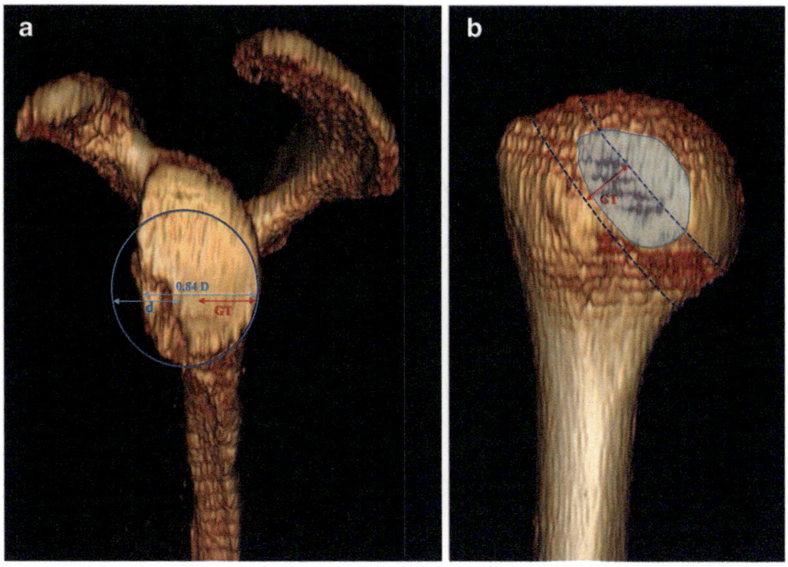

Fig. 31.1 The three-dimensionally reconstructed computed tomography of a patient with a bipolar bone loss defect illustrating the glenoid track concept; (**a**) a glenoid with a bony defect and (**b**) a humeral head with a Hill-Sachs lesion. D diameter of the anteroinferior glenoid, d glenoid bone loss defect, GT glenoid track: 0.84D—d

well as axial concerning the insertion angle. If not positioned 1–2 mm onto the glenoid surface, there is a risk of having created a functional ALPSA lesion [26].

- In magnetic resonance (MRI)-imaging, additional information relevant for the subsequent surgical stabilization can be extracted. An emphasis should be placed in the detection of labral avulsions, GLAD-lesions potentially affecting glenoid concavity, ALPSA/Perthes/HAGL lesions and a disruption of the labral continuity, labral hypoplasia, an increased capsular volume and further concomitant injuries such as LHB-pathologies, rotator cuff tears and cartilage defects (Fig. 31.1).

31.4 Treatment Options and Indications

- While in general treatment options at revision are comparable to techniques at primary stabilization, there remains substantial debate on the correct parameters warranting the respective indication in the setting of a soft tissue repair failure.
- Conservative treatment is of limited clinical relevance in the setting of a failed soft-tissue repair. It is reserved for patients older than 40 years with a low symptomatic burden, progressive glenohumeral instability arthropathy or patients with habitual instability associated to connective tissue disorders or functional shoulder instability. Individualized conservative regimens are aimed at mitigating the subjective symptomatic burden.
- Surgical decision making when addressing recurrent instability in the setting of a failed soft-tissue repair is guided by the patient-specific risk profile, with the portfolio including basic and adjunct soft-tissue based procedures or bone based augmentation (Fig. 31.2).
- Soft-tissue based procedures
  - Arthroscopic revision soft tissue stabilization for anteroinferior shoulder instability should include a minimum of three anchors at the 3:00, 4:30 and 5:30 position (right shoulder) in simple stitch configuration, inserted at an angle of 135° to the glenoid surface, performed with a concomitant capsular shift resulting in a bumper effect, providing additional glenohumeral stability [13].
  - In the setting of hyperlaxity with an increased capsular redundancy, a postero-inferior anchor should be introduced to reduce the capsular volume, while restor-

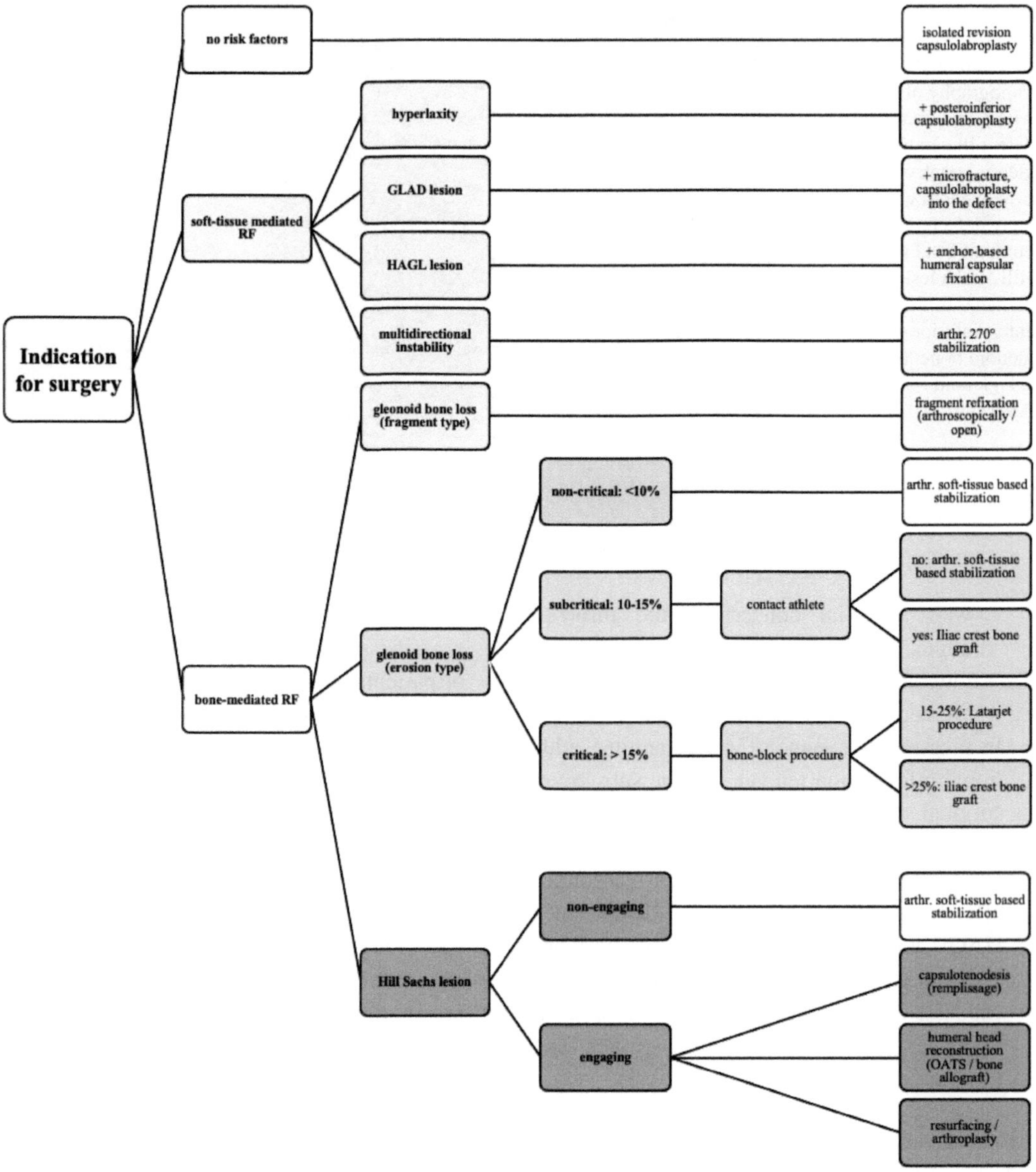

Fig. 31.2 Recommended decision making algorithm for revision surgical management in the setting of a soft tissue repair failure

ing physiological glenohumeral biomechanics [20].

– A concomitant remplissage procedure, which is mainly a capsulotenodesis of the infraspinatus tendon into the HSL to avoid engagement with the GLB area, may be evaluated in the setting of an off-track HSL with moderate GLB (bone loss pathology is predominantly humeral-sided) or in case the surgeon prefers not to penetrate subscapularis muscle with a non-anatomic bone block procedure.

– In the setting of multidirectional instability, an arthroscopic 270° stabilization (including 6–8 anchors inserted from 2 to 10 o'clock on the glenoid clockface of a right

shoulder) should be considered to comprehensively treat multidirectional pathology [14].
  - Special labral, chondral and capsular lesion configurations should be addressed adequately, with a special reference to GLAD-lesions affecting glenoid concavity, that can be addressed via a microfracture of the glenoid defect and a subsequent capsulolabroplasty into the defect [18] and HAGL lesions, the can be engaged via anchor-based refixation [3].
- Bone based procedures:
  - In the setting of a fragment-type glenoid bone loss/anterior glenoid rim fracture, after arthroscopic Bankart repair [16], a variety of options for fragment refixation are at the disposal of the surgeon. Arthroscopic procedure include anchor-based Bankart-bridge-like approaches [23] or combined arthroscopic labral repair and screw-based refixation techniques [24], with open reduction and screw-based refixation techniques being an option in more complex cases.
  - A bone-block transfer is indicated in a critical GLB of >15% to restore passive glenoid-mediated bony stabilization, with a variety of arthroscopic or open anatomical or non-anatomical surgical options available to the surgeon.
    - The non-anatomic coracoid transfer as described by Latarjet combines the advantages of glenoid reconstruction and the dynamical sling effect by the conjoint tendons in the vulnerable ABER position. Various technical options regarding the approach (open or arthroscopic) and bone block orientation (original technique or congruent arch), bone block placement (intra- or extraarticular) or capsular fixation have been described [11].
    - Autograft-based anatomic techniques such as modified Eden-Hybinette procedures employing iliac crest autografts have a relevance in larger degrees of GLB. In the recent literature, arthroscopic techniques relying on high tensile suture tape cerclage for bone block fixation are increasingly published in an attempt to avoid secondary screw protrusion after bone block resorption [10].
    - In attempt to reduce donor site morbidity, present experimental studies investigate the use bone allografts, most notably distal tibial osteochondral grafts, with non-inferiority trials and long term data on complications as well as investigations on bone union and potential upsides still pending [19].
  - In the presence of a substantial Hill-Sachs lesion not sufficiently adressable via a remplissage procedure, a posterolateral humeral head reconstruction is warranted:
    - Techniques of this bone-based augmentation include employment an iliac crest autograft or humeral head/femoral allograft, either harvested with an osteochondral autograft instrument or in block-shape, either introduced in a press-fit combination or via screw-fixation to restore native humeral morphology.
    - Focal humeral head resurfacing or hemiarthroplasty remain surgical options for the salvage situation.

31.5 Decision-Making Algorithm

31.5.1 Clinical Case

- Patient History
  - 29 year old male, previously involved in contact sports (judo), sedentary occupation, compliant to doctor's advice.
  - Index instability: 20 ant.inf. dislocations after judo-related index accident (adequate trauma mechanism).
  - Arthroscopic anteroinferior soft tissue stabilization at another institution 3 years ago: seven recurrent shoulder dislocations (inadequate trauma mechanisms), cessation of contact sport activity and impair-

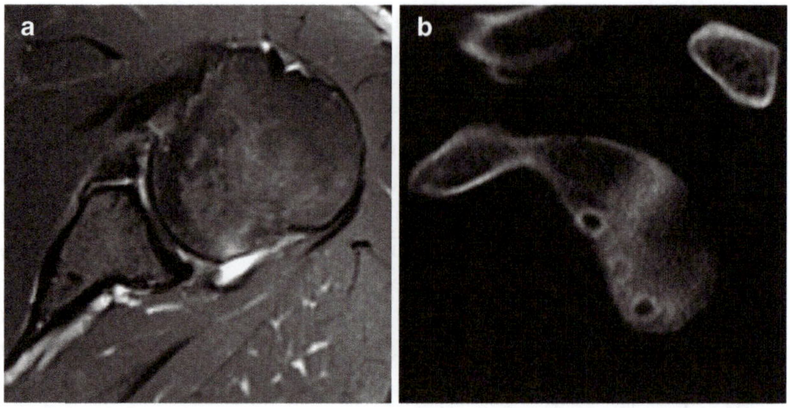

Fig. 31.3 Preoperative imaging including (**a**) magnetic resonance imaging showing an anteroinferior Bankart lesion with signs of erosive anteroinferior glenoid bone loss (GLB) and (**b**) computed tomography showing an anteroinferior GLB of 19% with anchors of index soft tissue stabilization in a slightly cranial position

ment in activities of daily life due to subjective instability at midrange ROM.

- Physical Examination
  - Instability tests:
    - Antero-inferior instability: Anterior apprehension test + (ABD45°, ER45°), relocation release test +, anterior load and shift test + (III°)
    - Posterior instability: Jerk-test -, Kim-test -, posterior Load and Shift test—(0°).
  - Hyperlaxity: HAT Gagey + (120°), Sulcus sign IR+ (I°)/ER + (I°), Beighton score 2, ER 90°.
- Surgical Documentation:
  - Imaging prior to index stabilization: MRI showing an ant.inf. Bankart lesion, no special labral tear configuration (APLSA/HAGL/SLAP/GLAD/Perthes), suspicious of erosive ant.inf. GLB; no CT to assess GLB was performed.
  - Fixation material: 3 ant.-inf. suture anchors, slightly cranial position.
- Preoperative Imaging (Fig. 31.3)
  - MRI: anteroinferior Bankart lesion, suspicious of erosive ant.inf. GLB, mildly enlarge capsule.
  - CT: 19% GLB, no bony Bankart lesion, non-engaging small post.sup. HSL.
- Surgical treatment:
  - Bone-based glenoid augmentation: Coracoid transfer according to Latarjet (Fig. 31.4)

Pearls and Pitfalls

- The physical examination (direction of instability, isolated or generalized hyperlaxity) is the key in the detection of soft-tissue based risk factors.
- The preoperative imaging (GLB, on/off-track HSL) is key in the detection of bone based risk factors.
- The patient history (functional demand, adequateness of trauma leading to recurrence of instability, severity of instability) can provide important information for decision making in borderline situations.

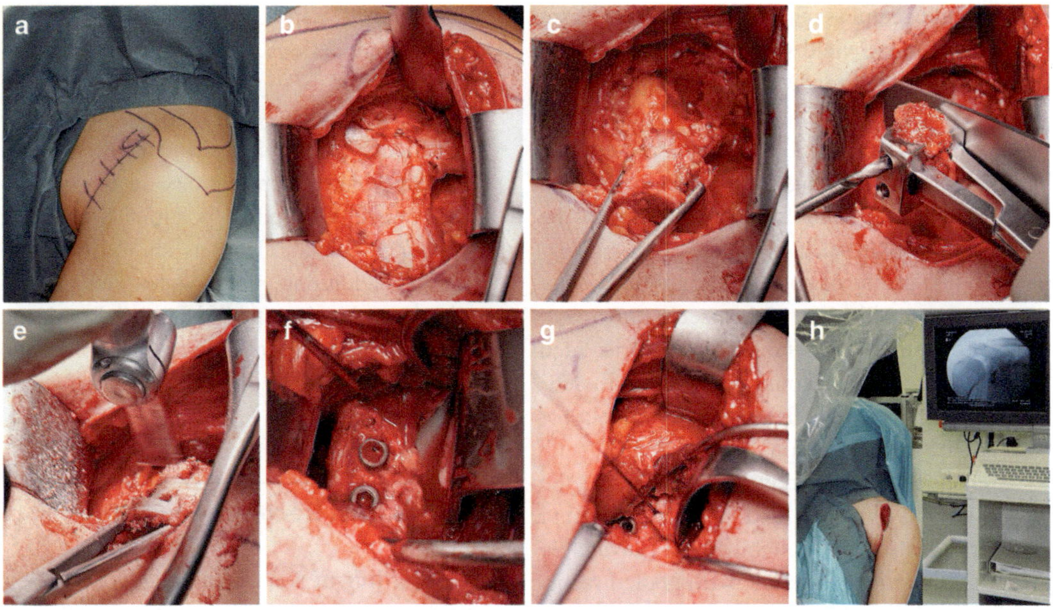

Fig. 31.4 (**a**) Placement in beach chair position with the arm draped free to allow abduction and external rotation, with landmarks annotated (acromion, clavicle, coracoid, limited deltopectoral approach); (**b**) coracoid preparation; (**c**) harvested 3-cm coracoid graft; (**d**) screw hole preparation with a 4 mm drill employing a coracoid drill guide; (**e**) decortication of inferior cortical surface with an oscillating saw; (**f**) coracoid fixation with 2× 3.75 mm cannulated screws; (**g**) capsular repair; (**h**) intraoperative radiographic control

31.6 Outcomes

- Results of revision soft tissue stabilization rates are heterogenous due to confounding by inconsistent documentation of preoperative glenoidal and humeral bone loss, hyperlaxity and concomitant procedures. With failure rates following revision soft tissue stabilization in the literature ranging between 0% and 26% [1, 21], a contemporary meta-analysis observed a recurrence rate of 15–16% [12, 27]. In terms of clinical outcomes scores, a clear postoperative improvement was observed (pre- vs. postoperatively: Rowe score: 69.9 vs. 85.3; Simple Shoulder Test: 7.1 vs. 10.3) [27]. Soft tissue stabilization as a revision procedure has been found to be valid especially valid in the setting of an adequate trauma prior to recurrency of instability, limited functional demand, non-critical bone loss, presence of arthroscopically treatable adjunct risk factors or verifiable technical errors at index procedure. However, patients expectations should be managed adequately, as patient reported outcomes tend to be inferior to primary stabilization [12].
- There is a paucity of outcome data of adjunct arthroscopic procedures in the revision setting and there exists substantial confounding by the presence of risk factors and combination of different procedures.
  - Techniques including rotator interval closure in the majority of the patients at revision are reported to achieve comparable outcome to arthroscopic revision Bankart repair, with failure rates ranging around 17% and score improvement (pre- vs. postoperatively: SST, 6 vs. 10) [6], however with associated loss of external rotation [5].

  - While remplissage procedures were demonstrated to yield satisfactory outcomes in the setting of moderate GLB and an engaging HSL after primary stabilization, failure rates in the revision setting are considerably higher (primary vs revision: 0% vs. 36%) [15] and should thus only be employed in selected patients.
  - While results of posteroinferior plication at index stabilization with success rates seem promising [4], no data on isolated arthroscopic concomitant plication the eligible hyperlax collective are available for revision stabilization.
- Among bone-based revision techniques, the most solid evidence in the revision setting after failed soft tissue stabilization is available for the Latarjet procedure, with pooled recurrent instability of 3.8% (0–16%) and improvement of clinical scores, as of a contemporary meta-analysis. In a comparative study using 25% GLB as the threshold relevant for decision making, the Latarjet as a revision procedure (GLB > 25%) has lower failure rates than revision Bankart repair (GLB < 25%) with 7.1% vs. 19% [9]. However, with a pooled rate of 12,3%, there is a considerable rate of adverse events, including delayed wound healing, infections, frozen shoulder, coracoid malunion and nonunion, and graft fragmentation. RTS seems to be inferior following the Latarjet procedure compared to arthroscopic soft tissue revision stabilization [2].
- According to the limited evidence for free bone blocks from the iliac crest or distal tibia in the revision setting, the weighted mean recurrent instability rate is 20.8% at a mean follow-up of 51 months [12]. Originating from case series reporting on complex scenarios describing salvage procedures, these results should however be interpreted with caution.

31.7 Potential Complications/Difficulties

- In borderline indications (20–25 year male with a GLB of 10–15%, mild hyperlaxity with a failure after soft tissue repair in an adequate technique) decision making is complex and the different options as well as associated outcomes should be openly discussed with the patient.
- In patients with high-demand labor or competitive athletes, expectations on the postoperative results including potential lifestyle or sport-specific modifications should be managed and additional prerequisites such as optimization of active stabilizers, full ROM and sport-specific training should be conducted prior to return to preoperative levels of sports or work.

31.8 Expert Recommendation

- In the setting of non-critical bone loss, a technical reason for failure of soft-tissue stabilization and the absence of concomitant risk factors, we recommend revision arthroscopic soft tissue stabilization.
- In the setting of non-critical bone loss and concomitant hyperlaxity, we recommend performing and revision arthroscopic soft tissue stabilization augmented with posteroinferior capsular plication.
- In the setting GLB > 15% after failed soft tissue stabilization, we recommend a bone based procedure such as the coracoid transfer according to Latarjet.
- In borderline situations (patient age 20–30, GLB 10–15%, mild hyperlaxity) we recommend to hinge decision making on the functional demand of the patient.

Take-Home Message

- The incidence of a failure after index soft tissue stabilization ranges around 13%.
- In the revision situation, emphasis should be put on evaluating the adequacy of the event leading to the failure of soft tissue stabilization with respect to the technical features of index stabilization and compliance during rehabilitation.

(continued)

- A thorough risk factor analysis—including lifestyle mediated, soft-tissue mediated and bone mediated risk factors—is the foundation of selecting the most adequate procedure for the individual patient.
- Surgical options in the revision situation include arthroscopic revision soft tissue stabilization with a portfolio of soft-tissue based (posteroinferior capsular plication), humeral sided arthroscopic (remplissage/McLaughlin, HAGL-repair) and open bone-based (Latarjet, iliac crest autograft, posterolateral humeral head reconstruction) procedures to adequately address the individual risk factors of the patients.
- In borderline situations, the indication for adjunct and bone based procedures is to be evaluated proactively.

References

1. Balazs LGC, Donohue MMA, Brelin CM, et al. Outcomes of revision arthroscopic anterior shoulder stabilization in a military population: a prospective cohort study. J Surg Orthop Adv. 2019;28:189–95.
2. Blonna D, Bellato E, Caranzano F, et al. Arthroscopic Bankart repair versus open Bristow-Latarjet for shoulder instability: a matched-pair multicenter study focused on return to sport. Am J Sports Med. 2016;44:3198–205.
3. Bozzo A, Oitment C, Thornley P, et al. Humeral avulsion of the Glenohumeral ligament: indications for surgical treatment and outcomes-a systematic review. Orthop J Sports Med. 2017;5:2325967117723329.
4. Chiang ER, Wang JP, Wang ST, et al. Arthroscopic posteroinferior capsular plication and rotator interval closure after Bankart repair in patients with traumatic anterior glenohumeral instability—a minimum follow-up of 5 years. Injury. 2010;41:1075–8.
5. Coughlin RP, Bullock GS, Shanmugaraj A, et al. Outcomes after arthroscopic rotator interval closure for shoulder instability: a systematic review. Arthroscopy. 2018;34:3098–3108.e3091.
6. Creighton RA, Romeo AA, Brown FM Jr, et al. Revision arthroscopic shoulder instability repair. Arthroscopy. 2007;23:703–9.
7. Defroda S, Bokshan S, Stern E, et al. Arthroscopic Bankart repair for the management of anterior shoulder instability: indications and outcomes. Curr Rev Musculoskelet Med. 2017;10:442–51.
8. Dvse. Untersuchungstechniken des Schultergelenks. Obere Extremität. 2012;7:1–67.
9. Frank RM, Mellano C, Shin JJ, et al. Clinical outcomes following revision anterior shoulder stabilization: arthroscopic revision stabilization versus Latarjet. Orthop J Sports Med. 2015;3:2325967115S2325900048.
10. Hachem AI, Del Carmen M, Verdalet I, et al. Arthroscopic bone block Cerclage: a fixation method for glenoid bone loss reconstruction without metal implants. Arthrosc Tech. 2019;8:e1591–7.
11. Hurley ET, Lim Fat D, Farrington SK, et al. Open versus arthroscopic Latarjet procedure for anterior shoulder instability: a systematic review and meta-analysis. Am J Sports Med. 2019;47:1248–53.
12. Lau BC, Johnston TR, Gregory BP, et al. Outcomes after revision anterior shoulder stabilization: a systematic review. Orthop J Sports Med. 2020;8:2325967120922571.
13. Lee SJ, Kim JH, Gwak HC, et al. Influence of glenoid labral bumper height and capsular volume on clinical outcomes after arthroscopic Bankart repair as assessed with serial CT arthrogram: can anterior-inferior volume fraction be a prognostic factor? Am J Sports Med. 2020;48:1846–56.
14. Mazzocca AD, Cote MP, Solovyova O, et al. Traumatic shoulder instability involving anterior, inferior, and posterior labral injury: a prospective clinical evaluation of arthroscopic repair of 270° labral tears. Am J Sports Med. 2011;39:1687–96.
15. Mccabe MP, Weinberg D, Field LD, et al. Primary versus revision arthroscopic reconstruction with remplissage for shoulder instability with moderate bone loss. Arthroscopy. 2014;30:444–50.
16. Nakagawa S, Hirose T, Tachibana Y, et al. Postoperative recurrence of instability due to new anterior glenoid rim fractures after arthroscopic Bankart repair. Am J Sports Med. 2017;45:2840–8.
17. Porcellini G, Campi F, Pegreffi F, et al. Predisposing factors for recurrent shoulder dislocation after arthroscopic treatment. J Bone Joint Surg Am. 2009;91:2537–42.
18. Porcellini G, Cecere AB, Giorgini A, et al. The GLAD lesion: are the definition, diagnosis and treatment up to date? a systematic review. Acta Biomed. 2020;91:e2020020.
19. Provencher MT, Peebles LA, Aman ZS, et al. Management of the Failed Latarjet procedure: outcomes of revision surgery with fresh distal Tibial allograft. Am J Sports Med. 2019;47:2795–802.
20. Rupp M-C, Siebenlist S, Scheiderer B, et al. Indication and technique for arthroscopic stabilization of anterior shoulder instability with multidirectional laxity. Obere Extremität. 2021;16:41–50.
21. Ryu RK, Ryu JH. Arthroscopic revision Bankart repair: a preliminary evaluation. Orthopedics. 2011;34:17.

22. Shin SJ, Koh YW, Bui C, et al. What is the critical value of glenoid bone loss at which soft tissue Bankart repair does not restore glenohumeral translation, restricts range of motion, and leads to abnormal humeral head position? Am J Sports Med. 2016;44:2784–91.
23. Sugaya H, Kon Y, Tsuchiya A. Arthroscopic repair of glenoid fractures using suture anchors. Arthroscopy. 2005;21:635.
24. Voleti PB, Camp CL, Sinatro AL, et al. Arthroscopic fixation of glenoid rim fractures after reduction by labral repair. Arthrosc Tech. 2016;5:e379–83.
25. Wasserstein D, Dwyer T, Veillette C, et al. Predictors of dislocation and revision after shoulder stabilization in Ontario, Canada, from 2003 to 2008. Am J Sports Med. 2013;41:2034–40.
26. Wiater JM, Vibert BT. Glenohumeral joint volume reduction with progressive release and shifting of the inferior shoulder capsule. J Shoulder Elb Surg. 2007;16:810–4.
27. Yon CJ, Cho CH, Kim DH. Revision arthroscopic Bankart repair: a systematic review of clinical outcomes. J Clin Med. 2020;9

Revision of Bony Reconstruction Failure

32

Juan Aguilar-Gonzalez and Emilio Calvo

Key Points

- Cause of previous bony reconstruction failure determines the appropriate revision treatment strategy.
- Bone block techniques, as well as soft tissue procedures such as remplissage and Extraarticular Capsular Reinforcement (ECR) are different available options for revision treatment.
- Coracoid graft status and Glenoid Track classification are key points when deciding the best revision technique.
- Computerized Tomography Scan is essential for preoperative decision and surgical planning.
- Physical examination must always rule out previous surgery neurological injury.
- Arthroscopic revision for bony reconstruction failure is a complex and challenging procedure due to the absence of regular anatomic structures together with the risk of severe nerve injury when working in the "out of the box" anterior space.
- Axillary and musculocutaneous nerve integrity is specially threatened and it is essential to know the exact anatomical relationships of the area.

Supplementary Information The online version contains supplementary material available at https://doi.org/10.1007/978-3-662-73064-5_32.

J. Aguilar-Gonzalez · E. Calvo (✉)
Hospital Universitario Fundación Jiménez Díaz, Madrid, Spain
e-mail: ecalvo@fjd.es

32.1 Introduction/Background

- The Latarjet procedure is a reliable and safe technique for the management of anterior shoulder instability, particularly in cases with significant bone loss, thanks to its triple blocking effect [1].
- However, Latarjet is not devoid of complications or failure. Complications such as mobilization or breakage of the screws, glenohumeral osteoarthritis, bone block resorption, restricted range of movement, infections, and neurological or vascular lesions, in addition to recurrent postoperative instability have been described [2–4].
- Latarjet failure is a term that specifically describes postoperative recurrence of instability, defined as subluxation or dislocation. Isolated positive apprehension sign is usually not considered as clinical failure if the shoulder is otherwise stable and does not interfere with daily activities.
- Range of motion (ROM) restriction or pain interfering with daily living or sports activities

L. Kovačič et al. (eds.), *Surgical Techniques for Anterior Shoulder Instability*,
https://doi.org/10.1007/978-3-662-73064-5_32

are also complications of Latarjet; however, those are not considered as failure.

- Since Latarjet is a non-anatomic technique, subsequent revision surgery can be seriously compromised not only by scar tissue obscuring normal tissue planes, but also by alterations of anatomic stabilizing structures. Furthermore, the number of published studies reporting the results of revision surgery after failed shoulder stabilization using the Latarjet technique is very scant [5–9].
- An algorithm to approach this challenging situation; based on the causes of failure and the type of lesions and anatomic findings can be a very valuable tool when planning revision surgery (Fig. 32.1).

32.2 Relevant Physical Findings

- The physical examination must include a 360° visual evaluation for muscle atrophy and scapular dyskinesia. Visual inspection of the skin looking for scars is also helpful for obtaining information about potential previous surgery modality.
- Neurovascular detailed examination is mandatory, with specifically assessment of the musculocutaneous and axillary nerves. Any suspicion of nerve injury justifies requesting electromyographic studies.
- An evaluation of passive and active ROM of the affected and unaffected shoulders is required.
- Shoulder hyperlaxity or undiagnosed multidirectional or posterior instability should be ruled out performing specific provocative maneuvers for shoulder instability.
- Any loss in ROM or pain within it should be noted, as coracoid graft osteolysis may lead to screw prominence causing interference with the normal gleno-humeral tracking compromising humeral head articular surface.

32.3 Relevant Imaging

- Anterior-posterior and scapular Y simple x-ray views are usually recommended, but computed tomography (CT) scan is the best imaging study after Latarjet procedure.
- CT scan is recommended at least at 6 months postoperatively after primary surgery in order to evaluate bone healing, graft position and presence of osteoarthritis.
- CT scan is mandatory in the planning of any revision of bony reconstruction failure as it is the best study to evaluate union, positioning, bone loss, osteolysis and graft viability.
- Glenoid Track (GT) classification measures should be performed preferably in CT scan or magnetic resonance arthrogram (MRA) in order to classify cases as on-track or off-track.

32.4 Treatment Options and Indications

- *Bone-Block Procedures*
  - Iliac crest bone graft (ICBG) has been traditionally regarded as the procedure of choice in patients with a failed Latarjet, but other options can be considered depending on the specific anatomic abnormalities.
  - ICBG is indicated in shoulders with off-track Hill Sachs (HS) lesion without a viable coracoid graft due to osteolysis.
  - There are different open and arthroscopic variations of bone block procedures:
    - Arthroscopic Eden Hybinette.
      - Preferred author's technique (Video 32.1)
      - Tricortical iliac crest autograft is commonly used.
      - Different arthroscopic techniques have been recently described [8–10] using different fixation devices such as cortical suture buttons.
    - Alternatively, distal tibia allograft can be reliably used for anterior bone block as previous studies have demonstrated favorable outcomes [11]. The use of distal clavicle autograft is promising but long clinical follow-up outcomes haven't been reported yet [12].
- *Coracoid Graft Repositioning*
  - Indicated in off-track HS with a viable but poorly positioned or avulsed bone graft.
  - The conjoin tendon insertion must be preserved without signs of osteolysis.

- The operative technique consists in bone graft dissection and repositioning on the anteroinferior glenoid rim. Osteotomy may be needed for repositioning the graft in case of poor position due to mal-union.

- Remplissage:
  - Indicated in off-track HS spite a correctly positioned and healed bone graft.
- Extraarticular capsular reinforcement (ECR) with isquiotibialis allograft [13].
  - Indicated in on-track HS with well positioned and healed bone graft, but with poor soft tissue quality. Very uncommon scenario, usually severe hiperlax patients in whom Latarjet is unable to restore stability (i.e., Eheler-Danlos).
  - Hyperlax patients show great range of horizontal extension that decreases the width of the glenoid track. Thus, in this subtype of patients, some authors believe that GT width is under the usual 83% and it should be adjusted by the range of horizontal extension. Using the adjusted GT width formula [14], these cases may actually be classified as off-track; however, ECR is the preferred technique instead of remplissage when hyperlaxity is present.
- Salvage procedures and nonoperative treatment:
  - Salvage procedures include shoulder arthroplasty and shoulder arthrodesis.
    - The indication of these techniques is very rare
    - Shoulder arthroplasty is reserved for old patients with severe osteoarthritis (OA)
    - Arthrodesis is usually reserved for cases with severe permanent brachial plexus injuries that compromise outcomes of other techniques.
  - Nonoperative treatment consists of initial immobilization rest period followed by an increasing muscle-strength conditioning and proprioceptive education to enhance dynamic stability.
    - It is an option when the patient does not consider undergoing additional surgical intervention.
    - The patient should be aware of the risk of recurrence of instability, development of arthropathy, and be willing to accept a modification of upper-limb-dependent physical activity.
    - There is some evidence that supports nonoperative treatment after failed Latarjet [15, 16].

32.5 Decision-Making Algorithm (Fig. 32.1)

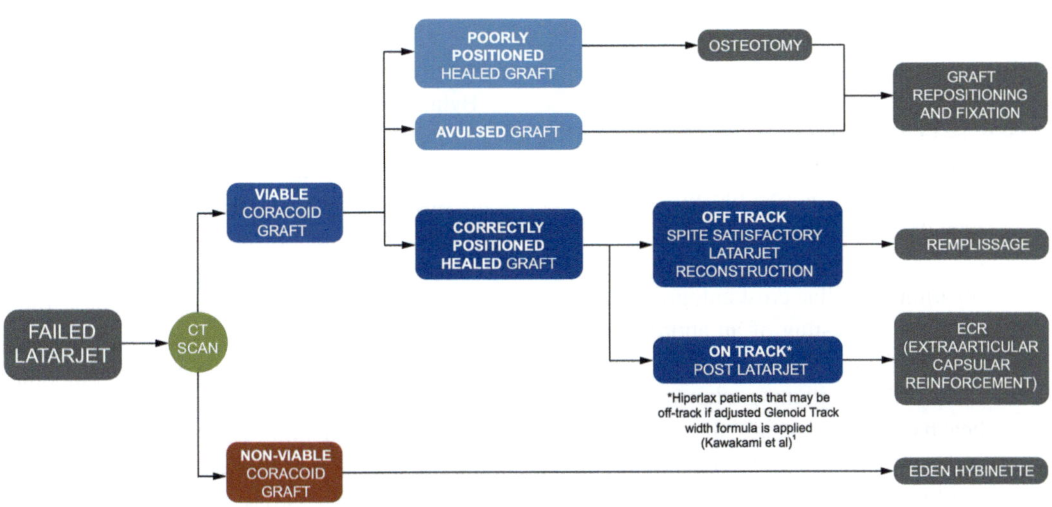

Fig. 32.1 Decision-making Algorithm [14]

32.6 Clinical Case/Example/ Preferred Treatment Option

- Twenty-nine-year-old healthy male.
  - Work: Plumber. Overhead activity.
  - Sports: Snowboard, motocross.
- Latarjet 6 months postoperative failure.
- Instability, painful and restricted range of motion.
- Physical examination (Video 32.1)
  - ROM: forward flexion (FF) 135°; external rotation (ER) 30° in abduction and adduction of the arm; internal rotation (IR) to the third lumbar vertebra (L3).
  - Passive and painful limitation of ROM.
  - Contralateral non-affected shoulder ROM: FF 180°; ER 90°; IR to interscapular space.
  - No muscular atrophies and normal neurovascular examination
  - No hyperlaxity
- Imaging studies:
  - CT scan (Video 32.1)
    - Non-viable coracoid graft
    - Bone osteolysis and resorption
    - Prominent screws
- Preferred Treatment Option:
  - Arthroscopic Eden Hybinette (Boxes 32.1 and 32.2)
  - Procedure is performed as soon as possible as the prominent screws due to bone resorption can damage the humeral head articular surface.

Box 32.1 Pearls in arthroscopic Eden Hybinette technique

- Pearl #1: Use of specific instrumentation designed for arthroscopic Latarjet [17] *(DePuy Synthes, Warsav, In)* when obtaining the iliac crest autograft facilitates the harvesting of an appropriately size and shape graft.
- Pearl #2: Positioning the patient in beach chair position initially with 45° of inclination and draping field both for graft procurement and shoulder arthroscopy permits access to the iliac crest while shortening the duration of the procedure.
- Pearl #3: Previous Latarjet portals can be very useful to serve as landmarks to obtain an orientation in the anterior shoulder space, due to the usual absence of other references.
- Pearl #4 Use of soft tissue blunt dissection instruments such as a Wissinger rod, switching stick, or arthroscopic scissor is safer the shaver or the radiofrequency probe when working in potentially dangerous areas.
- Pearl #5: Define subscapularis split level using a switching stick inserted through the posterior portal. The stick is directed to the tendon parallel to the articular surface. Medial extension of the split is carefully performed from posterior to anterior starting at this point. Medial extension of the split superior to 20 mm might pose the axillary nerve at risk and should be avoided.
- Pearl #6: Ensure that the trans-pectoral "M" portal is wide enough to avoid problems when introducing the graft through the muscle.

Box 32.2 Pitfalls in arthroscopic Eden Hybinette technique

- Pitfall #1: Absence of anatomic landmarks and presence of extensive soft tissue fibrosis obscure the identification of the brachial plexus jeopardizing its integrity.
- Pitfall #2: Visualization of the base of the coracoid is often not possible and it should be identified by palpation before starting soft tissue dissection.
- Pitfall #3: Failure to identify the superior border of the subscapularis and mistaking it for fibrous tissue may alter the

choice of the supero-inferior location of the split.
- Pitfall #4: Kirschner wire for primary fixation of the iliac crest graft does frequently coincides with the previous screw hole and needs to be rectified to ensure a good fixation.
- Pitfall #5: Lateral overhanging of the graft is common and should be identified. The use of a burr can help in restoring the articular surface-graft alignment if it is found to be overhanged.
- Pitfall #6: Capsular reconstruction over the graft is often not possible due to the poor soft tissue quality.

32.7 Outcomes

- Literature regarding long-term follow up outcomes after revision for bony reconstruction failure in anterior shoulder instability is very scant. Lunn et al. [5] reported a 18% recurrence rate and 48% of patients with persistent shoulder apprehension after a mean of 6, 8 year-follow-up.
- Arthroscopic revision recurrence instability rate has been reported between 14% and 17% [7–9]. This data should be carefully interpreted as it comes from studies that consist in small case series (seven, eighteen and twelve patients respectively).
- Similar to what happens in other revision scenarios, poorer clinical outcomes and a higher rate of complications may be expected compared with primary cases. This hypothesis needs to be confirmed with more future clinical studies.

32.8 Potential Complications/ Difficulties

- Severe nerve injury is the main potential severe complication of the procedure due to the proximity of the brachial plexus. Musculocutaneous and axillary are the most frequently involved nerves but cases of suprascapular nerve injury related to a wrong screw direction has also been reported [4].
- In contrast to primary procedure, identification of nerve structures or even other basic anatomic landmarks is extremely difficult sometimes and it is essential to know the exact anatomical relationships of the area to avoid unexpected iatrogenic injuries.
- Axillary nerve is specially at risk when performing the subscapularis split.
  - Axillary nerve medial distance from the glenoid surface is 19.8 mm [18]; but this distance could change depending on the supero-inferior level of the split and the rotation of the scapula [19].
  - The starting point of the split should be made with reference to the glenoid articular surface (Box 32.1: "Pearl #5")

32.9 Expert Recommendation

- Individualization of the treatment is based in the proposed decision-making algorithm (Fig. 32.1).
- Other soft tissue procedures different from remplissage and ECR, that are based on the anatomical repair of the capsulolabral complex or capsular shift are proposed by some authors when bone graft is preserved and correctly positioned [6, 7, 20, 21]. However, we find those techniques less reproductible and reliable due to the deformed anatomy and potential poor soft tissue quality, consequence of previous failed surgeries.
- Many grafts could be potentially used for the anterior bone block in the setting of a revision (ie. distal clavicle autograft; and distal tibia, glenoid, and femoral/humeral head allograft). Iliac crest autograft provides an excellent biological solution as it is versatile to reconstruct a variety of defects by shaping it to match the anterior glenoid neck surface without a significant morbidity on the donor site.
- Any option within the range of possibilities can be performed arthroscopically if the sur-

geon is sufficiently experienced with the technique. Otherwise, open surgery is preferred due to its complexity and the risk of severe nerve injury.

Take-Home Message

- Treatment for bony reconstruction failure should be individualized taking into account the cause of the failure, the status of the bone graft, the GT classification and the patient functional demands.
- Soft tissue techniques are indicated when a well-positioned and healed graft is unable to maintain shoulder stability. Remplissage or ECR
- Bone block techniques such as Eden-Hybinette are indicated when the previous graft is non-viable. If it is viable, but poorly positioned or avulsed, relocation of the graft is preferred.
- Revision of Latarjet is challenging. Arthroscopic techniques are complex, represent a high risk of severe nerve injury scenario, and require a learning curve and extensive experience in primary arthroscopic bone block procedures. Thus, open approach may be safer depending on surgeon experience.
- A
- Challenging arthroscopic technique. Only for expert shoulder arthroscopists.

Declarations of Interest

Juan Aguilar-Gonzalez

Declarations of interest: None

Emilio Calvo

DePuy, A Johnson & Johnson Company: Paid presenter or speaker; Research support

European Society for Surgery of the Shoulder and Elbow: Board or committee member

International Society of Arthroscopy, Knee Surgery, and Orthopaedic Sports Medicine: Board or committee member

Johnson & Johnson: Paid consultant

Journal of Shoulder and Elbow Surgery: Editorial or governing board

Smith & Nephew: Paid presenter or speaker; Research support

Stryker: Paid presenter or speaker

References

1. Mizuno N, Denard PJ, Raiss P, Melis B, Walch G. Long-term results of the Latarjet procedure for anterior instability of the shoulder. J Shoulder Elbow Surg. 2014;23(11):1691–9. https://doi.org/10.1016/j.jse.2014.02.015. Epub 2014 May 14. PMID: 24835298.
2. Bach BR Jr. Arthroscopic removal of painful Bristow hardware. Arthroscopy. 1990;6(4):324–6. https://doi.org/10.1016/0749-8063(90)90065-l. PMID: 2264902.
3. Strömqvist B, Wingstrand H, Egund N. Recurrent shoulder dislocation and screw failure after the Bristow-Latarjet procedure. A case report. Arch Orthop Trauma Surg. 1987;106(4):260–2. https://doi.org/10.1007/BF00450466. PMID: 3619608.
4. Sastre S, Peidro L, Méndez A, Calvo E. Suprascapular nerve palsy after arthroscopic Latarjet procedure: a case report and review of literature. Knee Surg Sports Traumatol Arthrosc. 2016;24(2):601–3. https://doi.org/10.1007/s00167-014-3075-5. Epub 2014 May 18. PMID: 24839042.
5. Lunn JV, Castellano-Rosa J, Walch G. Recurrent anterior dislocation after the Latarjet procedure: outcome after revision using a modified Eden-Hybinette operation. J Shoulder Elb Surg. 2008;17(5):744–50. https://doi.org/10.1016/j.jse.2008.03.002. Epub 2008 Jul 10. PMID: 18619868.
6. Boileau P, Richou J, Lisai A, Chuinard C, Bicknell RT. The role of arthroscopy in revision of failed open anterior stabilization of the shoulder. Arthroscopy. 2009;25(10):1075–84. https://doi.org/10.1016/j.arthro.2009.04.073. Epub 2009 Sep 6. PMID: 19801285.
7. Castagna A, Garofalo R, Melito G, Markopoulos N, De Giorgi S. The role of arthroscopy in the revision of failed Latarjet procedures. Musculoskelet Surg. 2010;94(Suppl 1):S47–55. https://doi.org/10.1007/s12306-010-0060-0. PMID: 20383681.
8. Boileau P, Duysens C, Saliken D, Lemmex DB, Bonnevialle N. All-arthroscopic, guided Eden-Hybbinette procedure using suture-button fixation for revision of failed Latarjet. J Shoulder Elbow Surg. 2019;28(11):e377–88. https://doi.org/10.1016/j.jse.2019.03.022. Epub 2019 Jul 19. PMID: 31331667.
9. Giannakos A, Vezeridis PS, Schwartz DG, Jany R, Lafosse L. All-arthroscopic revision Eden-Hybinette procedure for failed instability surgery: technique and preliminary results. Arthroscopy. 2017;33(1):39–48. https://doi.org/10.1016/j.arthro.2016.05.021. Epub 2016 Jul 16. PMID: 27432589.

10. Valenti P, Martinez-Catalan N, Werthel JD, Kazum E. Full arthroscopic Eden-Hybinette procedure using 2 cortical suture buttons for the reconstruction of anteroinferior glenoid defects. Tech Hand Up Extrem Surg. 2021; https://doi.org/10.1097/BTH.0000000000000348. Epub ahead of print. PMID: 33899824.
11. Provencher MT, Peebles LA, Aman ZS, Bernhardson AS, Murphy CP, Sanchez A, Dekker TJ, LaPrade RF, Di Giacomo G. Management of the failed Latarjet Procedure: outcomes of revision surgery with fresh distal tibial allograft. Am J Sports Med. 2019;47(12):2795–802. https://doi.org/10.1177/0363546519871896. Epub 2019 Sep 9. PMID: 31498688.
12. Tokish JM, Fitzpatrick K, Cook JB, Mallon WJ. Arthroscopic distal clavicular autograft for treating shoulder instability with glenoid bone loss. Arthrosc Tech. 2014;3(4):e475–81. https://doi.org/10.1016/j.eats.2014.05.006. PMID: 25264509; PMCID: PMC4175166.
13. Sanchez M, Cuellar R, García A, Albillos J, Azofra J. Anterior stabilization of the shoulder by means of an artificial capsular reinforcement and arthroscopy part I: surgical technique. J Long-Term Eff Med Implants. 2000;10:11.
14. Kawakami J, Yamamoto N, Etoh T, Hatta T, Mineta M, Itoi E, Isawa R. In vivo glenoid track width can be better predicted with the use of shoulder horizontal extension angle. Am J Sports Med. 2019;47(4):922–7. https://doi.org/10.1177/0363546519825629. PMID: 30870033.
15. Hovelius LK, Sandström BC, Rösmark DL, Saebö M, Sundgren KH, Malmqvist BG. Long-term results with the Bankart and Bristow-Latarjet procedures: recurrent shoulder instability and arthropathy. J Shoulder Elb Surg. 2001;10(5):445–52. https://doi.org/10.1067/mse.2001.117128. PMID: 11641702.
16. Hovelius L, Sandström B, Sundgren K, Saebö M. One hundred eighteen Bristow-Latarjet repairs for recurrent anterior dislocation of the shoulder prospectively followed for fifteen years: study I--clinical results. J Shoulder Elb Surg. 2004;13(5):509–16. https://doi.org/10.1016/j.jse.2004.02.013. PMID: 15383806.
17. Lafosse L, Lejeune E, Bouchard A, Kakuda C, Gobezie R, Kochhar T. The arthroscopic Latarjet procedure for the treatment of anterior shoulder instability. Arthroscopy. 2007;23(11):1242.e1–5. https://doi.org/10.1016/j.arthro.2007.06.008. Epub 2007 Oct 3. PMID: 17986415.
18. LaPrade CM, Bernhardson AS, Aman ZS, Moatshe G, Chahla J, Dornan GJ, LaPrade RF, Provencher MT. Changes in the neurovascular anatomy of the shoulder after an open Latarjet procedure: defining a surgical safe zone. Am J Sports Med. 2018;46(9):2185–91. https://doi.org/10.1177/0363546518773309. Epub 2018 May 24. PMID: 29792520.
19. Reinares F, Werthel JD, Moraiti C, Valenti P. Effect of scapular external rotation on the axillary nerve during the arthroscopic Latarjet procedure: an anatomical investigation. Knee Surg Sports Traumatol Arthrosc. 2017;25(10):3289–95. https://doi.org/10.1007/s00167-016-4224-9. Epub 2016 Jun 24. PMID: 27342985.
20. Mahirogullari M, Kuskucu M, Solakoglu C, Akmaz I, Pehlivan O, Kiral A, Kaplan H. Comparison of outcomes of two different surgeries in regarding to complications for chronic anterior shoulder instability. Arch Orthop Trauma Surg. 2006;126(10):674–9. https://doi.org/10.1007/s00402-006-0190-x. Epub 2006 Jul 29. PMID: 16896744.
21. Cuéllar A, Cuéllar R, de Heredia PB. Arthroscopic revision surgery for failure of open Latarjet technique. Arthroscopy. 2017;33(5):910–7. https://doi.org/10.1016/j.arthro.2016.09.017. Epub 2016 Dec 16. PMID: 27989356.

GPSR Compliance

The European Union's (EU) General Product Safety Regulation (GPSR) is a set of rules that requires consumer products to be safe and our obligations to ensure this.

If you have any concerns about our products, you can contact us on ProductSafety@springernature.com

In case Publisher is established outside the EU, the EU authorized representative is:

Springer Nature Customer Service Center GmbH
Europaplatz 3
69115 Heidelberg, Germany

Batch number: 10455847

Printed by Printforce, the Netherlands